W9-CNN-717

Contagious Divides

AMERICAN CROSSROADS

Edited by Earl Lewis, George Lipsitz, Peggy Pascoe,
George Sánchez, and Dana Takagi

# Contagious Divides

Epidemics and Race
in San Francisco's Chinatown

Nayan Shah

University of California Press
*Berkeley · Los Angeles · London*

University of California Press
Berkeley and Los Angeles, California

University of California Press, Ltd.
London, England

© 2001 by Nayan Shah

Library of Congress Cataloging-in-Publication Data

Shah, Nayan, 1966–
  Contagious divides : epidemics and race in San
Francisco's Chinatown / Nayan Shah.
      p.     cm. — (American crossroads ; 7)
  Includes bibliographical references and index.
  ISBN 0-520-22628-3 (alk. paper) —
  ISBN 0-520-22629-1 (pbk. : alk. paper)
      1. Chinese Americans—Health and hygiene
  —California—(Chinatown) San Francisco—His-
  tory.   2. Public health—California—(China-
  town) San Francisco—History.   3. Epidemics
  —California—(Chinatown) San Francisco—
  History.   4. Immigrants—Health and hygiene—
  California—(Chinatown) San Francisco—History.
  5. Chinese Americans—Health and hygiene—
  Social aspects—California—(Chinatown) San
  Francisco—History.   I. Title.   II. Series.

  RA448.5.C45 S53   2001
  614.4'9794'61089951073—dc21     2001027615

Manufactured in the United States of America
10   09   08   07   06   05   04   03   02   01
10  9  8  7  6  5  4  3  2  1

*For my parents*

# Contents

# Illustrations

## FIGURES

## MAPS

# Acknowledgments

I have depended on many mentors, colleagues, institutions, and friends to make this work possible. This project began as a dissertation at the University of Chicago and was guided by an engaging and challenging committee. Jan Goldstein, George Chauncey, and William Novak shared invaluable insights, offered research strategies, and expanded my conceptual horizons. I am especially grateful to Thomas C. Holt, who directed the dissertation project. The conversations we have had over the years have opened new worlds of interpretation for me and kindled an appreciation for the difficulties of rigorous scholarship. The warmth of his mentorship and the example of his intellectual daring and conscience have sustained me at moments when the enormity of this undertaking daunted me.

Archives and special collections throughout the United States have been invaluable to my research. I am indebted to the archival staffs of the Center for Research Libraries; the California Historical Society; the San Francisco Labor Archives and Research Center; the Bancroft Library at the University of California; the Asian American Studies Library at the University of California at Berkeley; the San Francisco History Room at the San Francisco Public Library; the National Archives in San Bruno, California; the San Francisco Theological Union in San Anselmo, California; Lane Medical Library at Stanford University; the Herbert Hoover Library; the University of California at San Francisco

Archives; the Holt-Atherton Department of Special Collections at the University of the Pacific in Stockton; the Presbyterian Office of History in Philadelphia; the Pennsylvania Medical College Archives; the National Archives in Washington, D.C.; the National Archives II in College Park, Maryland; the Oberlin College Archives; and the Special Collections of Knight Library at the University of Oregon in Eugene. Special thanks are due to Jeffrey Barr at the California Historical Society; Susan Parker Sherwood at the San Francisco Labor Archives; Wei-Chi Poon at the Asian American Studies Library; Dan Nealson at the National Archives San Bruno; and Aloha South at the National Archives in Washington, D.C. I have also benefited from the archival guidance and generosity of the historians Him Mark Lai, Theresa Mah, Peggy Pascoe, Lucy Sayler, Ling Chi Wang, and Judy Yung.

I received generous financial support for research and writing from the SUNY United University Professions; the Binghamton Foundation; the Mellon Foundation; the American Historical Association's Albert Beveridge Award; and the Mellon Foundation–University of Chicago Dissertation Fellowship. The revision of the book manuscript was supported by residential fellowships at the University of California Humanities Research Institute and the New York University International Center for Advanced Studies. I am grateful to Robyn Wiegman and Patricia O'Brien at the University of California Humanities Research Institute and the fellows in the Interdisciplinary Queer Studies group. Madelyn Detloff, Carla Freccero, David Gere, George Haggerty, Eithne Luibhéid, Lisa Rofel, and Sandy Stone challenged me to rethink the ethics and politics of queer formations in my work. My thanks as well to Thomas Bender and Barbara Abrash at New York University and the engaging fellows who joined me on the Project on Cities and Urban Knowledges during its inaugural year. Meske Brhane, Teresa Caldeira, Christine Choy, John Czaplicka, Farha Ghannam, Steven Gregory, James Holston, Mark LeVine, Louise Maxwell, Thierry Nlandu, John Rajchmann, Nicole Rustin, Smriti Srinivas, and Tracy Tullis enabled me to think capaciously about the cultural politics and tensions of divided cities worldwide. I am particularly grateful to John Chaffee, my department chair at SUNY Binghamton, for allowing me the time away from teaching duties to pursue intensive revisions.

Over the years many colleagues and friends read and offered generous commentary at different stages of the writing project. My thanks to Rifa'at Abou-El-Haj, Leora Auslander, Anne Blackburn, Katherine Bliss, Mary Pat Brady, Howard Brown, Kathleen Brown, Antoinette

Burton, Melinda Campbell, Patricia Chu, Deborah Cohen, Elizabeth Cohen, Nancy Cott, Susan Craddock, Katherine Crawford, Elizabeth Dale, Michael Davidson, Melvyn Dubofsky, Jill Dupont, Sarah Elbert, Yen Espiritu, Bud Foster, Dana Frank, Tak Fujitani, Alexandra Gillen, Lori Ginzburg, Gayatri Gopinath, Jessica Hagedorn, Judith Halberstam, Eleanor Hannah, Marta Hanson, William Haver, Chad Heap, Julie Hessler, Sarah Hodges, Trevor Hope, Miranda Joseph, Grace Kao, Elizabeth Kennedy, Daniel Kim, Elaine Kim, Alan Kraut, Philippa Levine, David Lloyd, Lisa Lowe, Theresa Mah, Martin Manalansan, Curtis Marez, Antoinette Chaurfauros McDaniel, David Morrison, Lisa Moses, Anne Elizabeth Murdy, Carl Nightingale, Gary Okihiro, Michael Omi, Tiffany Patterson, Vijay Prashad, Donald Quataert, Daniel Rodgers, Hannah Rosen, Charles Rosenberg, Dara Silberstein, Kathryn Kish Sklar, Thomas Sugrue, David Tannehaus, John Kuo Tchen, Leti Vollp, Michael Willrich, K. Scott Wong, Shelley Sunn Wong, and Marilyn Young.

I am fortunate to have had an extraordinary set of readers at the University of California Press. The American Crossroads series editors Earl Lewis, George Lipsitz, Peggy Pascoe, George Sánchez, and Dana Tagaki gave me spirited and challenging reviews of the book manuscript. In the final stages of revision George Lipsitz and Peggy Pascoe offered detailed comments and invaluable advice in shaping the book for publication. In addition, two anonymous readers helped me strengthen and clarify the book's key arguments. Finally, Monica McCormick has shepherded this book through many transformations, and I am grateful for her enthusiasm and confidence in the work. I also thank Bonita Hurd for her careful copyediting and Jean McAneny for bringing the book through production.

In San Francisco, a number of friends have opened their homes to me and invited me into their lives. I am grateful for the companionship of Elsa E'der, Shaffiq Essajee, Kevin Grant, Hima B., Dar Horton, David Jenkins, Pablo Jenkins, Ginu Kamani, Priya Kamani, Anna Karydas, Cathy Kudlick, Jasbir Puar, Greg Roberts, Sandip Roy, Hasan Shafiqullah, Rachel Sturman, Susan Tiemroth, and Lisa Trivedi. Several friends in Chicago and in Binghamton deserve special mention: Anne Blackburn, Adele Brown, Patricia Chu, Lisa Moses, Anne Elizabeth Murdy, Mahua Sarkar, Dara Silberstein, Dana Stewart, and Paul Venet have all provided impassioned support and given me their time and care when I have needed it most. In the last several years, Chandan Reddy's insights have stretched my own vision for this project.

My brother, sister-in-law, cousins, aunts, uncles, and grandfather have patiently waited for the birth of this book. Their good humor and interest in this never-ending project have made the pleasure of its arrival all the sweeter. Ken Foster has nurtured this book to completion. His spirited enthusiasm for the project, generous reading of the manuscript, and tender care have pulled me through.

Finally, I dedicate this book to my parents, Devyani and Bhupendra Shah. Their resolute faith in me, the generosity of their affections and the inspiration of their courageous lives have enabled my work.

# Public Health, Race, and Citizenship

A sudden and severe epidemic of smallpox struck San Francisco in the summer of 1876. By October, the epidemic had infected more than 1,600 and taken nearly 450 lives. Dr. John Meares, the newly appointed city health officer, acted swiftly to check the spread of the disease, instituting programs of quarantine of the infected and public vaccination of the uninfected. Meares blamed the spread and severity of the epidemic on the presence of 30,000 "unscrupulous, lying and treacherous Chinamen" living in the heart of the city and their "willful and diabolical disregard of our sanitary laws." The wanton and "malicious" defiance of hygienic conduct among "this infamous race," Meares feared, had made Chinatown a "laboratory of infection" that contaminated the rest of the city.[1]

Meares and his colleagues defined Chinatown as the material manifestation of the alien within the modern American city, emphasizing Chinese difference from, deviance from, and danger to white society and the American nation. Nineteenth-century San Francisco health officials and politicians conceived of Chinatown as the preeminent site of urban sickness, vice, crime, poverty, and depravity. The San Francisco Board of Health and the Public Health Department employees under its supervision took the lead in investigating health conditions citywide. Their reports produced extremely menacing conceptions of Chinatown, identifying it as a "plague spot," a "cesspool," and the source of epidemic disease and physical ailments. Health authorities readily conflated the physical condition of Chinatown with the characteristics of Chinese people. They depicted Chinese immigrants as a filthy and diseased "race" who incubated such incurable afflictions as smallpox, syphilis, and bubonic plague and infected white Americans.[2]

More than sixty years later, in 1939, the city health officer Dr. Jacob Casson Geiger pinpointed Chinatown as the epicenter of another rampant epidemic—tuberculosis. One-fourth of all city tuberculosis cases lived in Chinatown, and Chinese residents faced a tuberculosis infection rate three times the city average in a period when overall tuberculosis infection rates had tumbled. Geiger, however, did not characterize Chinatown as a threat to the rest of the city. Instead he blamed the deplorable tenement housing conditions that imperiled the health of the Chinese residents themselves.

In these tenements, Chinese residents faced a "conspicuous absence" of "hygienic standards," notably "community toilets, baths and kitchens" and dangerous "habits" such as the "common serving dish from which the entire family partakes of meals." In Geiger's assessment, a segregated housing market, rapacious landlords, and the fatalism of "older Chinese" bachelors who "refused . . . to admit that gross defects exist" all contributed to the dismal living conditions. However, Geiger saw hope for improvement in the commitment of "younger" Chinese families to transform their habits and adapt "Oriental customs to Occidental living," as well as in their eagerness "to participate in city-wide activities"—which evidenced their "desire to be good citizens." The healthy conduct and consciousness of young Chinese Americans galvanized the Public Health Department to redouble its efforts to test, track, and treat Chinese tuberculosis victims and enhance instruction in "healthy habits." In the 1930s and 1940s, health officials, along with white and Chinese business leaders, social workers, and civic activists, advocated that San Francisco's government should demonstrate its "civic responsibility" to Chinatown residents by making investments in public housing, clinics, and social welfare services in order to turn the tide of the tuberculosis epidemic.[3]

What accounts for this extraordinary switch from demonizing San Francisco's Chinese residents as a medical menace to assisting them as deserving citizens? Was it simply evidence of the progress of medical knowledge and evolution of public health practice that militated against the bias and opprobrium of an earlier era? Or was it further evidence of the process of inclusion in American society and the process of assimilation on the part of Chinese immigrants and their children to the "American way of life"? If the latter, what were the possibilities and the limits of liberal democracy's expansion of the privileges of citizenship in the twentieth century?

To see the Chinese Americans as the patient and fortunate recipients of the fruits of medical, social, and political progress would underestimate the remarkable agency of the San Francisco men and women, Chinese and white, who contested and rewrote the terms of political and cultural belonging and alienation in an American city. For Chinese Americans, the journey from menace to model minority followed a deep undercurrent of ideas about citizenship, conduct, and health. The idea that the Chinese were a people racially distinct and apart from other American immigrants and citizens was remarkably resilient, but the meanings of that difference and whether that difference could be accommodated or must be expunged were changeable. What unfolds is a remarkable and vexing tale of race, citizenship, and public health.

In the nineteenth century, lethal epidemics of cholera, smallpox, and bubonic plague struck locales with devastating force. These epidemics arbitrarily took lives and incapacitated and disfigured those who survived. European and North American public health officials, physicians, and scientists pursued a quest to understand the causes of these contagious and often fatal maladies. Public health investigation produced a repertoire of precautions and prophylactics to dampen the spread of contagious diseases.[4] Through strategies of sanitation, vaccination, and therapeutic care, public health extended human longevity, increased the chances of childhood survival, and suppressed epidemic disease. In fact, these tangible and benevolent results of public health were considered to be the hallmark of modernity's promise of progress, a triumph of technological and scientific innovation. Precisely because of public health's powerful influence in transforming social lives in the nineteenth and twentieth centuries and its centrality in definitions of modernity, how public health operated demands critical evaluation.[5]

Public health served as one of the most agile and expansive regulatory mechanisms in nineteenth-century American cities. Next to the police and tax assessors, municipal public health administrators assumed the most sweeping authority to survey and monitor the city and its inhabitants. Although municipal public health institutions often had small budgets and staffs, their legal authority to regulate property and people's conduct was considerable.[6] Public health's mandate demanded measurement of the welfare of municipal inhabitants and the removal of any threats to the general population's longevity, health, and well-being. The idea of securing the "health" of the population linked the condition and conduct of individuals with the vitality, strength, and prosperity of society overall.[7]

Measuring and maintaining health entailed a new way of thinking about persons and their lives in the environment and in society. In the early nineteenth century, sickness was no longer seen as an inevitable condition of living but rather as an avoidable flaw. Steadfast regulation of the body, conduct, and living environment became an increasingly crucial practice in guarding against the infiltration of disease. In the name of preserving life and protecting from disease, public health developed general regimens of personal hygiene and public sanitation. Voluntary associations and local government in the nineteenth century promoted hygienic care and sanitary management as essential to the modern project of ensuring human longevity, maintaining health, and managing the vitality of the population. Nineteenth-century bourgeois economic classes particularly valued the health benefits of self-care and contrasted their enlightened conduct and consciousness with the legions of the working poor and traditional agriculturists. Their models of proper conduct employed new categories of normal and deviant, which were dramatically defined and invigorated by putative race and class differences.[8]

Nineteenth-century San Francisco physicians and health officials feared that the mission of enabling human vitality was undercut by the reputed vile and disease-breeding qualities of Chinese settlement in the city. In the name of safeguarding the health of the entire population, public health strategies of surveillance, documentation, and quarantine generated new conceptions of Chinese behavior at odds with the standards of proper social conduct. The collection and interpretation of knowledge about the incidence of epidemic disease, mortality, and morbidity produced an ethnography of different groups and locations in the city, of their habits, and of their conditions. Public health agencies and physicians generated considerable "knowledge" about the living conditions and social conduct of Chinese residents in San Francisco. They assembled a broad array of cultural and social differences to account for epidemic transmission. At the turn of the century, medical explanations for the cause of disease shifted from miasma and environmental discharges to microbes, but the application of these scientific principles both shaped and affected cultural and political dynamics in the city. This medical knowledge of Chinese deviance and danger emerged in the context of a fervent anti-Chinese political culture and escalating class confrontations generated by the social tumult of industrialization, rapid urbanization, and tremendous migration into San Francisco.[9]

The focus of this book on San Francisco across a span of nearly a century allows for an examination of how formations of race have coalesced, changed, and reconstituted in politics, culture, and society. Through the prism of public health, this book connects practices of race-making to the regimes of knowledge and the discourses that give them legitimacy and plausibility. The local formation of Chinese and white "races" was molded and mobilized by political, social, and economic conditions. In mid-nineteenth- to mid-twentieth-century San Francisco, concerns about the Chinese "race" and Chinatown became central to the social classifications of racial danger, difference, and subordination. The meanings of race gathered webs of prevailing gender, sex, class, national, and religious relations and forged new systems of social identities and political divisions.[10]

My analysis of race follows the work of scholars who refute the notion that "race" is a biological fact that transcends time and historical context. Instead, race is better understood as a social and political category that persists because it offers a seemingly "natural" observable difference to explain social inequality and domination. Racial beliefs are persuasive and appealing because they claim to translate physical differences into markers of innate characteristics, talents, and dispositions. Differences in skin color, hair, eyes, and the size and shape of the body, supposedly provide visible clues to differences in human nature and capacities. Racial schema of the body are thought to explain perceived differences in intellect, character, physical capacity, and artistic abilities, as well as the inclination of cultural tastes and everyday activities.[11]

In order to understand the intensity of violence, fear, and fascination that racial distinctions have provoked, some social critics have charged that race and racism constitute an irrational, archaic legacy at odds with the rational and modern world. However, historians, anthropologists, and political philosophers have demonstrated that the ideologies of race are constitutive of modern rationality and its regimes of classification and regulation. The entanglement of race in modern science, governance, and morality reveals a paradox at the core of modernity itself. Modernity, on the one hand, promotes ideas of universality and, on the other hand, obsessively objectifies difference. In nineteenth- and twentieth-century science, social science, law, and political systems, this contradictory process employed race as a category to explain the bodies, behavior, and cultures that deviate from and defy presumably universal norms and standards.[12]

Projects promoting health and hygiene culled and remade social differences of race and class in locations across the globe in the nineteenth and early twentieth centuries. My study of San Francisco resonates with studies of public health in cities as varied as Cincinnati, Bombay, Atlanta, Paris, Rio de Janeiro, Cape Town, and Los Angeles. In each instance, contemporaneous physicians, politicians, and social critics attributed the spread of epidemic disease to the unsanitary habits and habitations of subordinate groups defined by racial, class, or national status.[13] The strategies of urban public health reform, with their heightened recognition of race and class boundaries and the possibilities of contamination, reinforced political trends toward segregation, enhancing and justifying the spatial and social division characteristic of early-twentieth-century cities in the United States and colonial Asia and Africa.[14]

My analytical contribution to these rich historical studies is to offer insight into the dynamics of public health in processes of inclusion and exclusion. In San Francisco, the constellation of race and public health pivoted upon systems of governance and citizenship. Over the course of nearly a century, the dynamic of public health transformed its role from that which produced standards of regulation in the nineteenth century to that which produced standards of entitlement in the twentieth century. The shift from regulation to entitlement reflects the development of the American state and marks a crucial period when racial ideologies were recast. In the nineteenth century, public health operated to exclude difference, whereas in the twentieth century, public health sought to accommodate difference. In nineteenth-century American cities, public health served as an expansive regulatory mechanism that produced the minimum standards or norms for the population. The work of nineteenth-century sanitary regulation was done by closely scrutinizing those groups and environmental factors that were viewed as disruptive to health norms, and then seeking to contain or exclude any such threats.

However, in the twentieth century these health norms regulating environments and social behavior became recalibrated as the minimum standards for the emerging system of social welfare and entitlements. In the twentieth century, "progress" was articulated by a range of public health–inspired welfare projects, including housing; health care for mothers, infants, and children; industrial health; and recreation. In contrast to the nineteenth-century policy of exclusion, this new entitlement system sought to sanitize and accommodate differences. There is a persistent congruence between the public health logic of normal and aberrant and the racial logic of superior and inferior and their reconfiguration over time. Racial difference as an organizing principle of society and state formation does not disappear in the entitlement system. Rather, race is remade from a difference that threatens, to one that can be modified and reconciled with the norms of society. The result is the development of separate and segregated infant clinics, foster care programs, and public housing institutions.[15]

The transformation from exclusion to inclusion opens up questions about the terms by which Chinese residents were recognized as participants in the governance of U.S. society. The question of governance complicates the issues of race discrimination and focuses attention on underlying processes of individual subjectivity and citizenship in modern liberal societies. I use the concept of citizen-subject to understand the mutual constitution of cultural and political attributes necessary for participation in society. The concept of citizen-subject combines the political status of liberal democracy with the social practices of modern disciplinary institutions. The idea of the citizen emphasizes the equality of the independent individual in political participation and in access to privilege and resources, while the subject is constituted in disciplinary practices in places such as schools, prisons, factories, hospitals, and clinics that inculcate the individual self with the norms of the population. The modern process of public health reform emerged within a web of social, political, and cultural linkages that produced a new conception of the human subject in the nineteenth and early twentieth centuries. Modern public health crafted a strategy of both state regulation and bourgeois self-regulation that linked the conduct and consciousness of the individual self with the vitality of society overall. The liberal vision of governance limited direct intervention in the lives of individual subjects and instead fostered a range of practical strategies to shape, guide, manage, or regulate individual consciousness and conduct. What was crucial to the formation of the modern self and subjectivity was the capacity to reason "correctly" and follow codes of "civilized" conduct.[16]

In liberal democracies, the concept of citizenship has established the meanings, expectations, and boundaries of full membership in society through claims of universal equality and access to political, economic, and social privileges, opportunities, and participation.[17] However, the history of U.S. democracy is littered with instances of citizenship deprived and of personal liberties and opportunities denied to various groups on the basis of race and gender. Different forms of citizenship— from nationality status to suffrage to property rights to the access to social provision—have been abridged, circumscribed, and repudiated based on gender, race, nationality, and economic standing.[18] The crite-

ria of both subjectivity and full citizenship converge in the recognition
of the capacity to reason and an expectation that certain manners, habits, and types of consciousness and socialization would foster the capacity for self-governance.[19]

The objective of liberal governance is to cultivate citizen-subjects
who can govern themselves. In this way the public conduct exhibited by
the citizen-subject reflects the subjective emotional and intellectual capacities of individuals and the ethical regimes through which they govern their lives. The process of fostering citizen-subjects does not emanate
from a coherent state program but emerges, haphazardly and unevenly,
through a variety of voluntary associations. It occurs largely through the
"proselytizing of independent reformers" who take up certain problems, such as epidemics of tuberculosis and infant mortality, and recode
them as "social" problems with consequences for national well-being
and which call for new forms of remedial attention. Liberal strategies of
governing have emphasized ruling at a distance—that is, granting authority to professionals who are licensed and empowered by the state
to create norms of individual conduct, make judgments, and administer
policies.[20]

At times the category of citizen-subject described what the Chinese
immigrants were not. At other moments it was held up as an aspiration
of acculturation and assimilation. Legal prohibitions against naturalized
citizenship for Chinese immigrants in the Chinese Exclusion Act (1882)
served as a substantial racial barrier against Chinese men and women
attempting to claim the political rights and privileges of citizenship. The
political status of aliens was amplified by certain norms of "civilized"
conduct that divided the civilized member of society from those lacking
the capacities to exercise citizenship responsibly. Government public
health and voluntary associations focused on the imputed failure of self-
regulation on the part of the Chinese immigrants. Their lack of sanitary
behavior, the condition of their residences, and their visible absence of
respectable domesticity demonstrated the failure to achieve the desired
standard of reasoning. These were grounds on which to count them out
of the American polity and indeed out of American civil society. Some
Chinese immigrants contested this denial of status and attempted to
prove that their conduct demonstrated an ability to reason properly. At
the same time, others sought to demonstrate their acculturation into society through their adoption of "hygienic standards" and their eagerness
to adapt to "Occidental living."

In San Francisco, white politicians, businessmen, clergy, social critics, and labor leaders dominated the debate in the public sphere on Chinese conduct and settlement. The rhetoric about the degraded and regressive space of Chinatown and the recalcitrant Chinese was so strident and deafening that it was difficult for Chinese Americans and their supporters to address this white American audience. Chinese Americans had to marshal the dominant discourse in order to intervene effectively in politics and participate in society.[21] From the nineteenth to the twentieth century the terms and tactics of effective participation in the public sphere changed dramatically. In the nineteenth century, Chinese business and community leaders communicated through intermediaries such as white attorneys in the state and federal courts and published memorials to Congress that highlighted the favorable testimony and affidavits of prominent white businessmen, journalists, ministers, and physicians.

The Chinese merchant elite and diplomats developed politically effective strategies in the late nineteenth and early twentieth centuries. They waged opposition to government policies and legislation through a combination of the press and the courts. They were able to mobilize judicial protections of economic freedom in the courts and recast the debates in professional medicine to their advantage. They became familiar with the principles of liberal government, democratic citizenship, and the moral ideals of American society in their often successful attempts to limit government interference in business and property. Their lobbying efforts and court cases sought to reduce the arbitrariness of immigration restrictions and the administration of public health regulations.

In the middle of the twentieth century, a class of second-generation Chinese American male and female professionals, businesspeople, physicians, and social workers emerged who became directly involved in the crafting of health policy and allocating of public and charity resources, rather than responding to onerous regulations. Through a range of civic and voluntary associations, these Chinese American women and men developed institutional sites for organizational learning and oppositional consciousness. They learned how to be heard and understood, how to define problems and solutions in line with the acceptable concepts of standards, nuisance, statistics, and rights. In the 1930s and 1940s, Chinese American activists were able to demonstrate that they were experts on themselves and their living conditions, and they made this self-knowledge a potent political claim. By engaging prevailing norms of conduct, Chinese American activists could argue for the worthiness of Chinese Americans to participate in and draw upon the resources of American society.[22]

These very struggles for effective political voice for Chinese Americans revealed divisions and disputes within the Chinese American community. On questions of bodily autonomy, mobility, and the legitimacy of public health administration, the turn-of-the-century Chinese merchant elite, diplomats, and community leaders diverged from the positions of Chinese American laborers and small merchants in the city and the detained immigrants on Angel Island. In the middle decades of the twentieth century, the political campaigns for housing revealed the breaks between elite businesspeople and community leaders, on the one hand, and second-generation Chinese American activists and professionals, on the other, concerning the strategies for representing Chinatown living conditions and for claiming entitlement. The full range of expressions of opposition—many of which have been ignored or distorted in the public record—outlined the parameters by which Chinese Americans became politically effective, the political and cultural avenues by which the social order was constituted, and the allocation of opportunities and resources.

The records generated by the dominant public sphere can only offer hints as to how Chinese Americans understood their bodies and their care. A number of historians and anthropologists of medicine have deftly examined the internal dynamics of traditional Chinese medical knowledge, as well as the mutual transformations and redefinition of both Western public health and Chinese traditional medicine in late-nineteenth- and twentieth-century China.[23] In cosmopolitan San Francisco, Chinese residents had access to a tremendous variety of therapies—herbal medicine, acupuncture, homeopathic medicine, and allopathic care—that far outstripped the options available in their natal villages. Medical historians have explored how traditional Chinese medical practice changed under competitive and regulatory pressure in the United States and reshaped its own avenues of legitimacy into professionalization in the twentieth century. However, the full cultural and social dimensions of how Chinese responded to these therapies and understood illness is far more difficult to assess from either the pharmacological records of Chinese herbal practitioners or the political and legal records of those who defended traditional Chinese medicine. From the records available, we can draw some inferences as to how Chinese selected and consumed different medical therapies and how their choices impacted their understanding of disease, health, and the care of their bodies.[24]

*Contagious Divides* explores how the production of Chinese difference and white norms in public-health knowledge and policy impacted social lives, politics, and cultural expression in San Francisco. The contestations and definitions of Chinese bodies, conduct, and spaces held immense significance for white Americans.[25] Health discourses and policy concerning the problematic "Chinese" or "Oriental" body revealed how whiteness and white identity is performed.[26] These definitions of racial identity and embodiment also gave racial boundaries to social space and geography. As the geographer Kay Anderson has argued, *Chinatown* was not a "neutral" description of urban settlers from China; rather, it was a potent "evaluative" designation that ignored any of the categories of representation employed by the residents of the territory. "Regardless of how Chinatown's residents defined themselves and each other—whether by class, gender, ethnicity, region of origin in China, surname, generation, dialect, place of birth, and so on—the settlements were perceived by Europeans through lenses of their own tinting," Anderson has noted. "Without needing the recognition of the residents, Chinatown's representers constructed in their own minds a boundary between 'their' territory and 'our' territory."[27]

The maintenance of spatial and racial boundaries intensified the fear of Chinese medical threats and generated scenarios of white victimization. The avenues of infection and the diseases were multiple and reflected the material conditions of everyday life in late-nineteenth-century San Francisco. The presence of Chinese people in the economic and social life was emphasized in infection routes traveled by Chinese-laundered clothes and Chinese-manufactured goods, in the intimate proximity of Chinese servants in white households, and in leisure activities with Chinese men in opium dens and Chinese women in brothels. What was crucial in these scenarios was not just the representation of Chinese presence in San Francisco as dangerous but also a concern that Chinese bodies and conduct undermined the norms of white American society and could therefore threaten its prosperity and vitality.

Historians, geographers, and sociologists have been drawn to the public health struggles and contestations experienced by Chinese Americans in San Francisco, and their studies have illuminated the social and political repercussions in San Francisco city politics as well as in regional and national arenas.[28] My approach draws on this research and examines the process by which racial meanings of health and citizenship become revised and redrafted into social policy and cultural expression in the wake of epidemic crises. I explore how the very entanglement of race, health, and citizenship that shaped the public health menace of the Chinese in the nineteenth century later provided a basis from which Chinese Americans could mobilize in an effort to reform the social conditions of their communities.

The health threats did more than demonize the Chinese: they also marshaled civic resources and attention that promoted widespread health instruction, sewer construction, vaccination programs, bacteriological investigation, and public health management of the city. In addition to government programs, the concept of public health also suggested a repertoire of strategies, concerns, and practices of health that were developed by civic groups, private charities, business and commerce, labor unions, community groups, neighborhood associations, and other interest groups. There was a partnership of government and private charities to mobilize wide-scale civic action and instruction and to adjust the population to health norms. These voluntary associations crafted health standards that were gathered under the slogan of "the American standard of living" and were part of its aspirations. The American standard of living embraced the health of individuals and the population in housing, schools, workplaces, and other civic institutions.[29]

*Contagious Divides* further explores the proliferation and potency of cultural concepts of health and nation. At the turn of the century, "health" and "cleanliness" were embraced as integral aspects of American identity; and those who were perceived to be "unhealthy," such as Chinese men and women, were considered dangerous and inadmissible to the American nation. Women and men, white and Chinese, reinterpreted their identity and their relationship to the nation through racially coded languages of hygiene and health. This racial coding was shaped and transformed by the norms of class through discourses of respectability and middle-class tastes and by the norms of marital heterosexuality through discourses of the nuclear family formation, adult male responsibility, and female domestic caretaking.[30]

Models and visions of domesticity anchored the terms of participation in American society. The portrayal of Chinatown as a nexus of infection, domestic chaos, and moral danger reverberated widely in the political and cultural life of San Francisco residents. Public health rhetoric about the contagion of Chinatown bachelor society provided both white middle-class female missionaries and white male labor leaders the necessary foil against which they could elaborate the vision and norms for nuclear-family domestic life and a sanitary social order. The lives of Chinese men and women were depicted as contrary to respectable domesticity and an ominous threat to ideal visions of American morality and family life. From the mid–nineteenth century to World War II, white politicians and social critics characterized Chinatown as an immoral bachelor society of dissolute men who frequented opium dens, gambling houses, and brothels, and the few visible Chinese women were considered to be prostitutes. As Jennifer Ting has argued, Chinese men and women were perceived to practice "deviant heterosexuality," in which their sexual companionship rarely qualified as conjugal marriage; more often men sought female prostitutes or concubines. In twentieth-century historiography and sociology of Chinese American experience, this behavior was interpreted as deviance and a sign of sexual maladjustment. This interpretation presumed that the social relations among Chinese Americans were both delinquent and deficient of normative aspirations.[31]

In white representations of Chinatown society, the models of respectable domesticity were considered impossible to achieve. Although many Chinese merchants in San Francisco had brought their wives and children from China, critics of Chinese immigration observed the absence of large numbers of nuclear families among Chinese laborers as evidence that Chinese men had no commitment to permanent residence and assimilation to American society. Few critics addressed how U.S. immigration restrictions, violent discrimination, and migratory labor recruitment made it difficult for Chinese male laborers to consider permanent settlement or encourage reluctant wives and dependent children to join them. This skewed gender balance persisted well into the mid–twentieth century, with females constituting barely 10 percent of the San Francisco Chinese population before 1920.[32]

Physicians, politicians, and travelogue writers feared that the peculiar spaces of Chinatown sociability, such as prostitute cribs, concubine apartments, bachelor bunkhouses, and opium dens, fostered perverse intimate relationships and bred contagion. The prevailing social arrangements of Chinese bachelor society produced several types of queer domesticity, such as multiple women and children living in a female-dominated household, the affiliation of vast communities of men in bunkhouses and opium dens, and common law marriages of Chinese men and fallen white women. The analysis of "queer domesticity" emphasizes the variety of erotic ties and social affiliations that counters normative expectations. Rather than viewing the term *queer* as a synonym for homosexual identity, I use it to question the formation of exclusionary norms of respectable middle-class, heterosexual marriage. The analytical category of queer upsets the strict gender roles, the firm divisions between public and private, and the implicit presumptions of self-sufficient economics and intimacy in the respectable domestic household. The models of spatial arrangements, gender, and sexuality in the ideal of respectable domesticity contrasted with the fears articulated in white representations of the perverse spaces, anomalous gender roles, and deviant sexualities that they perceived had license for expression in Chinatown. In missionary tracts, physicians' accounts, and politicians' speeches, these questions of space, gender, sexualities, and domesticity became punctuated and explained by sickness. The routes of infection and contamination informed the sexual and social dangers of Chinatown.

The judgment of particular social lives as unhealthy and immoral, however, reverberated differently among the various constituencies of San Francisco. Nineteenth-century Protestant women missionaries and early-twentieth-century women social workers weighed the same critique of Chinatown society as did physicians and public health agencies; however, the missionaries and social workers eschewed wholesale condemnation. The Protestant missionaries displayed optimism in the potential transformation of Chinese Americans to respectable domesticity. Protestant Christianity and the public health rationality of modernity converged in the practices and ideals that gave meaning to "civilized behavior." Hygiene and social morality offered overlapping repertoires and regimens designed to cultivate proper relations between the self and society in the modern world. In order for "civilized behavior" to thrive, missionaries and public health advocates insisted upon the "monogamous morality" of respectable domesticity, with its regular households, Christian marriage and morality, and nuclear families. Within such an environment it was possible to create self-regulating citizen-subjects. The attempts of white missionaries and social workers to train Chinese women demonstrated their confidence in the American Protestant vision of inclusion in a single model of self and social fulfillment.[33]

This vision of respectable domesticity framed the criteria of participation in Christian civilization as well as in the political institutions of the United States in the late nineteenth century and twentieth century.[34] Public health and Christian morality figured Chinese bachelors as threatening to American society's claims to marriage and middle-class domesticity and as disruptive to the respectable Chinese American community. The difference of Chinese male bachelors, who were married to women in China but who lived in homosocial networks in the United States, produced a sexual and social subjectivity incommensurate with American sexual typologies of heterosexual married life and homosexual isolation. On the borders of race and sexual relations, those relations that became illegal, immoral, and illicit sharpened the constitution of gender, sexual, and social norms. The norms of heterosexual marriage and respectable domesticity tended to curb social variety into a narrow expectation of domestic, social, and sexual arrangements that were acceptable, plausible, recognizable, and knowable. The immense heterogeneity of social practices, identities, and expressions became folded into the norm, its particularities forgotten, or else amassed under the broad category of deviant. Ideas of bodily hygiene and environmental sanitation contributed to the normalization of bodies, family, and community and became complicit in the reproduction of dominant discourses of heterosexuality, respectable domesticity, and race uplift within and outside of Chinatown.[35]

The outcome of the Chinese American community's claim to citizenship and cultural belonging depended upon the performance of normative hygiene and heterosexual family forms. In the arduous struggle to be perceived as "normal" in their social habits and living styles, Chinese American activists in the 1930s and 1940s proceeded upon a strategy of highlighting those Chinese persons who had adapted to middle-class norms in consumer tastes, hygiene, and respectable domesticity. This strategy had dire consequences for the bachelors, who were ignored in the quest for welfare resources and housing entitlements available to the Chinese American family community. This paradox demonstrates how the terms of assimilation that privilege nuclear family domesticity limit inclusion and enable the resilience of exclusionary strategies in the modern liberal state.

Scholars of ethnic studies and colonial studies have questioned how the political and scholarly usage of minority "community" tends to ignore diversity and differences within groups and subsumes incommensurate lives, acts, politics, and ways of knowing into a unitary category.[36] Scholars of Asian American studies have questioned the political categories of identity—nation, race, and community—which have shaped the writing of U.S. history. Asian American scholars have resisted writing histories that can be incorporated as subsidiaries of U.S. national history to provide the particular tale of discrimination and struggle for political rights that confirms the "progress" of American democracy. Instead, they have drawn critical attention to the dynamics of political and cultural power that shape the categories "citizen" and "alien."[37] My contribution to this critique is to pursue the processes of governance in U.S. society that can turn some aliens into citizens.

These terms of incorporation into American society redefine certain

Chinese immigrants as citizen-subjects by their demonstrations of respectable domesticity, economic stability, and proper conduct. These Chinese American citizen-subjects create a distinctive minority community identity—the community of Chinese American families. This process of incorporation distinguishes Chinese American citizen-subjects from both internal and external aliens but also emphasizes their perpetual difference from "true" white American citizens. Those who do not fit the model of Chinese family society—namely, Chinese bachelors and female prostitutes—are represented as threats and aliens to the American social order. In mid-twentieth-century San Francisco, as Chinese American activists consolidated a claim to entitlement and citizenship for Chinese fathers, mothers, and children in nuclear families, the lives, social networks, and cultural expressions of Chinese bachelors were represented as an archaic, distant legacy. When Chinese middle-class men and women occupied the public stage as a "community," they did not address either the fact that Chinese bachelors had created viable and supportive social networks in a hostile society or where these bachelors belonged within society. In the late 1960s and 1970s, Asian American youth activists championed the cause of Chinese and Filipino bachelors in San Francisco. They framed the erasure and neglect of these men as problems of race discrimination, but historians must consider how their erasure was an effect of race uplift as well.[38]

Assessing the exclusion of Chinese bachelors from both the history of American modernity and Chinese American community raises questions about the dynamics of modern power and knowledge. Health is one of several modern concepts that seek to order and make intelligible the relationship between the self and society through the tutoring of conduct and the reformation of space. Questioning the practices that create health norms and exclusions unleashes the immense variety of lives, spaces, and meaning compressed under narrow definitions. Attending to the process that set Chinese bachelors apart from Chinese American family society unravels tidy consolidations of identity and puts seemingly natural processes askew. Instead of writing a history of Chinese American community, this study raises questions and unravels assumptions about race, domesticity, health, and citizenship that shaped how and for whom San Francisco was governed throughout the nineteenth and twentieth centuries' convulsions of mass democracy.

# CHAPTER I

# Public Health and the Mapping of Chinatown

Nineteenth-century San Francisco journalists, politicians, and health officials feared an impending epidemic catastrophe festering in the tenements of what was then labeled as Chinatown. In the press coverage of public health inspections, newspaper reporters described the Chinatown labyrinth as hundreds of underground passageways connecting the filthy "cellars" and cramped "garrets" where Chinese men lived. In their salacious portrayals, journalists related how dozens of Chinese men slept on narrow wooden shelves squeezed into claustrophobic rooms, "which was considered close quarters for a single white man." Opium fumes, tobacco smoke, and putrefying waste pervaded the atmosphere in these windowless and unventilated rooms, and "each cellar [was] ankle-deep with loathsome slush, with ceilings dripping with percolations of other nastiness above, [and] with walls slimy with the clamminess of Asiatic diseases."[1]

Periodic public health investigations—both informal midnight journeys and official fact-finding missions—fed the alarm about the danger Chinese men and women posed to white Americans' health. Seizing upon the suspected causes of contamination, health officials emphasized the "overcrowded" tenements, "unventilated underground habitations," and stale "nauseating" air.[2] These investigations produced a "knowledge" of Chinese women and men's seemingly unhygienic habits, the unsanitary conditions in which they lived, and the dangerous diseases they carried. The widespread publicity of the horrors of percolating waste, teeming bodies, and a polluted atmosphere in Chinese habitations underscored the vile and infectious menace of Chinatown spaces. Almost at once the threat of illness became the legitimate grounds for the city government's intervention and shaped health policy toward Chinatown and Chinese residents.

How did these revolting images become the incontestable truth about Chinese residents of San Francisco? How did the descriptions offered by health officers and journalists achieve the stature of scientific knowledge and pervasiveness of common sense? In order to understand how quickly public-health knowledge came to identify a place and its inhabitants as dangerous, it is necessary to examine the process by which description became policy through scientific knowledge. The category of Chinese race and place created the field of study for investigations; strategies of scientific knowing generated the rich descriptive data that were then interpreted by medical reasoning. This formation of scientific knowledge shaped regulatory policy that in turn spurred further investigations, and the process of knowledge creation intensified.

The investigations targeted Chinatown, identifying its location and its boundaries and surveying the spaces within it. In the nineteenth and early twentieth centuries, "Chinatown" ghettos proliferated in both cities and small towns throughout North America. The generic naming of a Chinatown in some locations referred to a handful of buildings and in others to a set of streets. Although the physical boundaries of these "Chinatowns" constantly shifted, the name signaled a potent racial designation of Chinese immigrant inhabitation. The cartography of Chinatown that was developed in government investigations, newspaper reports, and travelogues both established "knowledge" of the Chinese race and aided in the making and remaking of Chinatown. The idea of Chinatown as a self-contained and alien society in turn justified "recurring rounds" of policing, investigation, and statistical surveys that "scientifically" corroborated the racial classification.[3]

The creation of "knowledge" of Chinatown relied upon three key spatial elements: dens, density, and the labyrinth. The enclosed and inhuman spaces of dens were where the Chinese lived. High density was the condition in which they lived. And the labyrinth was the unnavigable maze that characterized both the subterranean passageways within the buildings and the streets and alleys aboveground. These spatial elements established the basic contours of the representation of Chinatown and provided the canvas for detailed renderings of Chinese living styles, conditions, and behaviors. The investigations and the accompanying publicity not only established the Chinatown spatial elements of dens, density, and the labyrinth but also generated the stereotyped imagery that would be used more intensively over the decades and that illuminates how racial categories in the United States were produced in the late nineteenth century and persisted in the twentieth century.

Five government-sponsored investigations were both emblematic and politically pivotal in defining the Chinatown menace: the 1854 inquiry by the San Francisco Common Council (the precursor to the San Francisco Board of Supervisors) that reestablished the municipal Board of Health; the investigation that resulted in the 1869 report of the San Francisco health officer C. M. Bates; the 1871 investigation by Dr. Thomas Logan, the secretary of the California State Board of Health; the 1880 inspection by the Board of Health that declared Chinatown a "nuisance"; and the 1885 survey of Chinatown by the San Francisco Board of Supervisors. Although these expeditions were not always led by physicians, medical expertise shaped their findings and implicitly supported the "truth" they exposed. From 1854 to 1885, reports of every official investigation recycled these spatial metaphors and both consistently and uncritically channeled the imagery of "dense" and "enclosed" living conditions into the interpretive framework of epidemic danger for white San Francisco residents.

Over the span of forty years, four strategies of scientific knowing developed that transformed the knowledge of Chinatown. These strategies were scientific observation, standards of normalcy and deviance, statistics, and mapping. Scientific observation emphasized firsthand descriptions. These descriptions were offered in a realist style, evoking a travel narrative rich in visceral sensory details. The strategy of creating standards of normalcy and deviance was especially critical to evaluating density in residential space. This primarily involved the calculation of room dimensions in relation to the number of inhabitants. Against the yardstick of the middle-class white ideal, Chinese residential practices were, therefore, designated as deviant and a sign of inhumanity. The strategy of using statistics stipulated the frequency of health violations and census enumeration of the inhabitants. The enumeration demonstrated both the ordinariness and the extensiveness of the dangerous conditions in Chinatown. Finally, through the regularity and thoroughness of sanitary surveillance, the public health authorities developed a map that identified every business and residence in Chinatown.[4] It was the combined weight of all four strategies that enhanced the intensity of scientific knowledge formation and substantiated claims to objective truth.

By 1880, the understanding of Chinatown as the site of filth, disease, and inhuman habitation had achieved a pervasiveness in public discourse as both scientific truth and common sense. Political discourse, travel writing, journalism, and public health reports all shared these strategies of scientific knowledge and interpretation. Public health alone did not invent this knowledge of Chinatown but rather organized it. The persuasive power of public health knowledge was its capacity to identify, intensify, and relentlessly classify popular representations into a limited array of mutually sustaining racial and medical meanings. The shared knowledge of Chinatown produced explanations that tenaciously connected the Chinese race to place, behavior, and cultural differences and framed the endurance of the Chinatown ghetto as a living repository of the strange, peculiar, and unassimilable in San Francisco.[5]

## INVESTIGATING CHINESE SETTLEMENT

Medical interest and municipal investigation of Chinese settlement began in 1854, when it was first possible to see and describe a San Francisco street as being predominantly "Chinese." The Chinese population had grown rapidly from a handful in 1848 to more than 2,000 Chinese residents six years later. The first substantial number of Chinese immigrants had entered the port of San Francisco in 1849. Chinese men, mostly from the southeastern province of Guangdong, emigrated in large numbers to California in the early 1850s. In California overall, the Chinese population leaped from 450 in 1850 to 20,026 in 1852. The Cantonese men called their destination *Gamsaan,* or Gold Mountain. Lured by the 1848 gold strike in the Sierra, most Chinese men traveled to the hinterlands to seek their fortunes. Even so, Chinese men accounted for 12 percent of San Francisco's total population, and a visible cluster of Chinese businesses emerged on Sacramento Street, between Kearny Street and Dupont Street. Chinese residents and travelers themselves recognized the cluster of their compatriots' businesses and in time called Sacramento Street *Tongyan gaai,* or "Street of the Chinese." [6]

In August 1854 a local physician, Dr. William Rabe, was perturbed by the "filthy" conditions on Sacramento Street and demanded that the Common Council immediately investigate the Chinese settlement in the city. The unhealthy living conditions of Chinese residents aggravated council members' concerns about Chinese immigration.[7] The council's official investigation of the nascent Chinese district became the model for the next half century's expeditions. These expeditions presumed first that discrete racial territories existed, and then that their features could be known through direct observation and expert analysis. In 1854, city council officials enlisted a police officer to conduct a tour and ferret out the hidden dangers of the settlement. The party was accompanied by Dr. Rabe, who provided medical expertise to diagnose the territory's problems.[8]

The political atmosphere around the 1854 investigation was charged, however, with the tensions of escalating anti-Chinese politics and the specter of epidemic disease. The *Daily Alta California,* an avowed opponent of Chinese immigration and the leading daily in the city, claimed that the Chinese were "notoriously filthy," an assertion that could be validated by "taking a walk through any of the Chinese quarters of the City."[9] News of a cholera epidemic heightened worries about Chinese filth. The newspaper issued frequent reports of a national cholera epidemic, detailing weekly death tolls in major Eastern cities and the rapid spread of cholera westward.[10] This coverage revisited the history of nineteenth-century cholera epidemics; the October 1850 outbreak was responsible for forty deaths in San Francisco.

The *Daily Alta* editors warned their readers that despite overall improvements in sanitation, cholera could erupt in "filthy localities like the Chinese quarters" because "cholera delights in filth, in decaying garbage, and stagnant water, and dirty clothing and filthy bodies: particularly when all of these are united in crowded localities." The editors employed popularized medical knowledge about the causes of cholera— waste, contaminated water, and filth—and combined it with an abhorrence of "crowded" and impoverished localities and bodies. The wave of cholera epidemics in Europe and in the United States since 1832 had generated intense medical and popular debate about the causes and spread of the disease. Although there was recognition that social status offered no immunity to the disease, there was a widespread moral and medical belief that the living conditions of society's poor and marginal were responsible for the spread of cholera. The *Daily Alta* had characterized the spaces inhabited by the Chinese as "dirty, filthy dens" where "sickly" Chinese were "piled together like pigs in a pen." The editors called upon municipal authorities to enforce sanitary regulations to eliminate these "dens" and expel the Chinese population from the city.[11]

These images of filth, density, and sickliness reappeared in the Common Council's investigation. The report identified the most intense dangers as being in the boardinghouses owned by the so-called Chinese Companies and depicted them as the "filthiest places that could be imagined." In some of these dormitories "hundreds of Chinamen are crowded together . . . and the stench which pervade[s] the air is insupportable." The crowding and filth generated rampant disease and resulted in high illness rates that affected 10 to 15 percent of the occupants of each house on average. Physicians and middle-class commentators in the period perceived the unsanitary living conditions as both evidence of moral turpitude and as an incubator of fatal epidemics. The filth and density of the homes of the poor and working classes enfeebled the occupants, making them unusually susceptible to common illnesses and even more vulnerable to epidemics. The investigating committee concluded that the Chinese settlement posed a health menace to the rest of the city's inhabitants; for example, the "excessive" number of Chinese was "dangerous to the health of the inhabitants owing to the crowded state of the houses of Chinamen, the sickness which they introduce and the extreme and habitual filthy condition of their persons and their habitations." [12]

The Chinese were characterized repeatedly in terms of "excess"—of their number, of their living densities, of the diseases they spawned, and of the waste they produced. The references to excess and extremes stood in menacing contrast to the presumed norms of the white middle class. The danger of excess lay in its perceived capacity to expand across class and racial differences and spatial boundaries, carrying lethal contagion. The investigators feared that cholera would not only "make short work of the Chinese in their quarters" but also that it would strike "our own citizens." The differentiation between Chinese "aliens" and the municipal "citizens" enabled the committee to entertain the suggestion of taking "extraordinary measures" to suppress the epidemic by expelling the Chinese and thereby "removing from our midst the germs of pestilence." In their rhetoric, the committee members shifted from attributing the health threat to collective Chinese *behavior* to denouncing the Chinese as the very *embodiment* of disease. Their substitution revealed how effortlessly the classification of racial difference could shift from social to biological attributes. Despite the interest in radical removal, the committee endorsed a plan to revive the Board of Health, implement health regulations, and appoint a public health officer to enforce them. Although the committee failed to remove the Chinese population, whom they regarded as disease carriers, they demanded that the Chinese Companies make provisions to take "their sick countrymen outside the city limits." [13]

Early in the history of Chinese settlement, Chinese merchants took the lead in establishing associations, known in Chinese as *huiguan* (literally, meeting halls), which translated into English as "company." The immigrants from each of the districts of Guangdong province spoke different dialects of Cantonese and identified strongly with places of origin. The district *huiguan* served as a mutual-aid umbrella group that comprised various subgroups organized around village origins and surnames. These associations were run by elected officers, usually merchants, and they provided their members with accommodations, work and business opportunities, and when necessary, health care and burial assistance. Although relations between the district *huiguan* were often strained, these *huiguan* banded together to respond to local and national political, immigration, and legal challenges. In the 1870s, the coordinating council of six *huiguan*—the Zhonghua (Chinese) Huiguan—adopted a formal English name, the Chinese Consolidated Benevolent Association (CCBA), and was commonly known as the "Six Companies." [14]

In 1854 leaders of several district *huiguan*, who referred to themselves as "respectable Chinese residents," convened the day before the Common Council hearings to respond to the report's recommendations. Supporting the public health concerns about the deleterious relationship between filth, crowding, and disease, the Chinese merchants developed a series of resolutions intended to "remove the causes of complaints which have been made recently against the Chinese." These resolutions included assurances that boardinghouses would be "cleaned and renovated" and "excess boarders" immediately removed, that "all Chinamen present will take immediate steps to have their premises cleaned," and that a hospital would be built on the outskirts of the city. Seeking to develop moral distinctions within the Chinese population, these Chinese merchants invited the intervention of inspectors to "force" noncompliant Chinese to abate "nuisances." They were eager to claim that the merchants represented at the meeting were law-abiding and responsive to the concerns of the city government. The business elite represented at the meeting served to further establish its "respectable" status by differentiating its members from those merchants engaged in illicit business. They requested that the police suppress Chinese brothels and gambling houses, "which the meeting considers to be a great grievance to the Chinese residents." In every regard, the merchants who petitioned the city council sought to ensure that the "innocent shall not suffer with the guilty." [15]

The "respectable merchants" retreated from a class condemnation of the Chinese laborers living in boardinghouses. Instead they denounced the brothel keepers and gambling-den owners. They conflated the operation of illicit businesses with sanitary negligence. Since the respectable merchants operated the boardinghouses, they were eager to prove compliance with city regulations and their good intentions. In the mid–nineteenth century, service delivery in the city was uneven and garbage collection and even police protection were transacted privately by businesspeople and residence owners. Merchants complained that white police officers collected weekly payments from merchants on Sacramento and Dupont Streets to "clean their respective quarters" and provide protection, but these same merchants rarely received proper trash removal or sanitary services. They felt helpless to redress the police extortion and fraud in light of the absence of regular city services.

The Chinese merchants' pledge to build a "suitable" hospital for Chinese immigrants outside city limits raised questions about the civic ambivalence toward providing services to the Chinese and especially about the unwillingness to include Chinese residents in the body politic. The city council's unusual requirement that they build outside city limits expressed the fear that "sick Chinese" would radiate contagion and the belief that they must be removed beyond city boundaries. City council members further questioned the effectiveness of Chinese medical treatment and hospital care and in the end refused any plans for a Chinese hospital. These suspicions belied the unwillingness of city and state officials to take any responsibility for providing health care and for opening the public hospitals to Chinese patients. The *Daily Alta* editor argued that the state of California was responsible for ill Chinese immigrants. In 1852 the state legislature had passed a tax on passengers arriving at the port of San Francisco, in order to pay the costs of the State Marine Hospital in San Francisco and public hospitals in Sacramento and Stockton. Although Chinese immigrants contributed substantial tax receipts, these immigrants were not entitled to medical care and treatment in public facilities.[16]

The cholera panic quickly subsided in September 1854, and in its wake emerged a new city health authority in the revived Board of Health and a new perception of space, race, and contagion. The *Daily Alta* disingenuously criticized the "unnecessary alarm among the nervous portion of our citizens." Without acknowledging the newspaper's own responsibility in fanning the hysteria with reports of "authenticated [Chinese] cases" of cholera the week before, the *Daily Alta* editor admonished those who would rely upon "rumors."[17] The hysteria and rumors created fears based on a new articulation of space and race. Chinatown had become a singular and separate place that henceforth could be targeted in official inspections and popular commentary.

From a single block on Sacramento Street in 1854, the territory described as Chinatown expanded by 1885 to a fifteen-square-block region bounded by Kearny, Broadway, Sacramento, and Powell Streets. The growth to the west and north was shaped by the hilly topography, exponential population growth, and the rapid articulation of other zones of the city. The Chinese businesses and residences spread rapidly west up the hill to Powell Street and north to the relatively flat streets as far as Broadway. The sharp ridges on California Street limited the expansion south. Although in the 1850s the businesses and residences occupied by the Chinese immigrants were located throughout the city, by the 1870s these businesses and residences had been consolidated in the Chinatown zone. In the last third of the century, the borders of Chinatown abutted four defined zones of the city: the elite residential district of Nob Hill on the west; the main commercial and business districts on the south and east; and the Latin Quarter (which in the twentieth century became known as North Beach) to the north. (See Map 1.)

The number of Chinese residents remained stable during the decade of the 1850s, but like San Francisco's population as a whole, the number of Chinese residents climbed rapidly in the 1860s. The total population of San Francisco nearly tripled in size, to 149,473, and the Chinese population quadrupled to over 12,000 in 1870. By the 1880 census the Chinese population stood at 21,745 out of a total of 233,979. In the 1860s, Chinese commercial enterprises and labor contractors set up business in San Francisco. Workers often circulated through the city between work contracts for rural agriculture and construction. After the completion of the Central Pacific Railroad, Chinese immigrant workers migrated to San Francisco, where they found work in the growing manufacturing industries and service trades.[18] The Chinese were the largest racial minority group in San Francisco at the time. By comparison, the population of blacks hovered between 1,100 and 1,800 throughout the nineteenth century.[19]

Although throughout the late nineteenth century the area called Chinatown had a variety of inhabitants, the predominance of Chinese residents meant the entire location had only one racial identity. Businesses and residences occupied by Irish, Italian, Portuguese, Mexican, Canadian, and Anglo Americans continued to thrive in so-called Chinatown, but they were of little interest to the health inspectors. These

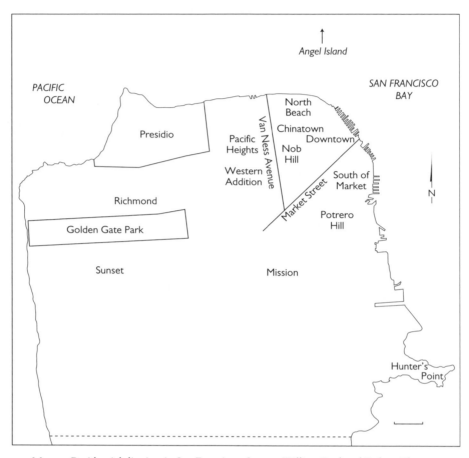

Map 1. Residential districts in San Francisco. Source: William Issel and Robert Cherny, *San Francisco, 1865–1932: Politics, Power, and Urban Development,* p. 59.

inspectors imagined the preeminent site of contagion as the spaces of Chinese residence, particularly the bunking houses of Chinese bachelor workers.

In the late 1860s and 1870s the increase in Chinese population exacerbated white fear of Chinese spaces. Health officials continued to identify Chinese behavior as the cultural cause of the perceived medical menace. In 1869 the city health officer C. M. Bates issued his report stating that Chinese "habits and manner of life are of such a character as to breed and engender disease wherever they reside." In the report, Bates warned that "unless their style of life is changed[,] . . . some disease of a malignant form may break out among them and communicate itself to our Caucasian population." Bates feared the perceived lethal consequences of Chinese living standards and styles: "As a class, their mode of life is the most abject in which it is possible for human beings to exist. The great majority of them live crowded together in rickety, filthy and dilapidated tenement houses, like so many cattle or hogs. Considering their mode of life, it is indeed wonderful that they have so far escaped every phase of disease. In passing through that portion of the city occupied by them, the most absolute squalidness and misery meets one at every turn. Vice in all its hideousness is on every hand." [20]

The "abjectness" of the Chinese "mode of life" was manifested in the comparisons to farm animals, feeding a perception not only of Chinese immigrants' inferiority but also of their inhumanity. In health reports and journalistic reports of health inspections, Chinese were likened to a wide array of animals, including rats, hogs, and cattle. The choice of animals underscored a relationship to waste and an imperviousness to crowding. As David Sibley has observed, rats and pigs especially have had a "particular place in the racist bestiary because all are associated with residues—food waste, human waste—and in the case of rats there is an association with spaces which border civilized society, particular subterranean spaces like sewers, which also channel residues and from which rats occasionally emerge to transgress the boundaries of society." [21] The insinuations that the Chinese were wallowing in cesspools and in possession of an instinct for crowded, decaying environments made the metonyms of reviled creatures all the more menacing and transgressive to the readers. Like pigs and cattle herded into pens, the living densities of Chinese "dens" demonstrated Chinese indifference to human comforts. Bates claimed that "apartments that would be deemed small for the accommodation of a single American [were] occupied by six, eight or ten Mongolians, with seeming indifference to all ordinary comforts." [22] The Chinese were presumed to relish these "miserable" circumstances of poverty, squalor, and filth.

As city health officer, a position created in the 1870 reorganization of the Board of Health, Bates held responsibility for the daily enforcement of sanitary regulations. Therefore, his pronouncements carried the weight of regulative authority. He carefully cultivated the professional objectivity of a physician to buttress this authority and distanced himself from the opportunistic "politicians and demagogues" who had manipulated hostility toward the Chinese for political advantage. Bates was particularly concerned that his conclusions would be dismissed by the city's business community and elected officials because they appeared similar to those of the Anti-Coolie Association, a white labor group who opposed Chinese immigration and settlement.

The tension between the white manufacturers and white laborers was exacerbated by a devastating commercial panic and depression in the late 1860s. After the completion of the transcontinental railroad, San Francisco's population increased 30 percent in two years, but manufacturing output plummeted once trade from the East Coast made the price of consumer goods plunge. Thousands of white workingmen were unemployed, and they blamed white capitalists and the Chinese workers for their troubles. The Anti-Coolie Association formed in March 1867 and coordinated boycotts of manufacturers who employed Chinese workers. The organization engaged in selective industrial sabotage citywide and persistently harassed and assaulted Chinese men. Its rapid growth and frequently violent mobilization of anxious white tradesmen and unemployed workers alarmed San Francisco's commercial elite.[23]

The Anti-Coolie Association deftly borrowed and elaborated upon the medical menace of Chinese settlement. In 1869 the organization outlined the threat posed by Chinese immigrants to white labor, national prosperity, and the general health of American citizens. The 1868 smallpox epidemic, which had left 760 dead in its wake, served as an ominous sign of the extreme health dangers posed by Chinese immigration. The virulent strain of smallpox "baffled the skill of our medical men" and was "unknown among the Caucasian race." The Chinese allegedly bred disease as a result of the "density of their population and their peculiar mode of living." To the medical causality that Chinese living densities and habits contributed to infection, the Anti-Coolie Association added the ominous assertion that Chinese immigrants carried peculiar disease strains.[24]

This problem of the Chinese possessing potentially innate dispositions to illness was taken up by Thomas Logan, secretary of the California State Board of Health and a nationally reputed physician who was elected in 1872 as president of the American Medical Association. For the California State Board of Health, Logan had commissioned in 1871 an investigation of San Francisco's Chinatown, charging not only that Chinese habits and living conditions had vital implications for all San Francisco inhabitants but also that Chinatown's conditions could "spread dismay and desolation throughout the land." Logan was attentive to environmental conditions and behavior but feared the contagious consequences of Chinese innate racial propensities. Logan predicted that their "hereditary vices" or "engrafted peculiarities" preordained the Chinese to chronic and unusual illness. In Logan's assessment, Chinese cultural behavior was not shaped by historical context but rather emerged from hereditary traits that were naturalized in their very bodies. This conflation of behavior and body as both the cultural and biological heritage of the Chinese "race" powerfully influenced the public-health knowledge of Chinatown and Chinese people.[25]

Logan's investigation not only contributed new explanations of medical causality but also advanced a key strategy of accumulating knowledge about the Chinatown "underworld." Logan popularized the eyewitness journey into Chinatown's dens and proclaimed the journey's narrative as the primary evidence of its hidden horrors. The vivid and visceral narration of the midnight journey through Chinatown became one of the standard forms of knowledge used in both medical and popular accounts to establish the truth of Chinatown as the preeminent site of vice, immorality, degradation, crime, and disease.[26] By visiting and surveying Chinatown, individual doctors, journalists, and middle-class tourists delineated the utter foreignness, exoticism, and evil of the place. The firsthand account and the narration of visual and olfactory sensations provided authoritative and seemingly transparent evidence of the true nature of the Chinese problem. The eyewitness account became indispensable to the social diagnosis and policy advanced by health officers like Bates, who had concluded that "nothing short of an ocular demonstration can convey an idea of Chinese poverty and depravity."[27] Investigators later in the century recommended a visit to Chinatown for skeptics in order to ensure that the official findings were not considered an "exaggeration" or a fictional "sketch." These investigators were confident that an excursion through the Chinatown labyrinth would produce sufficient "ocular and olfactory proofs."[28]

The question of "proof" and "evidence" shaped the procedures and itinerary of the eyewitness investigation and its narrative report. Logan's journey emphasized all the characteristic procedures and features of the investigation. Despite the confidence that visual scrutiny would provide proof, Logan and other investigators simultaneously held a keen appreciation that the "truth" of Chinatown was hidden from public view. The most revealing journeys, then, had to be conducted at night, when the "true character" of the quarter—with its gambling houses, opium dens, and brothels—revealed itself. Logan solicited the services of a police escort to navigate the serpentine and subterranean passageways—the labyrinth—and to provide physical protection from routine threats of violence. His party also included the local medical expert, Bates, who could interpret the consequences of "vice and abominations." Although the itinerary of the investigation could include the "tangled maze of narrow streets" and "dark alleys," the crucial objective was to penetrate underground and visit the labyrinth of bunking houses, opium dens, and barricaded gambling houses. Logan's itinerary ignored other Chinatown spaces—the merchants' homes, dry goods stores, temples, meeting rooms, and Chinese opera theaters included in other kinds of travelogues—since these more visible sites offered little evidence of filth, sickness, and pathology that demanded medical evaluation.[29]

The narrative of Logan's midnight journey dispensed with the posture of professional objectivity and disinterested observation. His narrative featured a dramatic selection of circumstances, details, and medical explanation that passionately yielded the author's own personal and immediate sensations and reactions. Logan offered his medical colleagues and the curious public some instances of his momentary disorientation, horror, disgust, and fascination. He described his visit to the "lowest dens of degraded bestiality," where he saw opium smokers, prostitutes, and furtive gamblers. The investigators crept through "foul labyrinthine passages" that would occasionally "open into a dimly lit room," where they saw "dusky human beings lying on tiers of broad shelves . . . with a foul opium pipe, and dirty little oil lamp used for lighting the pipe." In other rooms, female prostitutes "with painted lips and rosy-tipped fingers" solicited the visitors, or male gamblers would "hurry and scuffle to conceal" their illicit games. In their inspection of large lodging houses, Logan discovered tiny rooms that had been "cut up and divided into what might be called pens."[30]

Logan's medical authority transformed sensational observations into somber appraisals of environmental conditions that necessitated immediate public health surveillance and redress. His medical scrutiny fixed on the insupportable "stench" that made his party feel "enveloped in a physical atmosphere as tainted and disgusting, from superadded stale opium smoke, as the moral one was degraded." Logan conflated the unventilated physical atmosphere with the moral degradation of opium smoking, gambling, and prostitution. Unventilated space that locked in stale smoke and produced a horrible "stench" violated "sanitary law," requiring "immediate redress." The "absolute absence of ventilation" provided the pretext for the intervention of the health officials. Influenced by the miasma theory of disease that remained popular in the 1870s, Logan regarded Chinatown, with its "foul and disgusting vapors" and unsanitary conditions, as the primary source of atmospheric pollution.[31]

Logan was assured in his ability to faithfully narrate the "real" conditions and offer authoritative diagnosis of social ills. This self-confident medical authority made it possible for him to draw freely from both literary and political sources and to repackage fictional and partisan rhetoric into irreproachable medical diagnosis. For instance, he borrowed literary allusions to heighten the drama of an opium den encounter. In subterranean dormitory "pens," Logan encountered "half naked" Chinese "inmates . . . reposing on shelves—some sleeping, others blowing out curling puffs of narcotic fumes from their broad nostrils." The immodesty, lethargy, and unabashed narcotic addiction recalled for Logan the figure of the "opium-smoking hag" in Charles Dickens's novel *Edwin Drood,* which presented a "graphic instance of civilization touching barbarism." [32] The dramatic literary scene amplified the dangers of Oriental "barbarism" in the midst of the "civilized," modern city of San Francisco, particularly with the horrifying possibility of white American men and women being discovered among the addicts. Logan worried about both the physical and moral dangers to the body and society that opium addiction posed.

Logan's ready use of literary analogy did not confound his purpose of exposing the "real" conditions of Chinatown. Logan used realist narrative devices and evoked Dickens's "morally-ordered universe" to effectively communicate the hidden dangers of Chinese habitation. Nineteenth-century realist narratives appeared in a range of forms—newspapers, government inquiry, autopsy reports, and novels. The popularity of represented and sensationalized reality offered readers melodramatic experiences, naturalistic details, and the disclosure of private truth to a public world. Logan's description of sensations and realist narrative secured his authority as the eyewitness observer. His revulsion and his unfaltering judgment, however, demonstrated his distance from his object of study and bolstered his claims to comprehensive knowledge of the true nature of the Chinese residents. Logan applied both medical and moral discernment in his prognosis of the dens and showed little concern that his readers would mistake his literary allusions for the facts of Chinatown's dangers.[33]

Logan was equally unfazed by the potential taint of political partisanship. In a discussion of density in the boardinghouses, Logan supplemented his analysis with a quote from the Anti-Coolie Association deputation to the San Francisco Board of Health: "Some houses have five

hundred lodgers—some one thousand; and in the Globe Hotel—standing on ground sixty by sixty, and three stories high—there are twenty
five hundred tenants." Once Logan had marshaled the Anti-Coolie Association anecdote about the Globe Hotel, he propelled that description
into a popular and credible shorthand for the condition of all Chinese
boardinghouses and a poignant example of the degeneration that followed Chinese habitation of any site. White travelogue writers and labor politicians freely seized on the devolution of the Globe Hotel at
1001 Dupont Street from the most opulent hotel for Gold Rush pros-
pectors to a decaying and filthy tenement for the "flotsam and jetsam of
Chinatown." All the official and popular accounts of the Globe Hotel
shared a description of how, over the course of thirty years, the spacious
and luxurious accommodations had been subdivided into congested and
claustrophobic bunkrooms. Estimates of the number of inhabitants
ranged from eight hundred to twenty-five hundred Chinese "crammed"
inside.[34] The itinerary of this example—from Anti-Coolie deputation to
Dr. Logan's report to the myriad popular travelogues—raises questions
about precisely who investigated the building, what they saw, and how
they arrived at the wide range of estimates. Was it even important to distinguish between the facts and an exaggeration in this migration from
political anecdote to commonsense truth? The number of inhabitants
reported simply accentuated the shared idea that Chinatown boardinghouses were extraordinarily crowded and overpopulated.

The sensationalist imagery overpowered the range of estimates, and
all writers were quick to emphasize the typical and pervasive nature of
the problem of density and crowding. The Anti-Coolie anecdote in 1869
claimed that "Chinamen have burrowed dens, even beneath the streets,
holes that would 'not admit a coffin.'" The images of cramped, hidden,
and subterranean living quarters that resembled "pens," "dens," "cof-
fins" and "dungeons" was an imagery common to both physicians and
political activists, reflecting ubiquitous anxiety and an abhorrence for
crowded and dark spaces. These spaces were fit for animals, criminals,
and the dead, not for human habitation.[35] In 1886, the travelogue writer
Walter Raymond claimed that the general character of Chinese boardinghouses was a "noisome density in the atmosphere, which cannot
be received into the system without great nausea. . . . Here can be experienced all the horrors of a catacomb, packed with living, disease-
breeding flesh, slowly drifting into their graves."[36] The atmosphere
Raymond related gave white readers every indication of the experience
of being trapped alive in a grave. He detailed the horrors of visiting a

place that lacked light, oxygen, and free space, the opposite of the sun-drenched, ventilated, airy, and clean middle-class home—the presumed type of home inhabited by the visitors and the readers.

However, these startling assessments of unhealthy Chinatown conditions raise the question of why such "gross violations" had not resulted in more frequent epidemic disaster. Unbelievably, Logan explained that the city was blessed by natural ventilation: "Were it not for the strong oceanic winds which prevail during the summer months, San Francisco would . . . have suffered the heaviest penalties." Over the years, many of the city's public health officials and physicians would evoke the presence of good crosswinds to explain the city population's relative good health despite the dangers posed by Chinatown. This explanation demonstrated how the environment could both contribute to epidemic and suppress it. In the miasma theory of infection, festering waste would breed disease in enclosed rooms, and natural ventilation could air out rooms with windows. Yet it remained a mystery as to how winds could quickly de-contaminate the vapors that rose from the rotting waste in Chinatown's unventilated cellars before it infected its white neighbors in other parts of the city.[37]

The mysteries of infection and contamination had not, however, dis-suaded white labor politicians from elaborating on discourses of racial hygiene in their struggles for political power. In the late 1860s compli-cated relationships had emerged between white working-class political mobilization, anti-Chinese ideology, public health, and municipal poli-tics in San Francisco. These interests became increasingly entangled by the end of the decade. In 1877, at a moment of financial panic and the conclusion of a widespread smallpox epidemic, new political and social arrangements emerged that attributed economic distress and death to the Chinese "race." At the same time, workers organized the Working-men's Party of California (WPC), which appropriated this "knowledge" in their political rhetoric and action.

The party became an increasingly potent political force in local and statewide politics. By the September 1879 general elections, the WPC had absorbed much of the Democratic Party's electoral constituency and swept dozens of candidates into office. On the state level, the Working-men's Party and the Republican Party split election results; a Republican became California's governor, while a WPC candidate won the seat of chief justice on the California Supreme Court. In San Francisco, after an extraordinary mayoral campaign punctuated by assassination attempts and accusations of sexual impropriety, the WPC candidate and pastor of the Baptist Metropolitan Temple, Issac Kalloch, won the mayoral race.[38] Kalloch's campaign swept into office WPC candidates for sheriff, auditor, tax collector, district attorney, and public administrator as well. The labor organizer Frank Roney speculated years later in his memoirs that a deal had been made between the WPC and the bipartisan establishment to divide municipal administration. The Workingmen's Party won the mayoralty and a number of posts controlling patronage, while the real power centers—the board of supervisors and the police—remained in the hands of the establishment Republicans and Democrats. The divided administration created intractable government deadlocks.[39]

In his inaugural address, Mayor Kalloch outlined a WPC mandate to use the powers of city government to remedy the Chinese problem, provide relief for unemployed white workers, and reduce the tax burden by a voluntary salary cut for all elected officials. Although the work relief and tax abatement programs required the approval of the hostile board of supervisors, Kalloch could directly influence the Board of Health in his capacity of presiding officer. The health officer John Meares and the other state-appointed physicians on the board—Henry Gibbons Jr., William Douglass, James A. Simpson, and Hugh Huger Toland—were already sympathetic to the idea that Chinatown was a threat to public health.[40] Immediately after Kalloch's inauguration, Meares and Gibbons conducted a rapid investigation of Chinatown. The WPC was eager to supplement the findings of the official investigation; in January its Anti-Chinese Council commissioned a committee of physicians and other sympathetic members to conduct their own investigation of Chinatown's sanitary conditions.[41]

In the 1880 Board of Health report on the living conditions in the Chinese quarter, Logan's images of slime, filth, and underground habitations were reapplied with even more horrifying detail than before. Gibbons, Meares, and Kalloch had conducted the investigation, concluding that "unnatural overcrowding" was detrimental to the health of the Chinese and endangered the "health of the city." They gave a detailed description of several of the subterranean dwellings:

> Near the entrance to this underground den there are large waste pipes running from the water-closets and sinks of the building above ground, which empty into open wooden boxes above the sewer, and the mass of filth is so great that the sewer is frequently choked and the troughs run over. The crowded occupants of the underground regions are hardly to blame for avoiding such wretched apologies as their "water-closets" for the purpose of nature. . . . Amongst all this smoke and stench and rottenness, in rooms

barely 10 × 12 feet, 12 persons eat and sleep. . . . In another basement near by, thirteen Chinamen . . . live in a room eight feet square. In a room 6 × 6 feet ten Chinese men and women huddled together in beastly promiscuousness. . . . [These rooms] are absolutely without proper ventilation, and it seems unaccountable how human beings can live in them for a single night.[42]

These descriptions emphasized the sheer physicality of the "sickening filth" and "slime" and reiterated the animality and inhuman living density of the Chinese residents. In a boardinghouse where two hundred "Chinamen" lived, the report described "its inmates [as] having a ghastly look, and [they] are covered with a clammy perspiration. On the other side the rooms appeared to be filled with sick Chinamen, and ranged around the walls are chicken-coops, filled with what appeared to be sick chickens."[43] The equation of Chinese men with sick animals heightened perceptions of the intolerable, horrific living conditions and continued the comparison of Chinese to animals started by Bates.

The process of inspection and regulation of living conditions generated detailed knowledge of the location and nature of individual aberrations. Regulation, with its legal rules, standards, and threat of routine surveillance, generated knowledge that could be quantified and compared over time and against circumstances in other buildings and neighborhoods. The report catalogued dozens of health ordinances that the "Chinese people" habitually violated. During the 1870s, the city had passed ordinances regulating housing density, garbage disposal, the quarantine of contagious disease victims, the sanitary condition of food vendors, the condition of sewage systems, the construction of toilets, and the condition and location of hospitals. The report detailed a litany of stopped-up sewers, stench, and slime, all of which provided yardsticks by which to judge the unsanitary living conditions.[44]

When the committee catalogued the public health infractions in the Chinese quarter, they were quick to repudiate the idea that their investigation was biased by "race prejudice or class hatred," neglecting to consider how both race and class discrimination had forced Chinese immigrants to live in crowded and dilapidated tenements. They complimented some Chinese for "living quite decently and cleanly as any people could do who have to live under similar circumstances." The committee members emphasized that Chinatown—not necessarily the Chinese people—was a nuisance. The Board of Health unanimously adopted the report and the motion to declare Chinatown a nuisance to the public's health and welfare. The investigating members of the board

adamantly advocated that the "Chinese cancer must be cut out of the
heart of the city." They reasoned that such radical action would benefit "the Chinese themselves" as well as "our people." However, their
rhetoric revealed that their disgust of Chinatown actually did extend
to the "health-defying" and "law-defying" Chinese women and men
themselves.[45]

At the February 25, 1880, meeting, the Republican-dominated board
of supervisors initially supported the Board of Health's condemnation of
Chinatown as a "sanitary nuisance." However, the board of supervisors
expressed concern that the health notice would fuel an extralegal "in-
cendiary" response by white workingmen, and promptly gave orders to
the police to hire four hundred additional officers. Supported by the local business establishment, the board of supervisors feared a recurrence
of the 1877 riot, where a white working-class mob threatened to torch
Chinatown. Not only were the businessmen and the supervisors concerned with maintaining the general social order, many of the white
business elite were protecting their own interests: the majority of property leased by Chinese businesses and residents was owned by white
businessmen. The WPC suspected that the bipartisan establishment that
controlled the police would resist executing any orders that would eradicate Chinatown, knowing that East Coast capitalists feared that such
summary use of police powers would disrupt manufacturing and trade
on the West Coast. Sheriff Thomas Desmond, elected on the WPC
ticket, assured the party's rank and file that he would execute the Board
of Health's orders and warned that, if the police refused to comply, the
city authorities "would call on the Workingmen to clear out Chinatown." And the WPC issued resolutions warning that, if there were any
interference in the "abatement of the Chinese nuisance," the WPC
would "visit upon low-designing minions of power, backed up though
they may be by cowardly capitalists and corporations, a punishment
so swift and terrible that the reader of the history will shudder at the
record."[46]

In light of these threats, Kalloch had difficulty convincing the board
of supervisors that there was "nothing revolutionary or radical" in the
removal of the Chinese from the city center and the razing of Chinatown
for sanitary reasons. Many of the board's constituents among the elite
commercial establishment feared that property they leased to the Chinese
would be destroyed and they would lose their tenants. On February 28,
the board of supervisors decided to rescind its earlier endorsement of

the Board of Health's declaration of "Chinatown [as] a nuisance."[47] Although the mayor and the WPC organized mass meetings and pamphlet campaigns to marshal support for the Board of Health's order, the WPC rank and file remained orderly, and the city administration remained politically deadlocked—until the end of Mayor Kalloch's term and the dissolution of the WPC in 1881. No legal or extralegal action on the Board of Health's condemnation of Chinatown ever occurred. However, the Board of Health did continue to impose routine sanitary surveillance, vaccination campaigns, and fumigation of dwellings in Chinatown.

In 1882 the U.S. Congress passed the Chinese Exclusion Act, which disallowed Chinese workers to immigrate. Although the law exempted Chinese merchants, students, diplomats, and their families, it consolidated the disenfranchisement of all Chinese people by prohibiting any state or federal court from admitting Chinese immigrants to naturalized citizenship. Subsequent legislation virtually cut off Chinese immigration and that of other East and South Asian immigrants—as well as abridged opportunities to win citizenship and the right to political participation—by branding Chinese and other Asian immigrants as perpetual "aliens ineligible for citizenship." Throughout the western states, local white vigilantes drove out Chinese settlers. Many Chinese laborers sought safety in San Francisco along with the white laborers who flocked to the city because of a severe economic downturn in the eastern United States.[48]

Three years later, the Republican-dominated board of supervisors under the Democratic mayor Washington Bartlett revisited the issue of Chinese residents in San Francisco and commissioned a special committee to survey Chinatown. In May 1885, supervisors Willard Farwell and John Kunkler presented their comprehensive report to the public. They confined their investigation to the area bounded by California, Kearny, Broadway, and Stockton Streets, a twelve-block area. Although the supervisors recognized that the Chinese population had "drifted" into the blocks west of Stockton Street, they restricted the report to the popularly assumed boundaries of Chinatown because of fiscal considerations.[49]

The zeal of health officials to know the spaces within Chinatown culminated in a report that also produced the cartography of Chinatown. Nearly two decades of systematic surveillance and normalizing public health codes had aided in producing a map of the street-level Chinatown settlement. The special committee employed surveyors who accompanied them on visits of "every floor and every room." The detailed report

of the "conditions of occupancy of every room"—its use, number of inhabitants, and sanitary condition—enabled the committee to make a
map of the district, specifying the "character of occupancy" of the first
floor of each of the buildings as well as providing a detailed accounting of all the basements, the subbasements, and the floors above the
street level. Titled the *Official Map of "Chinatown" in San Francisco,* it
was color coded to distinguish "General Chinese Occupancy," "Chinese
Gambling Houses," "Chinese Prostitution," "Chinese Opium Resorts,"
"Chinese Joss Houses," and "White Prostitution." The "General Occupancy" sections were further identified by the type of factory, store, or
lodging, which were tagged by street number. The white sections sprin-
kled throughout the district and on its edges were identified as "white"
groceries, saloons, bakeries, and residences. (See Figure 1.)

This explicit map of Chinatown represented a new strategy of knowledge.[50] This cartography substantiated the 1885 report's goal of obtain-
ing a "correct idea of the general condition of things there and the ordinary mode of life and practices of its inhabitants" by providing precise
dimensions and visual representations of the extent of Chinatown. The
map ordered and made intelligible at least the street level of the hereto-
fore impenetrable and labyrinthine geography of Chinatown. Thorough
inventories of sanitary infractions, indices of manufactures, and cata-
logues of the secret exits and entrances of "barricaded gambling dens,"
in combination with the precise map of Chinatown, injected the "me-
dium of crystallized fact and the inexorable logic of demonstrated truth"
into the heated political debate about the condition of Chinatown. It
also served to further "crystallize" the seemingly transparent relationship between race and place.[51]

The map and inventories were the products and tools of extensive surveillance, but they also ensured that more intensive surveillance would
occur in the future. The report emphasized the scores of public health
violations throughout Chinatown, knowledge of which had been reaped
from the systematic investigation. The report presented an image of a
normative regulatory apparatus that employed inspectors, police, and
judges who forced all habitations in the city to comply with standard
regulations. Although the surveillance and investigation of Chinatown
were extraordinary, the violations were quite ordinary. A five-page catalogue of the most egregious, most frequent infractions merely cited in-
adequate plumbing and drainage, including clogged water closets, uri-
nals, and sinks; stagnant cesspools; and the lack of plumbing connections to street sewers. As a catalogue, however, these violations were no

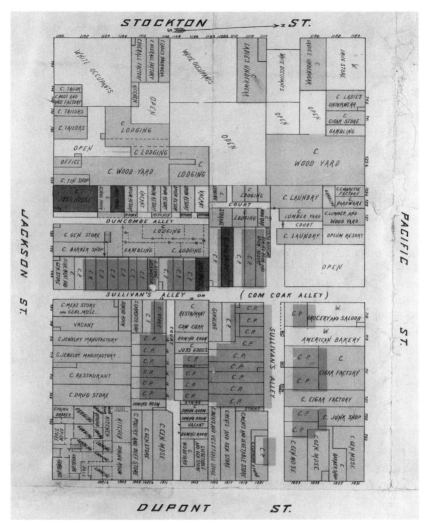

Figure 1. This detail shows a one-square-block section taken from the four-color *Official Map of "Chinatown" in San Francisco* (1885), which appeared in the San Francisco Board of Supervisors' *Report of the Special Committee of the Board of Supervisors of San Francisco on the Condition of the Chinese Quarter and the Chinese in San Francisco*. The original map showed twelve square blocks and pinpointed the precise location and purpose of each building and the race of its occupants. In this section some of the designations include Chinese prostitution (C.P), C[hinese] laundry], opium resort, C[hinese] general merchandise, gambling, w[hite] bakery, C[hinese] cigar factory, C[hinese] restaurant, and so on. Courtesy of the Bancroft Library.

longer individual or singular anomalies but were interpreted as a collective manifestation—evidence of collective behavior. They were perceived as evidence of "lawlessness" and resolute disregard by the Chinese population.

The precise mapping of vice onto Chinatown buildings and the perception of Chinese "lawlessness" inflamed fears of municipal corruption. For instance, in the early twentieth century an anonymous individual scribbled on one copy of the 1885 map of Chinatown a handwritten
annotation that demonstrated acute political cynicism and grave doubts
about police and public health enforcement: "This 'Official Map' of
Chinatown shows official knowledge of the illegal gambling resorts,
houses of prostitution, opium dens and houses of white prostitutes,
which by the payment of blackmail have secured immunity from prosecution etc. and continue collecting filth and unhealthy surroundings
which provided the ostensible excuse for the fraudulent quarantine
and plague scare of 1900 by the Board of Health." The accumulation of
knowledge through surveillance and mapping did not necessarily result
in effective prosecution and long-term reform. The anonymous critic's
allegations of police corruption also underscored a suspicion that the
Board of Health would overreact to its own negligence in enforcing sanitary regulations. During the 1900 bubonic plague crisis, according to
the writer's accusation, the Board of Health freely spent "public money
to clean up nuisances that it was their duty to compel owners and tenants to do at their own expense." The writer emphasized a breakdown
in governance, in which municipal officials were unwilling to curb vice
that bred both unsanitary conditions and lawlessness. For some investigators and political commentators, the evidence of unabated vice and
filth in Chinatown exacerbated fears of widespread government corruption and social anarchy that could spread beyond Chinatown borders.[52]

Officials had long worried that within Chinatown no respectable
society existed that put moral and social checks on the culture of vice,
lawlessness, and disease. The 1885 investigation included a population
census that numerically demonstrated this presumed absence of respectable nuclear families in Chinatown. The enumeration of persons, within
households and classified by their social relations, created an assessment
of Chinese society driven by statistical evidence, not anecdote. These
numbers revealed that the Chinese were at odds with the social structures and classification that organized the dominant white society. In
their tabulations of women and children, Farwell and Kunkler observed

that more than 40 percent of the women and more than 90 percent of the children were "herded together with apparent indiscriminate parental relations, and no family classification, so far as can be ascertained." [53] Like the late-nineteenth-century surveyors of urban England and colonial Africa who attributed disease and disorder to the improper social and spatial distribution of bodies, Kunkler and Farwell were horrified by the lack of distinctive and discernible nuclear families.[54] Many women and children lived together without the presence of a male head of household. And among "professional prostitutes," mothers and children lived "in adjoining apartments and intermingle freely," which for Farwell made it impossible to tell "where the family relationship leaves off and prostitution begins." This vision of middle-class domesticity and morality, which favored the presence of well-bounded and visibly distinct persons, families, and habitations, was widespread among European and American public health reformers in their imposition of proper sanitary practices.[55]

Not only did investigators want to prove collective activity, but they also intended to present the systematic nature of Chinese living conditions. In order to substantiate the assertion that the Chinese lived in "constant and habitual violation" of the cubic air ordinance, the report presented "some instances illustrating the *ordinary* habits of the Chinese laboring classes in the matter of sleeping and living accommodations," rather than providing "extreme cases" as investigators had repeatedly done in the past. Through statistical tables, the committee listed the addresses of more than two dozen locations, comparing the number of actual occupants with the allowable number of occupants. In every case, more than three times as many people lived in housing than could be legally accommodated. Farwell and Kunkler followed up their establishment of statistical "proof" with a more typically lurid and extreme description of an underground den. It featured all the conventions of previous medical travelogues; however, the statistical preface substantiated the description's claim to represent "ordinary" conditions:

Descend into the basement of almost any building in Chinatown at night; pick your way by the aid of the police-man's candle along the dark and narrow passageway, black and grimy with a quarter of a century's accumulation of filth; step with care lest you fall into a cesspool of sewage abominations with which these subterranean depths abound. Now follow your guide through a door, which he forces, into a sleeping room. The air is thick with smoke and fetid with an indescribable odor of reeking vapors. . . . It is a sense of a horror you have never before experienced, revolting to the last degree, sickening and stupefying. Through this semi-opaque atmosphere you discover perhaps eight or ten—never less than two or three—bunks, the greater part or all of which are occupied by two persons, some in a state of stupefaction from opium, some rapidly smoking themselves into that condition, and all in dirt and filth.

According to Farwell and Kunkler, the statistics and the description combined to provide authoritative "proof" for their assertion that the "mode of life among the Chinese here are [sic] not much above 'those of the rats of the waterfront.'"[56]

Following the now popular logic of medical discourse, the report predicted that dire health consequences would result from the presence of filthy, overcrowded, and inhuman conditions. These conditions presented "a constant menace to the welfare of society as a slumbering pest, likely at any time to generate and spread disease should the city be visited by an epidemic in any virulent form." Not only was Chinatown characterized as "the rankest growth of human degradation that can be found upon this continent," outstripping all other slums in "filth, disease, crime and misery," but, authorities suggested, no amount of cleansing would improve these conditions. The Chinese were expected to "relapse" into a "more dense condition of nastiness, in which they apparently delight to exist." Since its inhabitants were walking, seemingly unaffected, disease carriers, Chinatown constituted a constant and continual "source of danger." Disease was conceived as organic to every Chinese racialized space. Inhuman living conditions appeared to be "inseparable from the very nature of the race," and city authorities warned that Chinatown would remain a "cesspool" so "long as it is inhabited by people of the Mongolian race."[57]

The knowledge of Chinatown spaces, conditions, and social relations provided a material and representational terrain to explore the extreme contrasts between the "Chinese race" and the "American people." In public health reports the contrast fed the tension between aberrant and normal and the racial difference that separated the Chinese aliens from white Americans. In travelogues, this binary opposition of two irreconcilable peoples generated the underlying dramatic tension that propelled the narratives. G. B. Densmore's central "argument" that drove his *Chinese in California* travelogue was the "radical difference between Caucasian and Mongolian civilization."[58] These differences of civilization and "standard of living" emerged from the obsessive descriptions of

Chinatown as a space of difference antagonistic to the rest of the city. The editor of a local newspaper, Curt Abel-Musgrave, took the popular idea of Chinatown as a "subterranean world" to its logical extreme. In a bracing fantasy about a cholera epidemic unleashed in San Francisco, Abel-Musgrave conceptualized the territory of San Francisco as two distinctive cities—the "healthy paradise" of the true San Francisco aboveground and the "hell" of Chinatown underground. He explained that Chinatown below was impervious to the city's natural cleansing features: "Sunbeams that shine on us don't penetrate 50 feet deep into the pestilential dens of the Chinese population, and the fresh breezes which purify the air of our streets and our houses leave the sepulchres untouched in which for 30 years foul and disgusting vapors have been gathering."[59] Curiously, city officials offered detailed Chinatown maps to the street level only; it was up to travelogue writers to imagine and sketch out maps of the underground passageways and dens. Only Walter Raymond in his *Horrors of a Mongolian Settlement* offered a diagram of the subterranean roads and passageways of his journey.[60]

The public-health knowledge of dens, density, and the labyrinth cast Chinatown as a deviant transplantation of the traditional East in the modern Western city. This contrast emphasized the uneasy coexistence of growing, progressive San Francisco and decaying, regressive Chinatown. Chinatown was impervious to progress and was instead liable to rot and regress like the enervated Chinese empire across the Pacific. The environmental conditions of Chinatown could only harm the rest of the city.[61] The representation of the Chinese inhabitants was that of a race and culture apart and unaffected by the forces of modernity. City officials and travelogue writers represented the Chinese as burdened by the weight of an ancient civilization and impervious to beneficial change. These officials and writers conceived of time, in relation to Chinatown and the Chinese people, as a passage in which the physical environment was decaying and regressing while the residents lived without past or future. They perceived among the inhabitants of Chinatown ancient racial habits and proclivities that caused the Chinese to live in a "timeless present where all 'his' actions and reactions are repetitions of 'his' usual habits."[62] As with comparable racial formations, there was an insistent repetition of images that gave an ahistorical and unchanging quality to the represented reality of Chinatown and its inhabitants.[63] What propelled the endless, obsessive repetition of the idealized representation was the inherent impossibility to achieve the stereotyped racial category.

The project of naturalizing race identity involved the production of effects that posed as "reality," a daunting but compulsive task for those invested in the reproduction of racial "truths." [64]

In the racial formation of Chinese and Chinatown, medical discourses employed and adapted prevailing political and social discourses of Chinese "vice," "criminality," "immorality," "slavery," and "subversiveness" and, in turn, informed these popular discourses with the threat of Chinese "dirt" and "disease." [65] However, the reports of threats of disease originating in the social conduct of Chinese immigrants and the spaces in which they dwelled did not appear originally or exclusively in public health records or at the insistence of physicians. The *Daily Alta* newspaper and the anti-Chinese labor organizations from the very beginning of this period articulated concern about the unsanitary environment in Chinatown and the spatial elements of dens, density, and the labyrinth, which preoccupied city and state officials during the second half of the nineteenth century.

Medical discourse lent scientific weight to the project and turned every one of these stylized features of Chinatown into a cause of pathology and source of disease. The keepers of public health had broad powers, and over time they developed the authority to put these "ideas" about race into practice. Health officials and politicians justified the idea of Chinatown as inherently pestilent, and they invested this idea, through the accumulation of these stereotyped images in their reports and rhetoric, with the value of a natural truth.[66]

During the late nineteenth century, the imagery of Chinatown and the Chinese race as pestilent intensified to such an overwhelming pitch that any contradictions and inconsistencies were bent into and subsumed by the prevailing interpretations of the Chinese medical menace. The practices of "scientific" investigations and fact-finding missions persuasively defined the "truth" of Chinatown in terms of constricted, crowded, immoral, unsanitary, and unnavigable space. These discursive practices profoundly affected the lives of Chinese men and women in San Francisco. Disease-producing and death-engendering threats defined Chinatown as a civic problem and emboldened the nascent Board of Health to intervene decisively to regulate Chinese space and, more generally, to manage the environment and inhabitants of San Francisco. Race and public health had become inextricably linked, producing a combination that would have profound and far-reaching consequences for every inhabitant of the city.

# CHAPTER 2

# Regulating Bodies and Space

The image of Chinatown as a noxious and degraded space emerged in tandem with the Board of Health's ambition to make San Francisco the "healthiest city in the known world." [1] Creating a salubrious urban utopia became a political vocation and practical challenge for nineteenth-century city officials across North America. This agenda reflected a practical response to the problems besetting the cities undergoing explosive growth. Urban residents confronted the uncontrollable accumulation of garbage and sewage, exponential increases of persons, rapid spread of housing settlements and factories, and frequent eruptions of lethal epidemics. In the nineteenth century, city officials undertook massive public works projects and public health management with an interest in managing waste and limiting pestilence.

The city served as an intensive conduit of commerce and labor, and its compact territory became a key reference point for the capitalist nation-state. In the cities, governments experimented with measuring health, producing universal standards of human conduct and the physical environment, and applying sanitary science with the express purpose of securing freedom from disease. This agenda made the city an emblem of progress and an experiment in the perfectibility of modern society. This ambition of universal improvement, however, was set against daunting obstacles. For social commentators, politicians, and new professional experts, the ideal of the well-governed and healthy city confronted justifiable worries about civil unrest and social decay. In the middle of the nineteenth century, San Francisco's history as an American boom city, injected with the fortunes of gold and commerce, offered up equal shares of social turbulence and engineered growth.

During the nineteenth century, U.S. cities were legally and politically redefining their roles, constituency, and capacity to govern. The interests of capitalist development, industrialization, and rapid urbanization pressed municipalities to take on the responsibilities of a corporate, bureaucratic government and provide infrastructure, policing, education, and health services. Municipal governments across the country transformed their public images, becoming not governments that apparently served the needs and interests of property holders and businessmen only, but ones that apparently served all urban residents. San Francisco's consolidation of corporate bureaucratic control occurred at the very end of the nineteenth century. The Board of Health was one of several municipal departments that gradually grew in power, jurisdiction, and personnel during the latter decades of the nineteenth century.[2]

The reordering of the city coincided with new political values that championed the productive capacity of people as a measure of political strength. Measuring and maintaining the health of the city entailed a new form of thinking about the relationship of persons to, and their conduct in, the environment and society. Sickness was no longer seen as an inevitable condition of living but rather as an avoidable flaw. Disease was conceived of as flourishing outside the body and at a distance from those who exhibited proper moral rectitude. The very explanation and diagnosis of disease shifted in professional medicine from the early-nineteenth-century focus on interpreting the particular visible symptoms of a patient to a late-nineteenth-century practice of objectifying disease and evaluating an individual's deviation from the universal and normal healthy human. With the formation of contrasting categories of normal and deviant, medical therapy and public health instruction emphasized a repertoire of habits and civilizing norms to ensure health.[3]

Liberalism's practical vision of public health emphasized strategies of tutoring of inhabitants to regulate themselves. Vacillating between enforcing order and morality and sustaining liberty and economic activity, liberal government developed a rationale concerned with technologies of security not social control. Rather than controlling the territory and the body, liberal security sought to enable the vital and "economic processes of the population" through well-modulated interventions. Technologies of liberal security, primarily sanitary surveillance of buildings and the physical inspection of bodies, generated extensive data about diseases, bodies, and the environment. Experts developed authority out of a claim to process the myriad data into knowledge and to conduct their activities with professional neutrality and effectiveness. However, in liberal government there was a gap between what could be known and what could be done. Although in extraordinary moments of epidemics public health officials deployed the invasive techniques of fumigation, quarantine, and vaccination to contain disease, liberal public health emphasized the inculcation of normalizing practices. Health and therapeutics produced systems of advice and guidance to manage human vitality and the problems of living.[4]

The project of the healthy city encouraged its medical and engineering technicians to think in terms of a total and unified entity that connected population with territory. Health officials interpreted the vitality of the city principally as the aggregate of its inhabitants and as the system of its infrastructure networks. The city's inhabitants were represented as the "population," an aggregate whose total value exceeded the sum of its parts. Administrative technologies such as the census and vital statistics gave material heft to the concept of the "population." The vital signs of the population could be monitored by tabulating births, marriages, deaths, the causes of mortality, and the incidence of certain diseases. Population statistics did not banish distinctions of status, occupation, or group. In fact, statistical tabulation filtered this data of life, health, and death into classifications of locality, nativity, gender, age, and race. The nineteenth-century "vital conscience" found expression through medical statistics that did not flatten and equalize subjects but rather calibrated individual difference through group identity. Statistics became an instrument that organized territory, judged its inhabitants, determined individual difference, and regulated citizenship. In the quest for universal norms, the designation of racial differences in vital statistics could specify threats or provide yardsticks for improvement; it could identify the recalcitrant and untutorable, as well as chart those domains amenable to reform.[5]

Public health's agenda in San Francisco produced prophylactic mechanisms to ensure universal sanitary compliance but emphasized the health hazards posed by Chinese persons living in the city. Health officials justified the vigorous enforcement of sanitary regulations on Chinese persons and residences by stressing the vulnerability of the San Francisco population and the precariousness of universal health improvements. They applied public health technologies throughout the city to safeguard and promote the population's vitality and capacity for

growth. Surveillance, inspection, and quarantine, along with the installation of sewers, were not to be seen as instruments of invidious discrimination aimed mercilessly at the Chinese but were techniques applied
generally throughout the city. Nonetheless, the question remains: why
did the medical knowledge of Chinatown and the Chinese race become
inseparable from the operation of nineteenth-century San Francisco's
public health systems? The very discourses and practices that delineated
the pestilential Chinese generated the characterizations of extreme aberration and unsanitary conduct that would practically establish and con-
solidate sanitary norms. These norms functioned as the minimum standards to ensure that life would thrive in the physical environment. Since
liberal public health embraced the possibilities of tutoring and reforming conduct to ensure self-regulation, health officials, politicians, and
jurists vigorously questioned whether the Chinese residents were amenable to reform or so recalcitrant that they must be expelled so the rest
might thrive.

SYSTEMS AND POPULATIONS

The idea of the city's population corresponded to the conceptualization
of the urban physical topography as a system of networks. The "system"
model of the city emphasized the operation of the vital technological
"sinews" of a city, such as transportation routes, power grids, communication networks, and water and wastewater lines. This conception
naturalized the city as an organic body enhanced by technological mechanisms that would make the city a "smooth-running machine."[6] Engineering the health of the city required, for example, the smooth and efficient operation of water and wastewater lines.

In the nineteenth-century United States, cities faced twin crises of ob-
taining clean water and disposing of human waste. San Francisco, like
hundreds of other cities, commissioned a private company to pipe clean
and plentiful water into homes and businesses for drinking, cleaning, and
cooking. In 1858 the California legislature offered an exclusive franchise
to the Spring Valley Water Works Company to lay pipes in San Francisco. The company invested $15 million in pipes, pumps, and reservoirs
to meet water usage demands that accompanied the rapid installation of
indoor flush toilets, tubs, and faucets in the mid–nineteenth century.[7]
The phenomenal growth in indoor plumbing and water usage outstripped the overall increase in city inhabitants. Between 1865 and 1880

the city population doubled, but water consumption shot up by nearly a factor of eight, overwhelming the sewers.[8]

In San Francisco, health officers confronted a breakdown in waste disposal methods that one health officer decried as the "most wretched of any city in the civilized world."[9] As in cities across the nation, San Francisco residents lived among decaying filth. Garbage and wastewater accumulated and decomposed in alleys and backyards and on sidewalks and streets. Residents disposed of human wastes in backyard privy vaults that frequently overflowed into basement cesspools and into the streets.[10] Wastewater from surface sewers flowed into nearby ravines or collected in cesspools at the bottom of hills. Drawing on the miasma theory of disease origins in noxious gases, public health officials worried that decomposing "human excrement" in cesspools produced "gases" that "penetrated homes." The putrefying sewage also seeped into wells and contaminated local water supplies.[11] A local physician, Dr. Hastings Hall, envisioned apocalyptic consequences from "privies overflowing, the contents percolating . . . [and] the masses of putrid matter" that would surely generate a "magazine of fever" that would "cut us down like the sword of a devastating and relentless enemy."[12]

The urban filth crisis forced sanitary engineers to develop wastewater and sewage schemes. The engineers dreamed of building networks of underground sewers that removed sewage directly from buildings and sent it hurtling to the rivers and seas.[13] In San Francisco, sewer construction depended heavily on private capital, since the city government charter imposed fiscal limits on public works projects.[14] From 1858 to 1875, private landlords and the city authorities constructed seventy-four miles of sewers at a cost of $2.6 million. Although ordinances mandated that municipal inspectors regulate and review all sewer construction, city engineers complained that their specifications were ignored with impunity. The engineers dreamed of a "system" of public sewerage, but there was little political will to undertake massive public works construction. Fiscal constraints, however, did not stop engineers from dreams of "systematic, efficient and accountable" sewage plans. They favored underground, public sewer lines to improve efficiency and ensure uniform service that beset the capricious, unregulated, and hodgepodge disposal network in place.[15]

Subterranean sewers could create a greater nuisance than they eliminated because they were often difficult to clean and frequently became blocked, allowing filth to accumulate and decay. In the subterranean sewers, the refuse took a "sluggish course"; "open vents at every street corner" released a "volume of disease-bearing effluvia" into the atmosphere. In 1869, the health officer C. M. Bates worried that the acrid gases discharged by the cesspools and sewers could generate rampant epidemics of typhoid, dysentery, and cholera in the city.[16] For decades, engineers and health officials advocated gadgets and a variety of schemes to prevent "sewer gases" from backing up through the pipes into residences.[17] They also advocated mechanisms to ensure that fast-flowing water flushed out the sewers regularly and narrower sewer lines made the flushing more effective.[18]

The creation of a sewer system addressed the problems of removing wastewater and sewage, but like other cities San Francisco faced dilemmas with solid waste disposal. In the nineteenth century, residents and business owners hired scavengers to cart off trash and the waste in privy vaults.[19] Many of the scavengers were Italian and Portuguese immigrants. During the 1870s, the public health officials regularly complained that scavengers exacerbated the filthy condition of the city.[20] Health officials wanted to either regulate the scavengers or persuade city supervisors and taxpayers to undertake municipal garbage collection. The municipality did have responsibility for street cleaning, but often it blatantly ignored the condition of Chinatown streets. Both the influential physician Dr. Arthur B. Stout and the special police officer George Duffield testified that the city superintendent of streets ignored Chinatown streets despite tax contributions by Chinese residents.[21]

Municipal politics of growth shaped the districts and constituencies that benefited from technological solutions to the waste crisis. The miserly public outlays for services did not restrain San Francisco's growth to the south and west. In 1875, when city supervisors sold licenses for streetcar lines to the Mission and Western Addition Districts, the city more than doubled in physical size. The rapid construction of residential districts in the Mission and Western Addition and manufacturing developments in the Potrero District and South of Market area increased demands for utilities and infrastructure.[22] The mounting political pressure to address the sewer crisis in the Mission District demonstrated the power of white working-class voters to force a frugal board of supervisors to act. By the mid-1870s, swamps of refuse had choked Mission Creek. In 1878 working-class residents who were largely Democrats and Workingmen's Party male voters were galvanized to lobby the board of supervisors to allocate seventy-five thousand dollars for the city to fill in Mission Creek. The city constructed large sewer lines to relieve the demand for sewage disposal and mandated that individual owners connect their drains to the public sewer as well as fill in cesspools and swamps adjacent to Mission Creek. The health officer Meares praised the conversion of this "hot-bed of disease" into a comparatively pleasant and healthy section of the city.[23]

The transformation of the Mission District demonstrated how government resources were allocated to white homeowners without direct intervention into their private residences and property. The subterranean infrastructure of drains and sewers and the government mandate to fill cesspools ensured the security and the "sanitary integrity of the private home." Liberal styles of governing required that state intervention make limited demands on private property even as it recognized that the very category of the private was materially dependent upon public powers. The law protected rights to possess and use property without state interference. In liberalism, property possessed an intrinsic purity; however, property could be corrupted by its use. Nuisance law allowed government intervention to reshape human conduct in the use and habitation of property.[24] Nuisance law carefully catalogued baneful conduct, observed aberrations to environmental norms, and specified violations that required remedy. In order to prevent the environment from polluting human living spaces, nuisance legal strategy had to prove injury to public welfare, not just specific individuals. This extraordinary power to intervene into private property and private conduct sought to maintain the public good under the constraints imposed by a skeptical judiciary.[25]

San Francisco municipal authorities attempted to apply the profound power of nuisance law to regulate Chinese residence within the city. In 1854 when the Common Council committee declared the Chinese an "unmitigated and wholesome nuisance," they recognized the formidable power they conjured. They decried the public injury and health menace posed by the Chinese. If successful they could have ordered the "immediate expulsion of the whole Chinese race from the city," but judicial constraints prohibited obviously discriminatory targeting of the Chinese.[26] Thirty-five years later, in 1880, when the Board of Health declared the entire Chinatown District a "public nuisance," they embarked on a similar strategy to empty "this great reservoir of moral, social and physical pollution" that threatened to "engulf with its filthiness and immorality the fairest portion of our city."[27] (See Figure 2.)

Throughout the period, Meares repeatedly declared Chinatown a "cesspool" and "nuisance," which conflated the problem of poor and

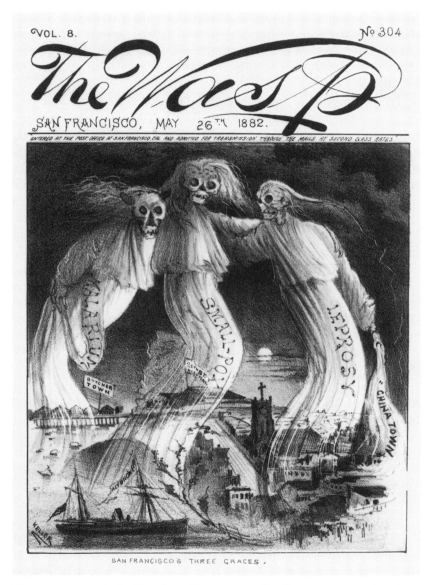

Figure 2. Captioned "San Francisco's Three Graces," this illustration appeared in *The Wasp,* May 26, 1882. Courtesy California Historical Society, FN-23702.

defective sewerage with the environmental condition of an entire district. As city health officer from 1876 to 1888, Dr. John Meares was the principal architect of San Francisco's system of health regulations and the spokesperson for the city's "vital conscience." Meares had been born in North Carolina, trained as a physician in Philadelphia, and served as a surgeon in the Confederate Army. He moved to San Francisco in 1871 and, within two years, was appointed San Francisco's quarantine officer. Three years later, in 1876, he assumed the position of city health officer. In all of his annual reports, Meares emphasized Chinatown as a totality that endangered the entire city: its crowded and filthy dens bred pestilence, contaminating both their inhabitants and the surrounding neighborhoods.[28] Public health officials could justify discriminatory regulation as necessary to prevent health catastrophe for the entire population. The commitment to health preservation and epidemic suppression enabled even skeptics to countenance drastic measures against individuals and locations that did not comply with emerging health standards.

San Francisco health officers' reports addressed sanitary conditions in all sections of the city, but when writing about other sections of the city, rarely did the health officers engage in the kind of invective and vilification they aimed at Chinatown and its residents. For instance, when Meares drew attention to the South of Market area inhabited by unskilled, young, immigrant European men as "cesspools reeking with fermenting and putrefying animal and vegetable matter," he simultaneously sympathized with the European "laboring classes" who were "obliged" to live in the "densely populated district" with "imperfect" drainage systems because they could not afford better accommodations.[29]

Meares issued blanket condemnations of the Chinese, whom he characterized as a subversive race with a "willful and diabolical disregard for sanitary laws."[30] The medical geographer Susan Craddock and the medical historian Joan Trauner have argued that San Francisco health officials and politicians scapegoated the Chinese, displacing blame for general sanitary conditions onto a vulnerable minority.[31] In San Francisco, no other social groups defined by race or nationality were unequivocally identified as health threats.

The impulse to expel the Chinese and remove Chinatown from the city animated the nuisance declarations. The practice of scapegoating the Chinese in San Francisco demonstrated the public-health strategy that specified aberrations in order to achieve reform. Health officials characterized the aberrant conduct of the Chinese and condition of Chinatown as polluting the entire city system and threatening the total population. The norms that governed public health reform materialized most vividly in specific aberrant sites. By putting the normative and normalizing agenda at risk, the nuisance demanded immediate remedy. Remedies could entail either reforming the conditions that produced the nuisance or destroying and expelling the nuisance from the site. The cataloguing of aberration and deploying of remedies demonstrated how widely or narrowly the norm was practiced.

The limits to the liberal strategy of declaring a nuisance also dissuaded its usage as wholesale condemnation. Judicial scrutiny of the municipality's police powers required the city government to enumerate specific violations of legal codes. After the 1876 smallpox epidemic, the board of supervisors hired health inspectors to place residences, businesses, and factories under regular surveillance and granted them powers to condemn houses. Meares expected the threat of condemnation to pressure Chinatown's "capricious or negligent landlords" to obey sanitary standards. However, white landlords owned the majority of property in Chinatown, and they readily complained that the condition of other zones of the city, such as the city dockyards, were far worse than Chinatown. Meares justified the special sanitary vigilance on Chinatown property because the aberrant conduct of its inhabitants required "constant surveillance."[32] Although other working-class sections of the city such as South of Market, the Mission District, the Western Addition, and the Latin Quarter experienced regular public health surveillance, Chinatown was the preeminent "notorious" site that presented the yardstick of sanitary aberration for the rest of the city.[33]

The health of the city was measured by counting the incidence of disease, debility, and death among its population. The collection of mortality statistics became a significant arena in which health officials could establish their authority in the assessment of public health problems. In gathering statistical data on the mortality and births of the municipality, they attempted to measure and record the health and welfare of the population. These documentation efforts provided legitimacy for public health programs while securing seemingly tangible evidence of "progress." Mortality rates indexed the vitality of the nation-state. The gathering of health statistics contributed simultaneously to the creation of essentialized social categories of age, gender, ethnicity, and race and to the constitution of the "general public."

Questions about the exact nature of Chinese deaths troubled the Board of Health once it began tabulating mortality rates in 1859. In many cases of Chinese deaths, officials expressed uncertainty in specifying the cause of death. Compared to other major cities in the East and Midwest, which were unable to specify the cause of death in less than 1 percent of their cases, San Francisco's authorities regularly faced higher figures, ranging from 2.9 to 9.4 percent. The health officer Henry Gibbons Jr. blamed these statistical inaccuracies on the behavior of Chinese immigrants. He accused immigrants of "secreting" their dead from city officials and blamed language barriers that made it impossible for public health officials "to get a correct description of the symptoms from the Chinese friends of the deceased," which was necessary in order to certify the cause of death.[34]

Even when Chinese practitioners did provide certification of deaths, city officials refused to accept them. Gibbons argued that certifications produced by Chinese practitioners were illegible and unintelligible.[35] Physicians trained in allopathic, Western medicine dismissed Chinese practitioners as ignorant of anatomy and physiology, incapable of surgery, and unschooled in proper treatments for epidemic disease.[36] In the 1870s, San Francisco's Chinatown offered the services of dozens of Chinese practitioners and pharmacists. Many Chinese physicians attracted prospective patients by advertising their treatments and specialties. Augustus Ward Loomis in 1868 described the variety of "sign-board" advertising: "Chinese doctors are not scarce. One hangs out a board, on which we read: Yeang Tsz Ying feels the pulse, and writes prescriptions for internal and external diseases; Dr. Ma U Yuk feels the pulse, and heals thoroughly the most difficult and unheard of diseases. Dr. Tseang Ling cures wounds [caused] by falling or being struck. . . . Another advertises to cure smallpox. Another proclaims the diseases of children are his specialty. Others announce to those suffering on account of their vices that they will be taken in hand." One of the wealthiest and most famous Chinese physicians, Li Po Tai, had a thriving practice located on Washington Street, where he reputedly served 150 to 300 Chinese and non-Chinese patients daily until his death in 1893. His popularity, however, invited ridicule from the city's allopathic physicians and the Board of Health.[37] Although the authors and editors of local medical journals expressed a lively fascination with Chinese techniques and treatments, writers of articles for medical journals regarded Chinese medicine as ruled by "superstition," "tradition," and an incomplete, "unscientific" understanding of the human body and the nature of disease.[38] Health officials mobilized these perceptions in their attempts to eliminate the potential competition of Chinese physicians. Furthermore, they undercut any inclination of the Chinese physicians to cooperate with municipal regulations by unilaterally withholding civic authorization of their practices.

The refusal of the San Francisco Board of Health to recognize Chinese physicians was characteristic of a larger national process of medical professionalization. The distinctions between professional and unprofessional physicians were only beginning to be systematically categorized during this era. In California, the process of the professionalization of medical practice through professional associations, certified medical schools, and licensing boards would continue well into the twentieth century. Medical men trained at select schools assailed the healing techniques and practices of midwives and homeopathic physicians, as well as Chinese practitioners of acupuncture and herbal treatments.[39]

Gibbons lamented that the "evil" of inaccurate mortality statistics was "unavoidable and must continue to exist while the Chinese form part of our population."[40] Since the Chinese were reluctant to involve public health officials in the supervision of their dead, and since health officials did not trust the judgment of Chinese physicians, a majority of the Chinese who died did not have an official cause of death. In the 1873–74 fiscal year, 73 percent of Chinese deaths did not have certification of a specific cause. However, these uncertified deaths accounted for only .4 percent of deaths in all races combined, according to Board of Health records.

The large number of deaths by unknown causes among the Chinese population unnerved Gibbons. He preferred to sidestep the statistical havoc by segregating Chinese mortality statistics from the overall mortality figures for San Francisco. By bracketing Chinese mortality statistics, he was able to make the city's mortality figures compare quite favorably with other major cities across the country. However, the repercussions of this temporary statistical maneuver were far more significant conceptually than the expected impact of comparative death rates. Although the Chinese did have high mortality rates in this period, which Gibbons estimated at 32.1 per 1,000 in 1873–74, and which declined to 23.8 per 1,000 the following fiscal year, deaths in the Chinese population made up no more than 9 percent of the total and, therefore, did not have a disproportional impact on overall figures.[41]

In cities during the nineteenth century, death statistics were generally unreliable, drew from patchwork data sources, and were prone to both exaggeration and undercounting. The San Francisco Board of Health, like other health departments nationwide, relied upon physicians and undertakers to help compile numbers and causes of death. Since health officials depended on these professionals' goodwill, they rarely prosecuted those who did not comply.[42] The purpose, then, of excluding the Chinese from mortality statistics had far deeper implications than alleviating the consternation at the high percentages of deaths from unknown causes (which in themselves were irrelevant in calculating aggregate mortality rates). If the task of these statistics was to measure the health of the population, the exclusion of the Chinese mortality rate revealed a refusal to consider the Chinese immigrants to be part of the population. Such removal paralleled contemporaneous arguments favoring the exclusion of Chinese immigrants. For public health officials, the Chinese represented an alien, unassimilable, and potentially subversive group that had to be excluded before their incorporation perverted the reality and "destiny" of San Francisco and the United States.

## EPIDEMIC SMALLPOX AND THE STRATEGIES OF CONTAINMENT

Setting the Chinese apart from the overall population also led to their being targeted and isolated during the smallpox epidemics. Smallpox epidemics in 1868, 1876, 1880, and 1887 shaped the establishment of an ensemble of public health regulations in San Francisco. Smallpox spread rapidly, produced painful and deforming symptoms, and resulted in incredibly high death rates. A tenacious virus that could survive outside the body, smallpox was communicated person to person through airborne droplets or by contaminated surfaces such as clothing, walls, and floors. The disease symptoms progressed from fever and chills to a dense rash of blisters and pustules. If the victim survived, he or she was likely to have severe scarring, particularly on the face, and could suffer the loss of eyesight.[43] The first two epidemics were devastating, claiming 760 lives in 1868 and 482 lives in 1876. The mortality rate for smallpox infection dropped precipitously in the 1880s. In 1876, nearly 30 percent of the 1,646 reported cases died; but in 1880 the deaths declined to 18 percent of reported cases, and in 1887 fell further, to 12 percent of reported cases.[44]

Public health officials attributed their success in combating smallpox to the implementation of public health technologies and to the epidemiological knowledge that traced the source of smallpox to incoming Chinese immigrants and to Chinatown. At first the health officer Issac Rowell did not ascribe the source of the 1868 epidemic to Chinese immigrants, but the Anti-Coolie Association blamed the Chinese for the virulent strain of smallpox that was "unknown among the Caucasian race."[45] Subsequent health officers, however, readily charged that smallpox either arrived from China or thrived in Chinatown.[46] They applied a series of public health technologies to contain the spread of smallpox. First, in order to arrest the "invoices of smallpox" from China, health authorities established a quarantine, the physical examination of passengers, and the fumigation of clothing and baggage at the San Francisco port. Second, addressing the fear that Chinatown conditions bred disease, the health officials conducted house inspections and insisted upon disease reporting and the isolation of the sick. Finally, in order to protect bodies from contamination, the health authorities conducted mass vaccinations.

After the 1869 smallpox epidemic, the San Francisco Board of Supervisors required the quarantine and physical inspection of passengers and cargo from Asia.[47] All vessels were directed to Mission Bay, where they anchored three miles from shore. A local physician was appointed quarantine officer, and he collected his salary from the fees levied upon shipping companies. If smallpox was found onboard, the ship, its crew, and its passengers were detained for at least fifteen days. The vessel would then be fumigated with chlorine and sulfur, and infected articles would be immersed in bichloride solution and washed with boiling water. While health officers fumigated the vessel and its cargo, the passengers were transferred to hulks, increasing the discomfort and potential danger to passengers.[48]

Public health officers traced the source of smallpox infection to steamships that had arrived from China. During the 1876, 1880, and 1887 epidemics, health officers and newspaper reporters scrambled to link the epidemic to a Chinese smallpox case detected through the quarantine process. However, it was just as probable that smallpox arrived with European and American migrants traveling westward by rail. Smallpox epidemics in eastern cities often preceded outbreaks in San Francisco by several years. Since the incubation period for smallpox was twelve to fourteen days, it was often easier to track and quarantine smallpox over the longer journey across the Pacific than by overland rail. By securing the source of smallpox in Chinese bodies, authorities redoubled the perception of danger in Chinese immigration and the foreign nature of the disease.[49]

Tracking the source of smallpox to Chinese passengers also heightened anxieties about the permeability of the quarantine net. These concerns erupted into public controversy during quarantine of the British

ship *Altonower* in April 1882. During inspection, smallpox was detected among one of the 874 Chinese steerage passengers. The ill passenger was removed to the City Pesthouse, but the other passengers were
forced to stay onboard for fifteen days, which was later extended by another thirty when additional cases of smallpox were discovered. In this
crisis, the American lawyer Frederick Bee, who had been hired as the
Chinese vice consul in San Francisco, aggressively protected the interests
of the quarantined Chinese passengers. Vice Consul Bee demanded that
the National Board of Health (precursor to the U.S. Public Health Service) intervene to alleviate the discomfort and danger in local quarantine
operations. Bee claimed that the passengers' treatment was "outrageous" and would have been considered intolerable if the immigrants
had been European.[50]

The editor of the *Berkeley Beacon,* a "bitter" opponent of Chinese
immigration, decried the inhumane conditions that required healthy
Chinese passengers to remain until the quarantine period was over:
"Think of the torture and despair of those condemned to live in the
midst of contagion and forbidden to fly from infection." Playing on
fears that defective quarantine could radiate disease rather than suppress it, the editor declared to the *Beacon* readers that "for the sake of
the honor of white men," the government should act quickly to "let the
undefiled be separated from the plague-stricken."[51] The San Francisco
Board of Health defended its actions but appealed to the federal government to build a permanent quarantine station to "intercept" smallpox brought by "Chinese coolies."[52] The National Board of Health
folded in 1883, however, and no federal financing for a permanent quarantine station was forthcoming until 1890.[53]

San Francisco quarantine officers developed a vigilant defense against
Asian epidemic invasion by instituting race-based precautions to com-
pensate for the lack of permanent and systematic quarantine facilities.
In 1888, smallpox fears prompted the quarantine officer to detain unilaterally all ships from Hong Kong for two weeks irrespective of the
health of their passengers. A local physician, Dr. C. J. Wharry, accused
the Board of Health of "ignorance" and an "outrageous abuse of
power."[54] However, the *Pacific Medical and Surgical Journal* exonerated
the board's zealous response by enumerating the archetypal traits of Chinese medical danger: "studied concealment," "deception," and a "systematic evasion of sanitary rules."[55]

In an earlier epidemic crisis Meares claimed that the "concealed"
cases accounted for the "hot-beds" of smallpox that spread "the germs

of contagion" throughout the city.[56] Public health regulations required
physicians to report smallpox cases, place individuals afflicted in isolation, and fumigate all affected residences and businesses.[57] The strategy
of house inspection, fumigation, and isolation were applied to the residences and individuals in Chinatown more thoroughly than in the rest
of the city. During the 1876–77 epidemic, health inspectors fumigated
every house in Chinatown, regardless of whether disease had been detected or not. During the inspection, fumigators discovered several
"concealed" cases of smallpox and a "large number who had recently
recovered from the disease." [58] Fumigation, then, both exterminated the
disease in an "infected" locality as well as imposed surveillance on the
Chinese.

Concealing cases from health authorities represented the most malev-
olent accusation leveled against Chinese immigrants. Public health officials and physicians blamed the persistence of epidemics on the refusal
of the Chinese to report cases of smallpox to the authorities.[59] For "per-
niciously and willfully disregard[ing]" regulations, Meares branded the
Chinese as "enemies of our race and people." The Chinese were accused
of incubating smallpox, which ruined white families, made children orphans, and struck down young men in the "bloom of their youth and
vigor." Meares's accusations of "wickedness" and "criminal neglect,"
combined with the litany of lethal assaults on white family members, in-
sinuated that the Chinese were engaged in nothing short of biological
warfare to destroy the lives and livelihoods of San Francisco's white
families. The redeployment of images of "unscrupulous, lying and treacherous" Chinese braided the medical threat into the political critique
that the Chinese were incapable of modern American self-regulation and
citizenship.[60]

The accusation of malice and race warfare ignored the concerns of the
Chinese community. Their reluctance to notify health officials did reveal
the distrust of Chinese men and women for the public health procedures, as well as their doubts about the ability of Western physicians to
cure the ill, but the problem may also have been that they did not approve of measures to segregate those afflicted with disease from their
friends and family. They perhaps recognized that once identified, those
afflicted with smallpox would be removed to the City Pesthouse, where
they were just as likely to die. Hospitalization in this period did not necessarily ensure recovery from a contagious disease. According to the statistics prepared by the Board of Health during the 1876–77 smallpox
epidemic, the fatality rate of reported smallpox cases was about the

same—a little less than 30 percent—for those hospitalized as it was for those who received care at their homes.[61]

The Chinese refusal to submit to health regulations became the most vexing issue for Meares, who readily contrasted Chinese behavior with that of European and South American immigrants, who were willing to "report" their cases of smallpox and who welcomed isolation procedures. Even when white individuals were identified as the source of a particular smallpox epidemic, they were not demonized but rather were characterized as the unwitting disseminators of a "loathsome disease." By contrast, the Chinese immigrants, as a whole, were considered deliberate and diabolical in their intentions to spread smallpox.[62]

The Chinese medical threat ensured the extension of normative public health regulations of disease reporting and the isolation of the sick. The public health declarations were consistent with the workings of an "epidemic logic," which justified the use of invasive measures and regulatory strategies to contain the threat that had already been discursively produced.[63] Meares's invective about the diabolical deceit of the Chinese and the horrifying sanitary conditions in Chinatown persuaded the board of supervisors to pass regulations that conferred direct authority on the health officer to condemn houses and remove smallpox cases, as well as to extend physicians' reporting obligations to other diseases, such as diphtheria, scarlet fever, and typhoid. Meares claimed that these new powers had effectively "stayed the spread of loathsome and fatal disease."[64]

Chinatown residents, nevertheless, continued to experience onerous treatment. The systematic fumigation and surveillance of Chinatown residences became an established policy during succeeding epidemics. A decade later, during the smallpox epidemic of 1887–88, the city Board of Health undertook a thorough fumigation and house-to-house inspection of the Chinese quarter in order to discover "concealed smallpox" cases and to ensure that all "suspicious and faulty houses" would be purified of their disease-breeding potential.[65]

During and between smallpox epidemics, the Board of Health promoted mass vaccination as the most reliable method for warding off the disease. Smallpox vaccination had been invented by Europeans in the late eighteenth century, but vaccine production was unregulated and it was frequently ineffective. In 1868 the health board hired vaccinators to combat the raging epidemic and hired a special inspector, Dr. Davis, to examine Chinatown and Chinese cases of smallpox.[66] At first, vaccination of passengers arriving from Asian ports was mandated, then, in

1872, vaccination was provided generally to the public free of charge.
Prominent physicians and health authorities advocated compulsory vaccination as a "duty of self-protection" and community safety.[67] During
the 1876–77 epidemic the Board of Health employed public vaccinators
to administer the bovine smallpox virus vaccine to all who applied.
Meares estimated that more than twenty thousand people were vacci-
nated, but few Chinese had voluntarily come forward. The reluctance of
Chinese immigrants, however, may have had much to do with their uncertainty about the cure offered by the city's physicians. Meares acknowledged that "vast numbers of intelligent persons are prejudiced
against and oppose vaccination, because of the known fact that the hu-
manized virus has conveyed syphilis." He claimed that this prejudice
was rapidly disappearing as use of the bovine virus proved effective
and free of noticeable side effects. Meares credited the bovine vaccination for clipping the smallpox mortality rate during the 1880 smallpox
epidemic, when only 64 people died, out of 507 reported cases.[68]

The board of education adopted a smallpox vaccination policy in
1876 that required vaccination certificates for every child entering the
public schools. In the first four years of the program, more than 34,000
children complied. Despite the school entrance requirement, the
"poorer classes" often delayed vaccination. In order to ensure compliance, Meares appointed "vaccinators" who would make "house visitations" to poor white neighborhoods, a power first exercised during the
1880 epidemic in Chinatown.[69]

The deployment of vaccination in Chinatown and in Asian ports of
departure gave added security to San Francisco health authorities. With
the curtailment of the immigration of Chinese laborers in 1882, Meares
believed that San Francisco had "great protection against any future
danger" of smallpox epidemics.[70] Such hopes underscored not only the
equation of "indiscriminate immigration" with disease flows but also the
health authorities' interest in controlling the movement and the disease-
incubating potential of Chinese bodies. In 1887, when smallpox re-
emerged in San Francisco, Chinese concealment tactics were again
blamed for the epidemic. The health officer took the opportunity to expand the public health vaccination campaign by offering free vaccinations for "several thousand" white workers in manufacturing and mercantile firms.[71]

The threat of "invoices" of smallpox from China, the concealment of
cases in Chinatown, and confidence in the bovine vaccine provided sufficient pretexts for the Board of Health to institute vaccination programs

in public school and work sites that applied to the entire population. The rhetoric and procedures employed to combat the Chinese threat of smallpox were extended into a systematic program of universally applicable health regulations. In European countries at the same time, compulsory and widely available smallpox vaccination became an early means for the medicalization of the entire population.[72] In San Francisco, however, the process of general medicalization necessarily implied disproportionate official anxiety about the role of Chinese immigrants in germinating and disseminating disease. The idea that Chinese people, practices, and spaces posed a public health threat provided medical professionals the opportunity to deploy technologies of public health on Chinese residences and bodies.

## REGULATION, SEGREGATION, AND REMOVAL

Public health officials and politicians anticipated ominous consequences for the movement of Chinese people beyond the boundaries of Chinatown. Politicians feared that the employment of Chinese servants in white middle-class homes was a lethal luxury because the Chinese would inevitably convey the diseases generated in "Chinatown pestholes" into "our homes." The city supervisor Willard Farwell claimed that Chinese cooks and servants masqueraded in "cleanly" appearance and "habits of decency" in order to acquire their positions. However, their racial "instincts" and ingrained habits were revealed when the servant "joyfully" hastened back to "his slum and his burrow." Though adaptable to the requirements of American domestic service, Chinese servants' moral character reverted back to the immutable "instinct of the race." The fetid slum of Chinatown defined the sinister and singular "truth" of Chinese character. These practices of filth and vice represented a perversion of the healthy habits undertaken by responsible, modern Americans.[73]

White labor politicians fixated on the medical monstrosity generated by the Chinese servants' daily circuit between the "American household" and the Chinatown slum. The traffic of Chinese servants produced a "perfect network of contagion[,] . . . a veritable octopus of disease, having its seat in Chinatown, and its infectious arms thrust into every home of the city." The metaphor of the "octopus of disease" conveyed a horrifying image of masses of faceless Chinese servants totalized into a monstrous disease machine, and it reframed the innocuous presence of "obedient" servants and laundrymen as the source of domestic contamination for the middle-class white family.[74]

Domestic service was only the most visible contact between Chinese and white persons. Meares feared the "daily contact with our citizens" of hundreds of Chinese laundrymen and laborers who manufactured "clothes, slippers and vermicelli . . . in the very house and very room in which a Chinaman was dying" of smallpox. Through their labor, Chinese workers cleaned the clothes of, and manufactured the consumer goods for, whites. Meares feared that since the Chinese were "poisoned with the contagion of smallpox," they inevitably would transform the seemingly pure material culture with deadly contagion.[75]

The alarming speculations that Chinese workers and servants were injecting disease into the white middle-class home prompted increased vigilance in regulating Chinese work sites and workers. Health officials' worries about the route of contamination of laboring bodies and manufactured commodities demonstrated obsessive concern with the leakage of seemingly strict borders between the traditional, dangerous, and recalcitrant zone of Chinatown and the rest of the modernizing city. Monitoring disease flows, public health officials worried about the physical sites, such as businesses, institutions, and residential areas, where the Chinese presence disrupted norms of white American modernity. City officials attempted to control Chinese conduct and presence in laundries, in public hospitals, and within the city itself. They raised questions of nuisance and threats to public health in order to regulate the conduct and presence of Chinese persons.

Chinese laundries were the most visible symbol of the Chinese presence in the local economy and outside the borders of Chinatown. In 1870 more than thirteen hundred Chinese laundry workers lived in San Francisco. Most of the washhouses were small joint ventures between several men, employing few workers and conducting all operations manually. White-owned laundry businesses were mostly larger, mechanized operations. White politicians' concerns mounted as it became known that nine-tenths of Chinese laundries were located outside Chinatown. Chinese firms located in the central business district and increasingly in the new residential neighborhoods that had emerged with the development of streetcar transportation. Since laundry workers and their owners lived in their shops, politicians anxiously speculated that the number of Chinese workers residing in white neighborhoods had grown to nearly one thousand.[76]

The municipal government had repeatedly attempted to regulate Chinese laundries since the early 1870s, but most ordinances were shot down by the courts. Court rulings narrowed the boundary for regulation down to nuisances that were proven health and safety hazards.[77] The Supreme Court case of Yick Wo in 1886 defined how municipal laws of health, safety, and nuisance could infringe on economic interests. The board of supervisors had passed ordinances that required a battery of certifications and rules of operation for laundries in the city's densely populated areas. Sanitary and safety conditions in the washhouses had to be certified by the health officer and fire warden. The rules of operation prohibited laundries from running at night or on Sundays or using scaffolding as drying racks, and it disallowed persons suffering from infectious diseases to lodge or remain in any laundry.[78] During the board of supervisors' 1885 Chinatown investigation, city authorities enforced the new laundry regulations in earnest, arresting nearly two hundred Chinese for violating the laundry regulations. Yick Wo, a proprietor who had operated his laundry for twenty-two years, had already received certifications from the health officer and fire warden. The board of supervisors refused to license the laundry and arrested Yick Wo for his use of scaffolding on the roof because it posed a fire danger. The Tung Hing Tong Association, the Chinese laundry guild, hired attorneys to submit a habeas corpus petition to the courts.[79] A parallel case was mounted in the federal courts in the name of Wo Lee on grounds of habeas corpus. The cases were joined in the U.S. circuit court, where Judge Lorenzo Sawyer remarked that the record of enforcement revealed that the ordinance's "necessary tendency" was to "drive out of business" all small Chinese laundries and give monopolistic power to large laundries established by "Caucasian capital."[80]

The U.S. Supreme Court ruled in favor of Yick Wo and Wo Lee. In the majority decision, Justice Stanley Matthews ruled that the supervisors arbitrarily enforced the ordinances and discriminated against all Chinese operators pursuing their "harmless and useful occupation," while eighty others who were not Chinese were permitted to carry on the same business under similar conditions. Matthews condemned the laws that had vested total and unrestrained licensing authority to a municipal legislative body. Matthews did not deny the authority of municipalities to regulate health and safety but demanded that the regulations be applied to all and be administered by nonpartisan professionals rather than the politically motivated board of supervisors.[81]

The Supreme Court judgment in the Yick Wo case protected economic freedom from legislative favoritism and limited the distribution of state burdens and benefits on the basis of race or citizenship. It also sharpened the judiciary's claim to supervise local and state governments'

exercise of nuisance and licensing powers. Since the Supreme Court's ruling in Slaughterhouse Cases in 1871, the prevailing interpretation of the
Fourteenth Amendment's prohibition of state laws that would "deprive
any person of life, liberty or property without due process of law" and
would "deny to any person within its jurisdiction the equal protection
of the law" upheld federal oversight of economic freedom over political
freedom. The Supreme Court nationalized federal protection of "civil
rights," which the judges interpreted as the pursuit of property rights
and economic interests, but allowed states to regulate individuals' "political rights," such as the right to serve on a jury, vote, and hold office.
This protection of property and business over safeguarding political enfranchisement allowed for the proliferation of African American disenfranchisement in Southern states and paved the way for the segregation of public accommodations under the "separate but equal" doctrine
in *Plessy v. Ferguson* in 1896.[82]

The economic freedom the court guaranteed to Chinese business
owners infuriated those who wanted to close Chinese laundries. The city
could not single out Chinese laundries for invidious regulation on the
grounds that they were Chinese owned and operated. The *San Francisco
Bulletin* editor feared that the ruling meant that San Francisco government could "do nothing to bridge the chasm which separates [the
Chinese] from modern races of men. We can do nothing to elevate or
reform them, for that would be discrimination, contrary to the 14th
amendment."[83]

The use of government powers to reform the conduct of the Chinese
to match that of the "modern races of men" required the aura of professional, nonpartisan bureaucrats, which was the hallmark of the Progressive era of municipal government. The regulation of the city by politically disinterested experts moved closer to realization with the 1895
mayoral election of the Progressive candidate James Phelan. Mayor Phelan championed accountability, efficiency, and the role of government in
managing society and development. Endorsed by the San Francisco Merchants' Association, Phelan shrugged off the budgetary stringency of the
1880s and financed ambitious public works and professional municipal
bureaucracy by issuing bond debt. From 1895 to 1899 the Public Health
Department dramatically grew in power, programs, jurisdiction, and
personnel. After years of subsisting on the stagnant appropriation of
twenty-six thousand dollars annually, the Board of Health received an
allocation of sixty-five thousand dollars for the 1896–97 fiscal year.[84]
These funds supported the expansion of the milk and food inspections

that enabled the Board of Health to establish and equip bacteriological laboratories for food examination and other investigations. The Board of Health also hired cadres of health inspectors for residential and business plumbing and for sewage investigations, as well as industry-wide inspections of bakeries, bathhouses, laundries, cigar factories, markets, butcher shops, and slaughterhouses.[85]

At the end of the nineteenth century, the Board of Health renewed its commitment to cleanse Chinatown through redoubled residential inspections. Working with the Chinese consul, the police, and the fire department, the Board of Health began a campaign to condemn buildings in Chinatown. Their campaign led to the immediate condemnation of twenty-eight houses, and they placed an additional thirty-eight, designated as "nuisances," under threat of condemnation. Although some property owners attempted to secure legal injunctions, the courts rejected the majority of petitions. The Board of Health celebrated its success in lifting the rights of "life and health" above those of "property." In conjunction with the Chinatown inspections, the board extended surveillance throughout the city by deputizing over five hundred police officers as ex officio health inspectors, empowered to investigate every building in the city. This ensured that the health inspectors' focus on Chinatown would not distract the city from conducting universal sanitary surveillance. In the course of the year, health inspectors and deputized police visited fifteen thousand houses across the city and pressured property owners to abate 402 "nuisance" charges.[86] The *Pacific Medical Journal* applauded the Board of Health for finally "purging Chinatown of its filthy and unhealthy structures" that had "too long been a menace to the health of this city."[87]

The Progressive era financing also made it possible for the Public Health Department to apply sanitary surveillance and regulation to all workplaces in any chosen industry. The administration of inspections and licensing satisfied judicial guidelines but also bolstered an official scientific judgment on the peculiar dangers of Chinese-operated businesses. In 1896 the Board of Health appointed William H. Tobin as chief bath and laundry inspector. From November 1896 to June 1897, Tobin and his assistants inspected over six hundred laundries in the city, two hundred of which had white owners; the remaining four hundred were Chinese operated. Tobin evaluated laundries on their appearance and use. He demanded that deficient laundries put cement floors in wash rooms and fresh coats of lime on the walls, and he strictly enforced regulations that prohibited workers from living in laundries. Tobin claimed that white owners of laundries cooperated with health inspectors, and that Chinese owners were unwilling to remedy "vicious evils" and opposed "all sanitary improvements" until threatened with the withdrawal of laundry permits. Tobin described Chinese laundries as overcrowded and unventilated and their workers as engaged in vile practices that generated disease.[88] Prior to the publication of Tobin's report, the Board of Health committee member Dr. H. Hart publicized the investigation in the *Pacific Medical Journal*. Hart championed the value of sanitary surveillance of laundries by highlighting the dangerous conduct in Chinese laundries. Chinese laundry workers made the workplaces their residences, confusing distinctions between public and private behavior. Hart observed that Chinese workers slept under their work tables, using "their patrons clothes for bed linens and pillows." He warned that the "consumptive Chinese" soaked their patrons' laundry with "dangerous mouth spray." This purported practice of Chinese workers preparing clothes for ironing by spraying water from their mouths onto the clothes became a signature feature of transfer of disease through suspect conduct. The supposed mouth spray exacerbated anxieties about the role of leaking Chinese orifices in spreading vicious contagion such as tuberculosis and syphilis. The innocuous Chinese laundry located in any part of the city became, through Hart's descriptions, transformed into the quintessential crowded, immoral Chinatown den. The "inmates" were packed "together like sardines," the stench of opium filled the air, and the denizens seduced "whites of both sexes" to come by day or by night. The recycled imagery of the immoral and filthy opium dens exacerbated fears that Chinese laundries throughout the city distributed narcotics. Fearing the contaminating power, Hart refused to "wear a Chinese-washed garment" because of his suspicions that "cases of consumption, syphilis or skin diseases existing in this community can be traced back to Chinese laundries."[89] (See Figure 3.)

The municipal government's attempts to regulate laundries demonstrated the limitations of public health interest in justifying legal and administrative practices. Targeting the Chinese laundries with the intention to abolish rather than reform them invited stern judicial rebuke. The Fourteenth Amendment's equal protection clause forbade special scrutiny of a particular group without similar investigation of all businesses of the same type. However, the courts never disputed the power of the municipality to regulate and manage the urban environment by public health agencies. At the turn of the century, when the Board of

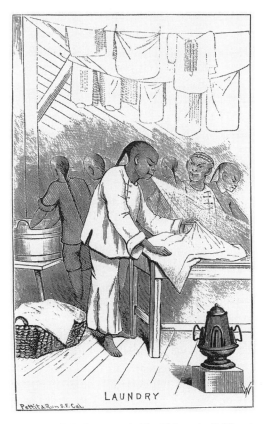

Figure 3. G. B. Densmore's *The Chinese in California* (1880) included this drawing captioned "Loathsome practice of mouth spray in the Chinese Laundries." Illustration by Voegtlin.

Health conducted systematic inspections of all laundries, the courts were not called upon to intervene, even though the rhetoric and intention of ordinances prohibiting "water-spraying" and "sleeping under ironing boards" was aimed predominantly at Chinese workers and Chinese laundries.

Equal protection under the law did not easily extend to the use of public accommodations, and little could be done to circumvent their discriminatory policies. Despite the perceived inadequacy of Chinese medical care and unsanitary hospitals, the Board of Health refused the admission of Chinese patients to the city's hospital. Instead, Dr. Meares advocated a policy of "separate but equal" facilities in his attempts to coax Chinese residents to report cases of smallpox during the 1876 epidemic. Chinese were allowed to enter only the special pesthouse for the quarantine of those suffering from smallpox or leprosy.[90]

An attempt to admit a Chinese man to the county hospital in 1881 pressed the Board of Health to make their policy of segregated hospital facilities explicit. The Chinese vice consul asked Dr. Silvers, a former police surgeon, to gain admission for Chun Chung, who suffered from tuberculosis and was destitute and "friendless." The superintendent of the county hospital rejected the application because it was not "customary to receive Chinamen in the hospital," and appealed to the Board of Health to set a formal policy. The debate revealed tensions between those who appealed for "equal rights" for the Chinese and those who objected that their intrinsic pathology would contaminate "civilized citizens." The board compromised and decided to "nurse and provide for diseased Chinamen" in an "out-house" at the Twenty-sixth Street Smallpox Hospital.[91] Ten years later, in 1891, Jung Lin, a Chinese man suffering from pulmonary tuberculosis, challenged the segregation policy. His attorney appealed to the Board of Health to admit his client "without prejudice to race" because Lin was a San Francisco resident and taxpayer. The board unanimously denied his application as well.[92]

In both cases board members and medical professionals equated all Chinese with "chronic" and "incurable" diseases, and this underwrote their exclusion from the city hospital and even the main wards of the Smallpox Hospital, which ministered to those suffering from epidemic disease. The board's actions reflected a refusal to consider Chinese residents as part of the city's "public"; they were perceived as the antithesis of "civilized citizens." Chinese "habits and mode of life" were considered unsuitable for admission into a hospital ward. No matter what the diagnosis, then, the Chinese were sent to the "out-house" of the Smallpox Hospital. Yet all others, including foreigners of other nationalities, suffering from the same diseases, smallpox and tuberculosis, were admitted to the county hospital. The board was reluctant to offer the full range of public services to indigent Chinese, despite the fact that the customs office at the port of San Francisco had, since the early 1850s, continued to collect a hospital tax from Chinese immigrants upon arrival.[93]

However, the medical establishment did sense a crisis occasioned by the two appeals for hospital admissions. The Chinese residents no longer accepted the city government's blatantly discriminatory status quo. The editor of the *Occidental Medical Times* suggested that if demand for city services increased, the city would be obliged to "establish wards or separate buildings for this special class of indigent sick." The Board of Health, which regularly condemned "makeshift" Chinese hospitals in Chinatown and refused to recognize Chinese physicians, also denied approval for the Chinese to build a modern medical facility. In 1888, when the Chinese consul general and Chinese Six Companies collected seventy-five thousand dollars, purchased land, and petitioned the board for permission to build a hospital outside the city limits, their application was refused. City authorities forbade construction on the grounds that the Chinese intended to use "objectionable Chinese systems of medical treatment," which would make a Chinese Hospital a grave "nuisance" to the rest of the city.[94] The San Francisco medical establishment feared that a Chinese Hospital would concentrate infection and radiate it throughout the city. This concept of Chinese contamination resonated with Meares's characterization of Chinatown as a "laboratory of infection" that would poison its surroundings.

The efforts to regulate Chinese laundries and deny admittance of Chinese patients to public hospitals encouraged city supervisors to consider legislation that would ensure residential segregation of all Chinese in the city. Their anxiety arose from a recognition that every time city inspectors demarcated the boundaries of Chinatown, a considerable number of Chinese fell outside their purview, living in the border zones where Chinatown overlapped with Nob Hill, the Tenderloin, and Telegraph Hill or further afield in the Western Addition, South of Market, and Hunter's Point. Even more disturbing were the numerous instances of non-Chinese, including Italians, Portuguese, Irish, and Mexicans, even white women, who lived within Chinatown. These pernicious social mixtures heightened worries about contamination. The leakage of the "Chinese race" beyond prescribed boundaries suggested the impossibilities of containment.[95]

The existence of social mixing and the enduring characterization of Chinatown as "a pernicious plague spot" galvanized city supervisors to legislate Chinese residential segregation. In 1890 the supervisor Henry Bingham sponsored an ordinance that required all Chinese throughout the city to move to the toxic industrial section of the city, where "slaughterhouses, tallow factories, [and] hog butcheries" were located. The ordinance made Chinese presence equivalent to that of businesses that harmed the "public health and comfort."[96] The ordinance passed, and the city attorney coordinated with the Chinese vice consul Frederick Bee to make a single arrest of a Chinese merchant in order to produce a legal test case. Infuriated that the city attorney was cooperating with Chinese leadership, Bingham zealously took enforcement of the law into his own hands. Accompanied by his personal lawyer, Bingham arrived at the local police court and demanded that it issue seventy-five blank warrants for the arrest of the alleged violators of the law. The supervisor and press corps then followed a police squad's raid of the Globe Hotel, the much maligned residential hotel, where they randomly arrested twenty Chinese men.[97]

The federal judge Lorenzo Sawyer condemned the ordinance for its blatant discrimination, seeing no plausible justification for the "arbitrary confiscation of homes and property." The authority of nuisance law did not apply since the ordinance was "not aimed at any particular vice, or any particular unwholesome or immoral occupation, or practice."[98] As the legal historian Charles McClain has noted, the ordinance was the first municipal attempt to impose residential segregation on the basis of race, and Sawyer's federal circuit court ruling condemned the legal imposition of "race ghettoization." (Curiously this 1890 legal precedent did not buttress the early twentieth-century decisions that limited the use of racially explicit zoning law.)

In San Francisco, as in other cities across the globe, residential segregation practices grew more conspicuous and organized in the twentieth century.[99] Municipal attempts in 1890 to use zoning law explicitly to segregate Chinese residences gave way, after 1910, to a more subtle combination of restrictive deed covenants and land use zoning, which served to protect high-income residential areas from the location of industry, commerce, and multifamily apartments.[100] In San Francisco, the formation of the San Francisco City Planning Council in 1917 institutionalized the implementation and regulation of zoning law in the city, providing legal mechanisms to segregate residential and industrial areas. Across the United States, zoning laws were designed to "reinforce existing patterns of wealth, status and power," and their implementation suggested a pattern of racial and class discrimination.[101] However, zoning could not directly segregate racial groups. In *Buchanan v. Warley*, the U.S. Supreme Court invalidated a Louisville, Kentucky, ordinance that established exclusive residential zones for blacks and whites on the grounds that it unreasonably interfered with the rights to sell and acquire property. The court granted that some zoning restrictions, such as those that differentiated among residential, business, and industrial uses, could be lawfully used to interfere with property transactions and development, but only in those cases where the government could justify "the exercise of police power in the interest of the public health, conveniences and welfare."[102] The use of restrictive deed covenants, however, was upheld by the U.S. Supreme Court in 1921 in *Corrigan v. Buckley*. Individuals had a right to make restrictive agreements and could not be compelled to sell or lease property to anyone. Blacks, Asians, Jews, Mexican Americans, and any other group commonly excluded in covenants could not appeal to the equal protection clause of the Fourteen Amendment, because it applied only to state action and did not restrict private individuals "from entering contracts respecting the control and disposition of their own property."[103]

Once the strategies of racial zoning were frustrated by the 1917 Supreme Court decision, white property-owners turned to restrictive convenants to create exclusively white residential districts.[104] In San Francisco, the completion of the Twin Peaks and Portal Tunnels made possible tram service to the outer Sunset District and encouraged the development of a number of exclusive residential neighborhoods. The race restrictions regulating St. Francis Wood were typical of those used in other exclusive residential developments: "No person of African, Japanese, Chinese or of any other Mongolian descent shall be allowed to purchase, own, or lease said real property, or any part thereof."[105] The developers of St. Francis Wood, Mason and McDuffie, explained the advantages of the restrictions on property as an effort to permanently protect homes and to increase land values. Mason and McDuffie argued that the restrictive covenants "ward off the blighting effect of stores, flats and apartments; they protect from the crowding together of houses and cutting off of view; they deny entrance to undesirable neighbors and ugly and inharmonious houses."[106]

The rationale of nuisance law underwrote the cultural logic of residential covenants. In the upper-middle-class residential developments, real estate developers defined the public good narrowly in terms of corporate interests in order to guard against threats to property values. In contrast to the mixed-use heterogeneity of older districts such as Chinatown, the new residential districts sought to create a homogenous, bucolic world by denying entrance to "undesirable neighbors" and strictly controlling the appearance and type of buildings constructed. Neighborhood associations cultivated this vision of order, security, and homogeneity and mobilized around issues of housing density and lawn maintenance. The efforts of white home owners and their neighborhood associations to maintain the visual signs of a prosperous quality of life used class codes to support racial exclusivity. The fear of "undesirable neighbors" collapsed images of dirt, disorder, poverty, and noise into that of the presence of nonwhite races.

These cultural codes of difference contributed to the management of exclusively white residential zones and the persistence of racial minority ghettos. As David Montejano and Kay Anderson have argued, the discourse of health and hygiene played a formidable role in cultural definitions of racial difference and the racial character of living conditions.[107] The practices of public health investigation in San Francisco served to name, document, and forbid Chinatown. Public health officials took the prevailing languages of anti-Chinese antipathy and reshaped them into justifiable medical aversion. Popular observations about filth and overcrowding were enfolded into medical conceptions of epidemic disease, health risk, and sanitary danger and then recycled back into popular discourse. The California senator Aaron A. Sargent explained on the U.S. Senate floor in 1876 how the unsavory unhygienic habits of Chinese people drove white residents out of San Francisco:

> Experience has shown that Chinese population expels all other, as inferior currency expels all better kinds. The process has been going on for years, notably in San Francisco. . . . A landlord will rent a single house on a street to Chinamen, who at once crowd it to repletion with their compatriots. They take ordinary rooms, say of ten feet in height, put in a false floor half way to the ceiling and crowd both floors with bunks, and as many human beings as can be pressed into the space sleep therein. The atmosphere becomes fetid, and a sickly smell pervades the neighborhood, which causes the tenants of the houses to the right and left to vacate. These houses cannot be again rented to white persons, the rents fall, and finally the Chinese get possession. This process goes on in each direction until the whole street is abandoned to the Chinese. The property has fallen in value, becomes dilapidated and offensive, and the street is as much dedicated to Chinese uses and lost to any other class of residents as if it were a street in Hong Kong or Canton.[108]

Sargent invoked the derisive, attributed signs of Chinese residence— overcrowding, filth, and "sickly smell"—to explain why "no class of population (the white, the Negro . . . the Spaniard) . . . can endure contact with these squalid denizens. . . . Even the lowest classes of society flee." [109] With his observations, Sargent participated in the circulation of these ideas, simultaneously explicating, inciting, and confirming the formation of the Chinatown ghetto. Not all non-Chinese residents fled Chinatown, as Sargent has claimed, but over time white residents were able to move to the new residential neighborhoods, which were exclusive according to class and race. However, Chinese and other nonwhite residents were constrained by custom and law and confined to racial ghettos.

## RACE AND DIALECTICS OF PUBLIC HEALTH

Clearly, race was deeply implicated in the state projects and professional practices of public health in the last half of the nineteenth century in San Francisco. From its inception in 1854, the Board of Health used the perceived medical threats attributed to Chinese immigration and settlement to justify its most aggressive efforts. These health concerns about Chinese immigrants enabled public health authorities to apply sanitary regulations throughout the city of San Francisco, thereby fulfilling public health's objective of maintaining universal norms for the population and environment under its management. Even when official anxieties about Chinese behavior and health resulted in the exclusive and vociferous enforcement of sanitary regulations in the cases of Chinese persons, residences, and workplaces, as well as resulted in the persistent regulation of Chinatown, these actions were authorized and necessitated by the general objectives of public health reform.

The reform project was animated by the relentless comparison of the Chinese to so-called normative practices, most clearly evidenced by the practices of the white middle class. In this way, public health reform, like other modern reformatory projects, first focused on shaping the behavior of the middle class and then on using their reformed conduct as the model for regulatory norms for the entire population. Physicians, public authorities, and social reformers did not implement public health reform projects out of a conscious malice against those who failed to comport themselves in accordance with these norms, but out of a fervent conviction that the reform of habits and environment would prolong life, ensure good health, and perpetuate the social order. However, the production of these norms relied upon the recognition and reproduction of social differences. In the United States, race was perceived as the most immutable difference that could be used to distinguish population subsets and that could also be easily finessed into the public health hierarchy of the normative and the aberrant. In order for a reform project to engage in transformation, public health required the conspicuous and indisputable identification of aberration from the so-called norm.

One may speculate that the articulation of a racialized aberration may have not been necessary to the establishment of public health. Certainly, the medicalized racial formation of the Chinese and Chinatown was not inevitable. However, in San Francisco the focus on the aberration of the Chinese race and of the racialized space of Chinatown was crucial to public health reform. In general, public health, like all norm-based government projects, thrived on the perceived threat that aberrant behavior—and in this case, racialized groups—posed to the general well-being, galvanizing public support for administering a range of socially invasive procedures.

By collapsing abstract aberration into racial difference, the San Francisco public health apparatus presented a formidable and potent rationale for its growing power. However, because public health advocates relied on presumably immutable racial difference, they found the task of reforming the entire population to a particular set of norms impossible. Racial difference itself was perpetuated through systems of public health practice and other government practices. The wide social dispersion of public health discourses and practices that substantiated the dangerous difference of Chinese-identified space contributed to the unequivocal realities of geographic separation and social subordination. Excluded from opportunities, contained within a tight geography, and burdened with a sinister collective reputation, Chinese American women and men would find it difficult to be considered "normal" in their health, in their habits, and in their social interactions.

CHAPTER 3

# Perversity, Contamination, and the Dangers of Queer Domesticity

In the prevailing nineteenth-century ideology, respectable domesticity enabled the proper moral and biological cultivation of citizen-subjects necessary for American public life to flourish. The formation of respectable domesticity connected practices of individual health and sexuality to collective social well-being. Modern, healthy society was conceptualized as a series of heterosexual married couples and their children, who, as middle-class families, perpetuated the race and enriched the nation. Sexual and social practices by which individuals sought intimacy outside the reproductive marriage were identified as disruptive to the family and were perceived as a perversion, betrayal, and distortion of "the race" and of racially defined communities. At the turn of the century, reproductive sexual relations became more stringently scrutinized within marriage, and sexual practices outside of marriage were perceived as a threat. In this way, sexual activity either served or imperiled the racial order and national power.[1]

Nineteenth-century white politicians and social critics characterized Chinatown as an immoral bachelor society of dissolute men who frequented opium dens, gambling houses, and brothels. In this transient working-class world, Chinese single men lived herded together in bunkrooms, and the few Chinese women who had immigrated were considered to be prostitutes. Together their lives were considered contrary to respectable domesticity and capable of undermining American morality and family life. Physicians believed that Chinatown's vice culture and leisure spaces fostered intimate relationships between Chinese and white people that accelerated the transmission of syphilis and leprosy to white Americans. These dreaded diseases galvanized physicians to scrutinize Chinatown's perverse spaces, deviant sexualities, and peculiar domestic arrangements for both the clues and causes of contamination.

In the historiography and sociology of nineteenth- and early-twentieth-century Chinese American experience, Chinese bachelor sexuality is represented as deviant because the presumed sexual relations of these men living in San Francisco were considered nonreproductive and nonconjugal. Most Chinese men in the United States were separated from their wives, who remained in Guangdong. The few Chinese women present were considered to exist in sexual slavery, either as concubines to polygamous merchants or as prostitutes serving Chinese and white men. Even sympathetic sociologists and historians have interpreted the behavior of Chinese men as evidence of sexual maladjustment under a discriminatory immigration system in the United States. This interpretation presumes that the social relations Chinese men and women did have were delinquent and deficient of normative aspirations.[2]

Contemporaneous white critics sustained and bolstered a particular norm of heterosexuality and respectable domesticity in their fears about the dangers of deviant sexualities and queer domesticity in Chinatown. Normative visions of domesticity were defined by the narratives and explanations of its perversion and destruction. By attending to the concerns and policies developed to contain the contaminating effect of the perverse Chinatown social relations on the white public, historians can also observe a plurality of queer domestic arrangements, from female-headed household networks to workers' bunkhouses and opium dens.[3]

At the turn of the century, normal or respectable domesticity became increasingly defined by a self-contained household that had at its center the married couple's pursuit of reproduction. The space and social relations of queer domesticity countered or transgressed these normative expectations. It included emotional relations between men and women that upset normative heterosexual marriage, as well as homosocial and homoerotic relations. In urban subcultures of the time there existed a variety of sexual, social, and gender relations that could not easily be slotted into the emerging binary of "heterosexual" and "homosexual"—categories that were invented and became popular in the late nineteenth century and twentieth century. Sexuality was not a fixed set of acts, behaviors, and identities but rather a set of formations that encompassed a variety of social relations and sites. Exploring deviant sexualities and

queer domesticities allows us to conceive of alternatives that do not fun-
nel all valued erotic and sensual relations into heterosexual marriage and
reproduction.[4]

The perversity of Chinatown sociability threatened white society because it provided a constellation of options to respectable domesticity.
The social and leisure spaces of Chinatown could lure white men and
occasionally white women into a social world that presented a viable
substitute to the expectations of an incipient middle-class society.

Public health officials, politicians, and travelogue writers emphasized
figures of Chinese immorality and infection who imperiled white society. First was the mercenary prostitute who infected white boys and
young men with syphilis. Second was the sensuous and depraved "Chinaman" who lured unwitting white men and women into opium dens.
Third was the abject leper who represented the disintegration of the
body that would be the fate of American society after years of intimate
contact and miscegenation with the Chinese. These stereotyped and mute
figures of moral and physical peril served as ciphers for the insistent
worries of white officials and physicians. The process of knowledge formation focused on the deviant sexuality of these figures, paying careful
attention to their conduct, their bodies, and the perverse spaces they inhabited. This local production of deviant sexualities, queer domesticity,
and perverse geography provided a schema of the dangers of Chinatown
and Chinese residents to middle-class white society in San Francisco and
beyond.

## PROSTITUTION AND SYPHILIS

In the mid–nineteenth century, white politicians, missionaries, and physicians castigated Chinese female prostitution as a leading threat to the
moral and social order. Female prostitution and concubinage supposedly demonstrated the Chinese male disregard for marriage and respectable womanhood. The charge that Chinese female prostitution was an
"offense to public decency" accumulated a web of moral and medical
meanings. Critics of Chinese immigration emphasized how Chinese
women were kidnapped or sold into "sexual slavery" to prostitution
procurement rings run by criminal syndicates called "tongs."[5] At first,
when Chinese female prostitutes were perceived as providing sexual services exclusively to Chinese men, white critics viewed them as merely
immoral. But once they were believed to solicit white males, their presence was considered even more dangerous. The moral condemnation

intensified, as critics presented narratives of Chinese prostitutes as the cause of venereal disease and gender transgression. In the mid-1870s, physicians made ominous predictions about syphilis transmission from Chinese female prostitutes to white male clients and their families. Politicians quickly latched onto this catastrophic health scenario and, in their diatribes against Chinese immigration, reduced all Chinese women to the menacing stereotype of the syphilitic prostitute.[6] Although the medical threat was potent and pervasive, it did not eclipse the moral condemnation of Chinese prostitution in political discourse. Political critics freely combined both perils in their critiques of Chinatown society. The San Francisco supervisors Willard Farwell and John Kunkler characterized Chinese prostitution as "the most abject and satanic conception of human slavery" and the "source of contamination and hereditary diseases."[7]

Police and political knowledge about Chinese female prostitutes concentrated on their public visibility and danger to San Francisco's social order. Although women of many nationalities engaged in commercial sex, the activity of Chinese women came under careful scrutiny by white politicians, officials, and commentators.[8] As early as 1854, moral reform groups and the police singled out Chinese prostitutes for their visibility on major thoroughfares such as Dupont Street, which linked residential neighborhoods with the downtown commercial district. The police and moral reformers sharply criticized Chinese women who solicited out of open windows and doors on street level. Unlike streetwalking, which prevailed in East Coast cities as a dominant form of solicitation, many Chinese women worked out of "cribs," which were small rooms, often no larger than five feet by six feet, on street level. From these "filthy holes," women were most likely to solicit white males who worked in the downtown business district and traveled through Chinatown between work and home. The Chinese women who inhabited these street-level rooms were branded as prostitutes, irrespective of any other aspect of their lives or labor.

Police and politicians equated the presence of Chinese women in street-level rooms with sex solicitation. And, they confidently sought to fix the identity of these Chinese women as prostitutes. In this era, across the globe, the process of policing prostitution began with branding a permanent and inflexible identity on a woman who exchanged sex for money as one of a series of activities to acquire money for herself or her family. Knowledge of the activities of working-class women in public emphasized details and scenarios that heightened suspicions of sex solicitation. The variety of work that Chinese women did as seamstresses or piece-workers for manufacturers was dismissed in light of the conviction that the selling of sex was the only true activity of these women and the sole way of understanding their lives.[9]

In the mid–nineteenth century, police harassment decisively reshaped the urban geography and the social lives of women who were presumed to solicit sex.[10] From 1854 to 1865 the San Francisco police conducted aggressive campaigns to drive "crib prostitutes" away from the high-traffic thoroughfares of Jackson and Dupont Streets. The police chief demanded that the cribs be moved to the alleys and that screens be constructed to "hide the degradations and vice . . . from the view of the women and children who patronize the streetcars." [11] He encouraged the public health authorities to devise a plan to "herd" Chinese women to a distant location where they would "not offend public decency." [12] After the 1865 harassment campaign, which the police chief boasted drove hundreds of Chinese prostitutes from the city, brothel owners and police reached a settlement that pushed Chinese prostitution to side streets and alleys hidden from public traffic. The city council ordered that the "location and sanitary regulation of Chinese women" would fall under the jurisdiction of the city health officer.[13]

By the 1880s, Chinese prostitutes' cribs and brothels were located in the alleys between Jackson and Pacific Streets. According to the maps generated by the board of supervisors 1885 report on the condition of Chinatown, Sullivan's Alley, Bartlett Alley, and Stout Alley had the greatest concentration of Chinese prostitution. On the other side of Chinatown, white prostitutes served customers on Spofford Street west of Washington Street, on Waverly Place, Sacramento Street, and the alleys in between.[14] The intense harassment had made many women even more vulnerable. They required increased protection from the tong criminal syndicates to survive, and they could not access other forms of employment, such as sewing or piecework manufacturing without the assistance of tong middlemen. By branding women as prostitutes, the police and reformers limited their possibilities for work and made them far more identifiable for police harassment. For the white public, however, the removal of the cribs and brothels from public view heightened their distance from, and ironically, the danger they posed to, white marital domesticity. Secrecy and removal from view only amplified anxiety that immoral and wicked activity transpired outside of public oversight.

Visibility presented multiple dangers to the viewers, their relatives, the officials, and those under observation. In political rhetoric, the sight

of immorality could "offend" the dependents of white male citizens—
their wives and children. However, offending the moral sensibilities of
respectable women and their children might also have unpleasant rico-
cheting effects for their male relatives. The visibility of prostitutes could
readily inform married women of the variable sexual privileges exercised by men outside of marital domesticity. Although much of the opprobrium was leveled specifically at the female prostitutes, the thriving
sex trade might convince married women to dispense with white male
prerogatives of sexual independence and refuse to countenance sexual
betrayals. On the other hand, the visibility of the women from the streets
made them vulnerable to police harassment as well as available for re-
munerative encounters with clients. Official efforts to remove women
from public view disguised the sexual register of public activity and
made the transparency of these social transactions more difficult. Push-
ing illicit sexual activity to semipublic resorts and dens in the alleys and
side streets made the activity less amenable to surveillance. The frustration galvanized investigators to redouble their efforts and develop new
techniques of surveillance and new knowledge about that which politicians and police forced out of view.

The new techniques of surveying and census enumeration generated
a system of knowledge that would fix the identity of the women in question and ensure accurate police surveillance. The urgency in targeting
Chinese prostitutes, however, unleashed confusion in identifying the
signs of prostitution and distinguishing a professional prostitute from
other women. The motives, location, and conduct of Chinese women
had to be deciphered and classified. In the 1850s and 1860s, police singled out women who were observed peering out their windows or standing outside a door, or who worked in small, first-floor rooms. Police
presumed that in these rooms women allowed the frequent arrival and
departure of seemingly anonymous men. These women were interpreted
to be crib prostitutes. However, there were also women who lived in
more secluded, upper-story apartments who lavishly entertained regular
clients, primarily Chinese merchants. These women were identified as
courtesans who charged premium prices for the entertainment and companionship they provided.[15]

The social lore about these two distinctive types of Chinese female
prostitution, however, was not readily amenable to census tabulation.
U.S. census enumerators in 1870 and 1880 faced the daunting task of
classifying the inhabitants of Chinatown boardinghouses, in which an
average of seventeen individuals lived, into groups that conformed either

to definitions of family or of distinctive types of prostitution. Typical dwellings were inhabited by Chinese men and women of all ages. The 1870 U.S. census used a definition of "family" developed in 1850: "In whatever circumstances, in whatever numbers, people living under one roof and provided for at a common table, there is a family in the meaning of the law." One enumerator, William Martin, faced with boarding-houses containing on average seventeen Chinese female and male residents would divide the inhabitants by gender. Martin often recognized two "families" in such a dwelling—one family of female "prostitutes" and the other of male "laborers." In his tabulations, he identified 90 percent of all Chinese females over the age of twelve as prostitutes. Another enumerator, Henry Bennett, an editor and federal pension agent who was sympathetic to Chinese immigration, counted in his ward a greater number of families per dwelling and recognized a variety of married couples, children, male boarders, and female bonded servants *(mui tsai)* as distinct families.[16] In his overall calculations, only 53 percent of Chinese females over the age of twelve were designated as prostitutes. The 1880 census guidelines recognized the necessity for more elastic definitions of family, particularly in the "tenement houses and flats of the great cities," and instructed enumerators to record "as many families . . . as there are separate tables." The schedules themselves demanded that enumerators identify marital status and family relationships among members of a "family" group. These changes resulted in a greater number of identified families in each dwelling and a decline in the number of female prostitutes.[17]

The fact that a variety of households and domestic arrangements existed was seized by city officials as definitive evidence that typical Chinatown domesticity contradicted the nuclear family ideal. The 1885 board of supervisors' investigation of Chinatown counted only 57 women who were "living [in] families" with merchant husbands and legitimate children. According to this report, many merchants had several wives or concubines to "minister to animal passions" rather than to procreate. At the other extreme, there were 567 "professional prostitutes"—some of whom raised children—87 children were counted—as their "associates and perhaps protégés." The majority of women, over 760 living with 576 children, were "herded together with apparent indiscriminate parental relations, and no family classification." Their apartments, the investigators concluded, indicated that their lives existed in "a middle stratum between family life and prostitution, partaking in some measure of each." The complicated social relations between women and children in these houses frustrated white officials, who insisted on firm boundaries in family relationships. The surveyors observed that "prostitutes," women (who apparently were not professional prostitutes), and children "live in adjoining apartments and intermingle freely," which meant for the surveyors that prostitution did not result in pariah status in the Chinese community. The multiple roles of mothering and caretaking that several women undertook for a set of children made it impossible for the surveyors to mark "where the family relationship leaves off and prostitution begins." [18]

These versions of queer domesticity exposed the implicit expectations about gender roles, household numbers, and spatial arrangements in conventional domestic definitions of public and private. The surveyors' definition of domesticity was challenged in the attempts to single out a conjugal couple and their progeny. The investigators found it difficult to understand why caring and nurturance would develop between several women and children without clear kinship or maternal ties. They could not respect as a domestic option the cohabitation of several women and children without a man at the helm, so they ridiculed a white woman who lived among a large number of Chinese women and children for "berating" the surveyors for "invading their citadel of domestic rights." The absence of a family composed of a male patriarch, a sole wife, and their children made the claim of "domestic rights" appear ludicrous to the surveyors. There was a clear limit to which persons could deploy the "privacy" of social relations of domesticity to shield themselves from state intrusion into sexual activities and social affinities. The multiple women and children living together did not produce a reassuring transparency of gender roles and social affiliations of intimacy for the surveyors. For the occupants, however, the living space could be shared by dozens of people and yet produce privacy and clear webs of care and attention.[19] Prostitution and concubinage cast suspicion on all domestic relations and allowed city officials to persistently violate domestic spaces not conforming to their norms. For white observers, Chinese houses seldom possessed domestic features of intimacy, gender roles, or rights of privacy that characterized the white middle-class domestic ideal.

The policing of prostitution shifted from being a local effort to being a much broader one, with national immigration restrictions on Chinese and Japanese women. On the state level, from 1870 to 1874 the California legislature criminalized the entry of "lewd and debauched" Asian women into California, which in practice meant the state threatened steamship companies with heavy fines for transporting unmarried women. When challenged in the state courts, the San Francisco district attorney argued that California had jurisdiction in intervening in immigration regulations in order to exclude "pestilential immorality" from its cities. The debate over jurisdiction led the federal courts to overturn California immigration restrictions. In 1875, however, the U.S. Congress followed California's lead and passed the Page Law, which prohibited the immigration of Chinese, Japanese, and "Mongolian" women for the purpose of prostitution.[20]

The immigration bar was immediately raised at the borders to all women without husbands or fathers to claim them. The suspicion of prostitution made them uncommonly vulnerable to immediate deportation. These barriers to entry, coupled with police harassment, caused the Chinese female population in San Francisco to stagnate. Although, according to the census, the overall number of San Francisco Chinese nearly doubled, from 12,022 in 1870 to 21,745 in 1880, the population of Chinese women hovered at 2,000. The vitriolic political campaigns against Chinese prostitution made many women vigilant about being categorized as prostitutes, and the census figures for Chinese female prostitutes declined sharply: the proportion of "prostitutes" among all Chinese women shrank from 79 percent in 1870 to only 28 percent in 1880.[21]

Although police and politicians vilified and harassed Chinese female prostitutes, they readily deferred to medical authority in regulating the Chinese women's "loathsome contagion."[22] In 1871, when the San Francisco Board of Supervisors considered proposals for medical inspection of female prostitutes citywide, the local medical profession remained undecided, fearful of appearing to endorse the "safe" functioning of commercialized sex. Christian leaders deplored the regulation plan, which they perceived as condoning vice, and women's suffrage activists criticized the hypocrisy of the legislation, which singled out women for inspection and harassment but ignored their male clients. Like similar legislation proposed in other American cities, the San Francisco attempt at European-style military and colonial medical regulation went down in defeat.[23]

Although many physicians were ambivalent about regulating prostitution, some energetically developed knowledge about the effects of the Chinese prostitute on society. In the mid-1870s, at the height of the anti-Chinese political debate, physicians expressed fears about the spread of syphilis from Chinese prostitutes to the white population. During the California State Senate investigation of Chinese immigration in 1876, the senators questioned physicians about the prevalence of syphilis among

Chinese prostitutes and the ramifications for white society.[24] The most
famous testimony came from Dr. Hugh Huger Toland, a member of
the San Francisco Board of Health and founder of Toland Medical College (which subsequently became the University of California Medical
School). Dr. Toland reported that he had examined white "boys eight
and ten years old" with venereal diseases contracted at "Chinese houses
of prostitution." These boys neglected their condition and hid it from
their parents. When Toland diagnosed the disease as syphilis, the boys
enlisted his assistance to "conceal their condition from their parents."
Toland estimated that "nine-tenths" of all syphilis cases in white boys
and young men were attributable to Chinese prostitutes: "When these
persons come to me I ask them where they got the disease, and they generally tell me that they have been with Chinawomen. They think diseases
contracted from Chinawomen are harder to cure than those contracted
elsewhere, so they tell me as a matter of self-protection. I am satisfied
from my experience, that nearly all boys in town, who have venereal disease, contracted it in Chinatown. They have no difficulty there, for the
prices are so low that they go whenever they please. The women do not
care how old the boys are, whether five years old or more, as long as
they have money."[25]

A discourse on race, prostitution, and medical cure was prefigured
in Toland's account of his patients' testimony. According to Toland, the
doctor-patient confessional relationship yielded the true source of the
boys' afflictions. Out of a desire for a cure, patients eagerly accused Chinese women. The boys' candor stemmed from an already prevailing notion that "diseases contracted from Chinawomen are harder to cure."
The circulation of such a belief suggested a developed system of associations between Chinese prostitution, disease, and medical cure. The boys'
visits to Dr. Toland demonstrated a knowledge that Chinese prostitutes
transmitted specific diseases, for which medical men like Toland had
developed special cures. Toland's testimony quickly became the master narrative of the medical menace of Chinese female prostitutes. During the decades that followed, politicians, medical professionals, and
popular writers repeatedly invoked Toland's observations of the extreme
youth of the victims and the peculiarly virulent venereal disease.[26]

Toland dismissed the possibility of the boys having access to multiple
sexual partners who were diverse in race or gender. In order to mark
Chinese women as the white boys' exclusive sexual partners, Toland
elaborated an economy of prostitution in San Francisco. In this economy, Chinese prostitutes were available to white boys because their ser-

vices cost less than their white female competitors. Emphasizing pre-adolescent boys as the clientele of Chinese prostitutes heightened the depravity and danger of Chinese women. Toland brushed aside any notion of male responsibility in this economy and any hint that adult men frequented brothels. He reversed the power dynamic between Chinese female prostitutes and their white male customers by characterizing the women as powerful, manipulative, and mercenary. White men were framed as the passive victims of the Chinese women's sexual lure; Chinese women, then, would "syphilize" or "inoculate" the men, unilaterally acting upon them, depositing disease in white men's bodies. The perversity of sexual encounters with Chinese women was underscored by the women's active role and domination, reversing prevailing social expectations.[27]

Dr. J. Campbell Shorb, a fellow member of the Board of Health, inserted "white girls" into these circuits of infection. He argued that the "excessively cheap" prices charged by Chinese women gave "these boys an opportunity to gratify themselves at very slight cost." The boys, then, would take their "'windfall' and go among white girls and distribute these diseases very generously."[28] The Chinese female prostitute became the economic counterpart of the Chinese male laborer—both characterized by "excessively cheap labor." Like the "coolie" who appealed to capitalists with his low wages, but whose employment could result in the degradation of American democracy, the Chinese prostitute offered sexual services for a bargain price that would later haunt the client, his spouse, and his progeny with venereal infection.

The medical narration of syphilis remade the signs of the unhealthy body.[29] Syphilis was a "secret scourge" that could persist without visible manifestations and could be conveyed from generation to generation. As a covert disease that could be transmitted from one to another without the knowledge of the sick or of the infected, syphilis was unlike such epidemic diseases as cholera and smallpox, which had immediate, visible, and lethal effects. Dr. Mary Sawtelle, a local physician and editor of the *Medico-Literary Journal,* dramatized the difference between the two diseases and their impact on the individual and society:

> Small-pox is nothing. Suppose a few hundred people are destroyed by it. We might as well frighten ourselves with ghost stories. It may kill its victims, but death comes kindly. It may contort his features into a hideous deformity, but it does not lap over from one generation to another; does not eat away at his flesh and crumble his bones to ashes, and still leave him among his fellows to destroy and contaminate everything he touches or breathes upon as syphilis

does; and every ship from China brings hundreds of these syphilitic and leprous heathens. They sit in the streetcar beside our wives and daughters. They
are a stench. Their mean stature, their ugly faces and their imbecile nastiness
mirrors to us what syphilis will do for a nation.[30]

Sawtelle's descriptions of syphilis were marked by national and racial references that relentlessly implicated Chinese immigrants as the source of
all infection. Chinese physical features and behavior became the indications of syphilitic conditions. The indications of disease were enfolded
into the physical signs of racial difference—odor, size, facial features—
and estimations of mental traits: intelligence, morality, and character.
The grave danger of syphilis infection was its transmission through the
contaminated but seemingly healthy carrier. Sawtelle determined that
Chinese immigrants were not only the transmitters of disease but also the
cause of disease and the signal of its presence—by virtue of the "stench."

Sawtelle's discourse on syphilis created nightmares of proximity between the diseased and the healthy. She ventriloquized the male citizens'
fear of "our wives and daughters" sitting next to "syphilitic and leprous
heathens" on the streetcar. By escalating the earlier fears of Christian
reformers and the police regarding the Chinese prostitute being visible
to white women and children from the streetcar, Sawtelle revealed
that any spatial barrier on the streetcar itself had been eliminated. Her
description of the heathen Chinese body suggested a body that was un-
containable and that released contagion and odor to those around it.
Like the "grotesque body" that figured in European descriptions of the
carnivalesque, Chinese people were never "closed off from either their
social or ecosystemic context." The focus on orifices and openings opposed the norms of the bourgeois body, which was discretely ordered,
bounded, and sanitized.[31]

The marking of race and disease on the body became even more striking in the medical indications of syphilis infection on the skin and in the
body. Syphilis infection was considered a generic condition of the Chinese race. According to Sawtelle, as syphilis became situated in the body,
"ulcers" ate away at internal organs. The disease would first consume
"the flesh and then the bones" and "copper-colored blotches" would
appear on the skin.[32] The coloring of the skin became synonymous for
the endemic syphilis in the Chinese race. Sawtelle speculated that white
Americans would possess "that copper colored syphilitic skin" after the
race had degenerated to the Chinese "level."[33] Her commentary on the
transformation of white skin folded the degenerative consequences of
race-mixing into the disfiguration and destruction of the body.

Since syphilis infection was imagined as emblematic of the Chinese race, its transmission was not restricted to sexual contact with Chinese women. Chinese men, in their capacity as domestic servants, were just as liable to infect white families. Since women represented a tiny proportion of the Chinese population and lived physically restricted in Chinatown, the threat Chinese men could pose in disseminating disease was far more ominous. This possibility diverted attention from the presumed role of white males in conveying syphilis from Chinese prostitutes to white wives to children. Instead it focused suspicion on Chinese "houseboys." Sawtelle claimed that "half of the Chinese servants employed in the families of the wealthy" were "reeking with this venereal virus." She highlighted the intimate nature of the contact between Chinese servants and their white employers by noting that Chinese men served as "chambermaids, house servants and nurses for Caucasian babies. They mouth the pap bottle for our innocent little ones." She castigated wealthy white employers for replacing Irish women workers with Chinese workers: "Those who think it economy to have their food cooked and their children nursed by this class of help may, when it is too late, find it an expensive luxury." [34] In Sawtelle's medical horror story, the Chinese domestic servant became a contradictory figure who was simultaneously responsible for household cleanliness and the devious transmission of venereal disease. By insinuating that syphilis was conveyed by oral contact with a baby's bottle, Sawtelle saddled Chinese servants and their lethal child care with the responsibility of syphilis transmission.

Chinese "houseboys" represented a gender inversion of household service that made questionable their intentions, their care, and their manliness. Chinese men's role in nursing babies gave a curious gender inflection to the widespread bourgeois worries of hiring female nursemaids in European metropolitan as well as colonial and slave societies throughout the globe. Nineteenth-century household manuals and medical guides warned of the moral and physical consequences for white bourgeois children in developing intimate relations with a socially subordinate surrogate mother. Nursemaids were often accused of transmitting disease to their charges through leaking orifices such as nipples, noses, and mouths. In San Francisco, similar concerns of contamination heightened suspicions about the presence and role of the Chinese houseboy. [35] Some publications warned mothers of the dangers of unsupervised "Chinamen" who tended white children, "particularly little girls." These warnings, insinuating that Chinese men might sexually molest white girls, in addition to the concerns about possible syphilis transmission while nursing babies, redoubled white fears of the health and sexual dangers of employing Chinese male servants.[36]

The purported syphilis infection of Chinese houseboys drew questions about their social and sexual activities when they returned to the dens and bunkhouses of Chinatown, as well as about their racial inheritance. Among white physicians and critics, there was little consensus as to how Chinese men were infected. On the one hand, Dr. Thomas Logan, secretary of the California State Board of Health, believed that there was "infrequent evidence of syphilitic disease" transmission between Chinese women and men. The peculiar "physiology" of the "Asiatic race," particularly the "epilatory condition of the genital organs" and the absence of facial hair, indicated the "absence of strong and enduring sexual appetite."[37] On the other hand were those who speculated that Chinese men had more perverse tastes in sexual partners. Thomas H. King, a San Francisco merchant who had lived in China for ten years and served in the U.S. consulate in Hong Kong, reported that sexual activity between Chinese males was common on ships: "Sodomy is a habit. Sometimes thirty or forty boys leaving Hong Kong apparently in good health, before arriving here would be found to be afflicted about the *anus* with venereal diseases, and on questioning by the Chinese doctors to disclose what it was, they admitted that it was a common practice among them."[38] Locating disease on the body, even by nonmedical informants, emphasized the growing popularity and power of medical narratives of examining and mapping the body. Reports of sodomy offered by other San Francisco informants detailed variations that involved lurid descriptions of genital mutilation and bestiality.[39] Speculations of sodomy, however, were only entertained when questioning the syphilis infection of Chinese men. In considering the syphilis infection of white males, the avenues of transmission were limited to heterosexual sex with Chinese female prostitutes, ignoring any possibility of white males having "infectious" sex with other men. The narratives of Chinese male "degenerates" and "mercenary" Chinese female prostitutes placed both as a threat to white American married heterosexual couples and their families.[40]

## PERVERSE ENCOUNTERS IN OPIUM DENS

Chinese servants were not alone in traveling between white homes and Chinatown opium dens. White men and occasionally white women also experienced the web of perverse social relations, ambiguous sexuality, and queer domesticity in the Chinatown opium dens. The semipublic resorts became legendary for seducing white tourists with the "gentle harmony of their weird social intercourse."[41] The organization of space and the practice of smoking opium generated the possibilities of sexual relations and social intimacy across race and class lines. Opium smoking was considered to transpire in "every sleeping-room in Chinatown"; the white writers and physicians focused their scrutiny on the "public opium resorts" that supplied opium equipment and "sleeping bunks" for Chinese and white smokers alike. The opium dens were often small, subterranean rooms with shelves on all sides that accommodated a dozen bunks.[42] Health officials feared the role of opium dens in transmitting syphilis and leprosy between the Chinese and "white persons." Opium dens became the emblematic semipublic site of bizarre social communion, moral degradation, and vice. Together with brothels and gambling houses, the opium dens generated a sociability and atmosphere that was liable to destroy the "very morals, the manhood and the health" of white Americans.[43]

The common method of smoking opium encouraged a special intimacy. The bunks could accommodate a pair of opium smokers who would lie facing each other with their heads resting upon blocks of wood or tin cans. Between them would be a lamp and a pipe with a sixteen-inch bamboo stem connected to a ceramic bowl. The preparation for smoking opium was elaborate and required instruction. The smoker dipped a needle into a container of prepared opium and then held the needle above the lamp's flame, where the opium bubbled and swelled to several times its original size. Once it was properly "cooked," the opium was transferred to the pipe's bowl, where it was rolled into a small "pill." This pill was forced into a hole at the center of the bowl and heated. The pipe was tilted and held over the flame, and the smoker drew in the fumes.[44] (See Figure 4.)

The investigators identified most of the smokers as Chinese men but were acutely aware of dens that catered to white men and women. Dr. H. H. Kane speculated that the first white American was introduced to opium smoking in 1868 in San Francisco, and that the habit proliferated rapidly among white gamblers, sporting men, and prostitutes. Kane naively ignored the fact that American merchants and sailors had ample opportunity to partake in opium consumption as participants in nineteenth-century trade with China. The consumption of opium became widespread in Asia because of the heavy commercial traffic of opium be-

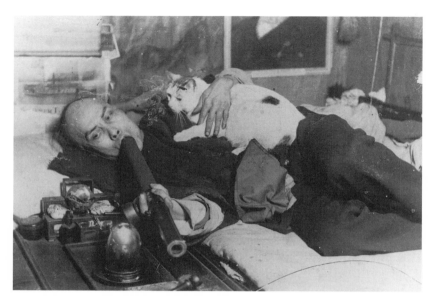

Figure 4. This photo shows the interior of a Chinatown opium den, circa 1905. Courtesy
California Historical Society, FN-15982.

tween British India and China, which was forced by the British military
to accept narcotic commerce.[45]

The techniques of observation and documentation of the illicit activity in the opium dens shifted from the textual to the visual with the use
of new photographic technology to depict the dens during police raids.
Isaiah West Taber and Company, famous for pictorial tourist photographs of San Francisco and the scenic West Coast, produced a series of
images of the Chinatown opium dens in the early 1890s. In style and
captions, they were more comparable to twentieth-century journalistic
photographs than either tourist shots or the pictorialist art photographs
of the period. Taber and other photographers used a magnesium flash
and a dramatic viewpoint shot that provided the "you-are-there" quality of the images. Practical photographic flash was invented in the 1880s,
and Taber quickly adapted the use of a flashlight or magnesium flash
gun to produce dramatic interior shots. The caption writer concocted
the dramatic, surprise entrance into the opium den and emphasized the
heroic flashlight photographer who shot the pictures while a detective
guarded the door. The textual cues demanded that the viewer ignore the
substantial time needed to set up the camera, focus in semidarkness, and
light the flash powder. Technically, the photographer's overexposure of

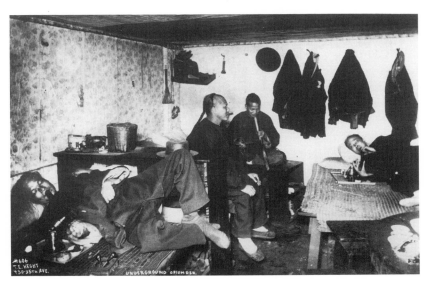

Figure 5. The photo *Underground Opium Den*, by T. E. Hecht, was taken circa 1900. Courtesy San Francisco History Center, San Francisco Public Library.

the foreground objects and the surprised expressions of the Chinese subjects emphasized the drama and speed of the shot.[46] (See Figure 5.)

Although the photography depicted only Chinese subjects in opium dens, medical reportage and travelogues detailed the disturbing repercussion of cross-racial social liaisons in the dens. The bunks were occupied at all hours of "night and day" as smokers puffed and dozed. Dr. W. S. Whitwell witnessed "ten to a dozen half-dressed American men and women and young girls, and perhaps two or more Chinamen. . . . Cheek by cheek, jowl by jowl, American men and women and Chinamen are smoking and dreaming the hours away." [47] The journalist George Fitch anticipated that "when a man or woman falls under the bondage of opium, self-respect is lost." Their social inhibitions were lowered by opium smoking and they were vulnerable to moral turpitude and immoral sexuality.[48]

The drug catalyzed a peculiar social communion. The very idea of opium "joints" entailed the image of a convention or congress of smokers affiliated with each other, not by status, religious belief, or occupation but by a shared pleasure in the drug. The allure of the opium den was that it promised withdrawal from the agitation of ordinary life, but it also made the attention to social distinction irrelevant. Opium smoking disrupted the sense of refinement and taste that distinguished the respectable from the lower classes. The failure to recognize and sustain cultural markers of demeanor and association ran counter to the expectations of people of "good repute." As a social setting the dens permitted mingling without regard for the social distinction of either class or race, creating the fraternity and egalitarianism of vice that undermined the republic of virtue and status distinctions.[49]

Moreover, the spectacle of white women in opium dens horrified white male observers. Kane argued that "many females are so much excited sexually by the smoking of opium during the first few weeks [that] . . . many innocent and over-curious girls have thus been seduced." The San Francisco physician Winslow Anderson described the "sickening sight of young white girls from sixteen to twenty years of age lying half-undressed on the floor or couches, smoking with their 'lovers.'"[50] The opium habit resulted in the "downfall of girls and the debasement of married women." Addicted white women often prostituted themselves in exchange for the drug, often seeking Chinese opium den operators as their principal clients. The damage to white women's virtue was irreversible from the perspective of physicians and journalists. The women were dismissed as "disreputable" and "fallen" by their very presence in a semipublic lounge and considered lost to good society.[51]

The psychic and material danger to white men, however, preoccupied the attentions of physicians and travelogue writers. The travelogue writer B. E. Lloyd was fascinated by the opium den denizens he counted as "our own respectable sons and brothers, who move in good society, and are of 'good repute.'"[52] The social intimacy between races in opium dens presented ominous perils to respectable men. George Fitch reported seeing a "very fastidious" man, who had "acquired the opium habit, lying side by side with a dirty coolie, each taking alternative puffs at the same pipe."[53] However, unlike a white opium addict, the neophyte was far less sanguine about receiving a pipe from the lips of a Chinese man. Allen Williams, a freelance reporter, related his own first experience of visiting a Chinatown opium den in New York. Williams described his ease in resting his head on the "shirt bosom" of his opium-fiend companion, Frank, and his "involuntary shiver of horror" when Tun Gee, "a cadaverous Chinaman," climbed into the same bunk facing him. Although Williams attributed his discomfort to Tun Gee's resemblance to a "certain Chinese leper," he was assured by his white companion that Tun Gee was one of the "best natured Chinaman" and a "thoroughly good cook" of opium. Lying in close proximity, with nothing to separate the reporter's face from the Chinese man except the opium smoking equipment, Tun Gee prepared the opium pipe for the two white men. Williams refused to take another draw of the pipe after Tun Gee smoked from the same pipe and prepared it for several other rounds for his companion, Frank. His narrative emphasized both the extent and the limits of "careless" physical intimacy in the opium den. The physical intimacy of a white man reposed on the "breast" of his white male companion and the close proximity of a Chinese opium cook were considered acts of bizarre but not disturbing intimacy. The prospect of actively sucking the same pipe as the Chinese cook, however, created intense revulsion and panic. Williams worried that "an opium pipe, when passed in short succession from lip to lip, must be a not infrequent conveyance of disease. An efficient ally it is in extending the sway of that arch-enemy to the bones and tissues, Syphilis." He suspected contagion not from the mouth of his white companion but rather from the Chinese cook with the "cadaverous visage." [54]

The revulsion at sharing the same pipe amplified speculations of "loathsome contagion" that could be passed unwittingly from one smoker to the next. Kane believed that an opium smoker was most likely to contract syphilis "from the pipe-stem," which was passed from "mouth to mouth a hundred times a day for months and years." He detailed several instances of unsuspecting smokers contracting syphilis from the pipe, including a "respectable young man" who contracted a "syphilitic chancre of the lip." [55] Suspicions about the virulent disease's transit emphasized the danger in sharing the pipe, an instrument of both oral pleasure and contact. The panic of ingesting the residues of bodily fluids and of sucking a pipe shared by multiple, anonymous mouths emphasized the promiscuous orality of the experience. In the circuits of smoking, the anonymity of the mouths that sucked on the same pipe provided no occasion for the exclusive possession of the instrument of pleasure. The pipe, the residues of saliva, and the act of sucking focused on a shared fixation on the pipe itself and the other mouths that took pleasure from it. The queer relations produced here could be ascertained by following the relays of erotic fascination though the unregulated, semipublic space of opium dens.

Starting in 1875 San Francisco and California passed laws prohibiting opium smoking and aggressively closed down Chinatown opium joints, but consumption of smoking opium continued to increase. Opium resorts proliferated outside the boundaries of Chinatown, and an estimated forty-five thousand pounds of the drug was imported into San Francisco annually in the 1880s. The legal importation of smoking opium ceased in 1909.[56] The extensive police raids on opium dens in San Francisco drove the white smokers out of Chinatown, but many other resorts and "lay-outs" emerged in boardinghouses in the nearby South of Market and the central business districts. With the proliferation of opium resorts outside of Chinatown, one police officer feared the spread of opium smoking to "schoolboys and clerks who would never have gone into a Chinese den," and who instead were "learning to like the habit" in "respectable places."[57]

Although the process of affiliation that developed around smoking opium resembled the creation of consumer taste and culture, it was not seen as a productive capitalist activity. The addiction to opium resulted in lethargy, diminished productivity, and the waste of time and capacity. The idea of addiction was an extreme example of the cultivation of consumer taste, because consumption was unmanageable and unproductive to the accumulation of capital.[58] Physicians tried to understand opium's "tranquilizing" effects, in which hours could be spent in exploring "pleasing hallucinations bordering on sweet oblivion." Rather than falling asleep, the smoker experienced the "dreams of wakefulness" that could be enjoyed quietly and within the opium den, "free of the annoyances of daily life." Practitioners and even some physicians believed that if such an experience could be harnessed and managed, then it would provide a useful "luxury" if taken in moderation. Dr. Flemming Carrow, who had practiced in Hong Kong, believed that smoking opium could be used to "stimulate the faculties, to awaken and sharpen them," if used sparingly. Dr. Carrow saw the value of such a stimulant for "gentlemen tired of business or a student weary from prolonged mental effort [who] retires to his opium couch, where after one or two whiffs at his pipe, he is rested and consoled and ready for his work again." But most physicians believed that the insatiable craving opium produced could not be managed, and once addicted one was obliged to "spend certain hours a day" smoking. The result was an overwhelming "fascination with indolence" and the disintegration of individual health: the addict's "appetite gives way to anorexia, nausea and dizziness, the muscular system degenerates and [the] smoker becomes pale, nervous and emaciated, and entirely unfit for his vocation."[59]

For aspiring bourgeois men, the requirements of earning a living were achieved only by constant vigilance against multiple temptations or against premature exhaustion. This tension sometimes drove people toward activities that promised surcease to these demands for self-discipline and self-denial. The stringent moral rectitude required of the respectable classes was the obverse of an urban landscape of saloons, red-light districts, dance halls, and opium dens. The lure of the opium den was understood in terms of the wasting of time and moral energy. The threat that opium smoking posed to the nation was viewed in terms of its capacity to vitiate the life of the youth and to compromise the vigor of the users whose productivity, biological and economic, would be lost to the nation.[60] While the saloon of the new European immigrant and white working class was characterized by disorder and boisterousness, the opium den was quiet and its "inmates" were subdued. The sociability of the dens created an intimacy far different from that in the saloons. In saloons, drinkers remained standing or sitting; in the dens, smokers lay side-by-side in the bunks. While the saloon seemed to have a corrosive effect upon a solid home-life, the opium den promoted an indiscriminate intimacy that could be construed as a substitute for the prized intimacy of the middle-class home. The opium den of the immigrant Chinese presented a substitute more ominous than the saloon of the immigrant European, since Chinese immigrant men were perceived as conspicuous in their lack of affiliation with nuclear families.

## LEPROSY AND CAUTIONARY TALES OF MISCEGENATION

The alleged sexual transmission of disease intensified fears of race degeneration. In nineteenth-century theories of race degeneration, there were two avenues of danger. The first emphasized the deterioration of the individual body, which was emblematic of health of the collective race, and the second focused on the fact that cross-racial reproduction produced defective, hybrid progeny. Both these scenarios bolstered the movement for social and legal prohibitions against heterosexual alliances between races.

Miscegenation law sought to regulate heterosexual marriage within racial bounds and finessed the perpetuation of racial purity in procreation.[61] Nineteenth-century California law developed injunctions against specific race mixing in marriage. As early as 1850 the state prohibited marriages between "white persons" and "Negroes and Mulattoes."[62] Injunctions against marriages between the Chinese and whites developed after a referendum proposed at the 1878 California Constitutional Convention. A delegate to the convention, John F. Miller, speculated

that the "lowest, most vile and degraded" of the white race were most
likely to "amalgamate" with the Chinese, resulting in a "hybrid of the
most despicable, a mongrel of the most detestable that has ever afflicted
the earth." [63] The ominous, apocalyptic pronouncement adapted scientific discourses of racial "hybrids" to stoke fears of cross-racial marriage
among white people.

In the mid–nineteenth century, ethnologists had developed experiments and theories about the mixing of human races, using analogies
from the crossing of plant species. Scientists believed in the existence of
pure and superior races that would be contaminated by the hybrid progeny, who would have diminished physical and intellectual capabilities. In
1862 Dr. Arthur Stout feared the infusion of "bad blood" from the inferior "Mongolian" race to the superior "Caucasian" race. Stout argued
that mixed-race men were "inferior to the pure races" and made the
"worst class of citizens." [64] Race degeneration held grave consequences
for the fitness and health of progeny over generations, and the proliferation of "degenerate hybrids" would "poison" and "undermine" both
national strength and economic prosperity. [65] Stout's conclusions became a facet of the public health debate in 1871. Logan feared the
"evils" that would occur with "the intermixture of the races and the introduction of the habits and customs of a sensual and depraved people"
in the midst of a white population. However, Logan believed that the
"intelligence" of the white race would prevail and limit "any serious risk
of race degradation." [66] Yet, the outcome of hybrids was always subject
to change because of the possibility of beneficial crosses between the
races, which had already justified the valued mixture of northern and
western European "races" as constitutive of "American civilization." In
this vein, Stout revised his findings and suggested the value to American
civilization that would accrue "if a first-class Chinese woman and a first-
class white man would marry," a considerable improvement over the in-
termarriage of white men to "Negro" women and Indian women. [67]

Despite Stout's confidence of the advantages of selective elite mixtures, in 1880 the California legislature prohibited the licensing of marriages between "Mongolians" and "white persons." [68] However, for
twenty-five years, the legislature did not amend the marriage statute
itself to forbid marriages between whites and Asians. In the last quarter
of the nineteenth century, journalists, officials, and missionaries occasionally reported that in San Francisco there were marriages between
white women and Chinese men, three to twenty of them, according to
the different reports. [69] Although the marriages provoked derisive com-

ment from white men, legislators were not eager to invalidate the marriages. In 1905 at the height of the anti-Japanese movement, the legislature finally sealed the breach between the license and marriage laws and invalidated all marriages between Asian and white spouses.[70]

Syphilis and leprosy and narratives of their cross-racial transmission became become both the metaphor and the material threat that contaminated the middle-class nuclear families and transgressed the boundaries of race and nationality. The Chinese leper's "invasion" of the United States began in 1871, when San Francisco public health authorities diagnosed Hong Tong as a leper and set him to the Smallpox Hospital, where all infectious disease patients were detained.[71] In five years, the Board of Health put a dozen Chinese lepers in indefinite quarantine. The pace of the public health incarceration of Chinese lepers fed the political hysteria about the disease. In testimony to a U.S. congressional committee in 1876, local physicians, politicians, and labor leaders argued that leprosy in California was an "inherent" condition of the Chinese race, and its rampant spread in the United States was inevitable with continued Chinese immigration.[72] The medical theory that leprosy was an "essentially Chinese disease" necessitated the social and sexual isolation of Chinese lepers from the diseased of other races. Over time, health authorities proposed to remove Chinese lepers from the Smallpox Hospital. Plans to place consumptives and lepers together were defeated by assertions that, despite the economy of the plan, it was inconceivable to condone the mixing of the "Mongolian race" and the "Caucasian race."[73] The solution was to segregate patients by disease and race; for lepers this resulted in the construction of one shack for "white lepers" and another for "Chinese lepers" on the edge of the Smallpox Hospital's property.[74]

Political pressure to solve the Chinese leper problem mounted. At the height of congressional inquiry into Chinese immigration in August 1876, the San Francisco Board of Health approved the deportation of dozens of Chinese lepers to Hong Kong.[75] From 1871 to 1883, the Board of Health confined seventy-nine lepers in the Smallpox Hospital and deported forty-eight of that number. Public health officials had unequivocally identified leprosy as an alien disease. For Chinese immigrants the policy of deportation for leprosy narrowed the health standards for continued residence in the nation.[76]

The deportations also exacerbated suspicions that any Chinese immigrant could be infected with leprosy, which the Workingmen's Party leaders played upon in their anti-Chinese campaigns. In one particularly sadistic act of street theater, the Workingmen's Party sympathizers drove disfigured Chinese men, alleged lepers, around San Francisco to display the physical manifestations of the disease. The street theater of the medically grotesque provided instruction in the dreadful consequences of Chinese settlement.[77] In travelogues and political speeches, the body of the leper became a horrifying spectacle. The decay and disintegration of the leper's body were painstaking detailed in the descriptions of "ulcerated hands," shedded "scales," "putrefying sores, " and "blue limbs."[78] The "swollen and repulsive features" of the leper's body combined with the knowledge that lepers were doomed to a slow and painful death did not inspire compassion. The mystery of their disease and the possibility that their condition was communicable contributed to calls to confine and expel the "intensely revolting" leper from American society.[79] The leper was literally less than human, a perception that justified the removal of diagnosed lepers from everyday social relations.

Although most of the lepers incarcerated were Chinese, a small but significant number were white. The cases of white lepers renewed worries about the contagiousness of the disease. Popular reports circulated on both coasts of white men catching leprosy through intimate contact with the Chinese or through the consumption of cigars allegedly wrapped by Chinese lepers. In order to quell growing public hysteria about leprosy, public health officials claimed that leprosy was limited to the Chinese and transmitted only through inheritance.[80] However, a vocal minority in the California public health circles disagreed and argued that sustained contact with a leper could also result in infection. The social-contact theorists argued that leprosy had been unknown in Hawaii before the Chinese immigrated there and disseminated the affliction to the Hawaiian natives.[81] Both the theories of inheritance and of social contact focused on racial origins. In the United States, the race of the leper depended on the dominant race of immigrant lepers in the region. So on the Pacific Coast, leprosy was "essentially a Chinese disease," but in the eastern and southern United States, leprosy was considered a Greek or Norwegian disease.[82]

Since heredity and sexual contact were considered the source of disease transmission, fears of leprosy mixed with fantasies of miscegenation and illicit intimacy. The moral taint produced by narcotic addiction and extramarital sexual relations was transmuted into physical contagion. In this economy of perversion and race degeneration, Chinese bodies were considered to be saturated with loathsome contagion that spilled into the white bodies with whom they shared intimate physical contact. At Board of Health inquiries and medical society discussions, physicians offered examples of young white boys becoming infected by "leprous Chinamen" who served them food or shared their beds. Other leprosy cases had an explicitly sexual origin, such as the instances of European sailors who had "illicit" intercourse with Chinese female prostitutes in China or Hawaii. In all these scenarios, Chinese women and men were conceived of as the original source of leprosy. Even when leprosy was attributed to native Hawaiians, the Chinese figured in as the original "inoculators."[83]

With the focus on intimate contact, leprosy easily became analogous to syphilis. The similarities between the two diseases, with their long incubation periods and disfiguring physical manifestations, led the health officer John Meares to conclude that "the so-called leprosy [that the Chinese] have here is simply the result of generations of syphilis, transmitted from one generation to another."[84] Nearly two decades later, Dr. Henry Brown examined lepers under city care and expected that lepers would also exhibit a syphilis infection. He too believed that the Chinese were the source of both diseases. In each case study, Brown relentlessly pursued any hint of sexual and social contact with the Chinese in order to ascertain how someone who was European, native Hawaiian, or American Indian had contracted leprosy.[85]

Social relations outside the hospitals and asylums, however, were far less amenable to medical regulation. Meares believed that in the domain of sexual relations, medical interests had to be served by the powers of moral persuasion and legal regulation. Public health officials emphasized the devastating health consequences of "illicit" interracial sexual relations and hoped that moral policing would prevent respectable whites from sexual relations with the Chinese. Meares feared that this moral policing could lose its power with the social rehabilitation of the Chinese and their entry into American society. Such a collapse would make the stigma of miscegenation less onerous, and in the course of years, Meares speculated, "marriage between the Chinese and people of all nationalities will become a more frequent occurrence."[86]

Meares could only hope that the identification of Chinese lepers as inhuman, the publicity announcing the removal of these "creatures" from society, and their eventual deportation would feed the social aversion necessary to keep the races apart. By equating leprosy's disfiguration, disintegration, and dehumanization of the body with Chineseness, medical discourse intensified notions of incommensurate racial difference. Meares recognized that differences based on language, custom, and living standards could be narrowed and overcome with instruction, time, and circumstances.[87] The presumption that all Chinese were potential lepers, however, made the diseased body the immutable racial difference. Meares employed the rhetorical exhibition of Chinese lepers as a kind of public instruction, similar to that used by the anti-Chinese labor activists, to isolate the Chinese population and to make their integration into American society impossible. For medical men like Meares and for the politicians they persuaded, the failure to contain social interactions held grave consequences. In their nightmares, the price of Chinese assimilation was nothing less than the transformation of the United States into a "nation of lepers."[88]

The medical, travelogue, and legal narratives concerning the transgression of racial boundaries were considered to be material and metaphorical symptoms of the unhealthy fluidity and dangerous freedom in the cities. The suspicions of moral degeneration, sexual perversion, and loathsome disease in the Chinatown opium dens, female-headed houses, and bunkhouses generated a sense of revulsion for the white reader. By contrasting the danger of Chinatown sociability, the white physicians, politicians, and journalists sought to tutor the conduct of wayward white males and inculcate habits of domestic discipline to promote compulsory heterosexual family life. For males of the respectable and aspiring classes, the habits of fastidious self-denial and the strict observance of social distinctions were expected to eliminate the desire for sensuous pleasures with, and the accompanying contaminating contact with, Chinese males and females. The medical and moral narratives characterized these spaces of cross-racial sociability and sexual ambiguity with revulsion and horror.

Heterosexual identity, marriage, and respectable domesticity made claims for privacy and demanded defined sexual and gender roles for men and women. In contrast, the queer domestic spaces and relations perceived to thrive in Chinatown could guarantee neither privacy nor rigid sexual and gender identities for the inhabitants. The intimate relations in the apartments of Chinese women and children, in the opium dens, and workers' bunkhouses generated alternative social possibilities and knowledge of social relations. In defending respectable domesticity and the intensity of their revulsion for queer domesticity, white physicians and critics left little space to explore these queer domestic arrangements on the terms of their own viability. We have but hints of the erotic, social, and ethical relations and their meanings for Chinese immigrant men, women, and children as they related to each other and to the non-Chinese women and men who joined them in the spaces of opium dens, bunkhouses, and apartments. We can recognize that, in the apartment households led by Chinese women, parenting and caretaking relations developed differently than in nuclear-family household models. Many unrelated women might share caretaking duties of children, and children might develop affection and draw on social guidance from a variety of adults. In the opium dens, social status, profession, and race might be irrelevant to comfort, harmony, and community among those men and women who congregated to smoke opium. Rather than feature exclusive couplings of intimacy, the opium dens encouraged an ethics of sharing pipes, beds, and bodily contact among strangers or informal acquaintances.

In the medical rhetoric on Chinese female prostitution and opium dens, syphilis infection was presumed to alarm and dissuade the presumably healthy from contact with the potentially diseased. However, the presence of persons with disease, even incurable conditions such as leprosy and syphilis, need not provoke aversion, fear, and the severing of social ties. For Drs. Meares, Sawtelle, Toland, and Kane, incurable disease conveyed presumably by sexual intimacy or heredity had to be avoided at all costs to ensure the health of the individual and the respectability of family and society. These doctors promoted a particular ethics of public health that expected the person with a dreaded disease to remove himself or herself from social contact or be forcibly ostracized for failure to comply. Their concern emphasized the vulnerability of white individuals who would be contaminated by Chinese bachelors or female prostitutes. As a result of the zeal to protect white men, women, and children from potential contamination, the diseases of syphilis and leprosy hung like racial status for Chinese immigrants, amplifying their pariah status and justifying an embargo of care, affection, and affiliation. The exclusive pursuit of health, privacy, and defined gender and sexual roles for some was paramount to the organization of respectable domesticity.

Neither the medical menace nor miscegenation law succeeded in dissuading men and women from intimate relations across racial lines, however. Illness or the fear of infection could not prevent white men from frequenting opium dens, or white families from hiring Chinese servants, or white women from living with Chinese women or Chinese men. These men and women, Chinese and white, developed different kinds of subjectivity, expressions of social affiliation, and participation in communities that were ignored and devalued by those eager to buttress their own ideas of respectable domesticity. Since queer domesticity produced alternative environments and relations of intimacy and social ethics, it was perceived to be a formidable threat to the norms of respectable domesticity. In order to flourish, these queer communities did not need to be organized by marriage and heterosexual identity, by race or class status.[89]

# CHAPTER 4

# White Women, Hygiene, and the Struggle for Respectable Domesticity

The achievement of American cultural citizenship for Chinese immigrants rested on proof that Chinese women were engaged in respectable domesticity and motherhood. However, in the nineteenth century, Chinese women in San Francisco were perceived as either mercenary prostitutes infecting white boys with syphilis or as sequestered and uneducated merchant wives unable to further the progress of their families. Both images presented a reversal of the prevailing gender ideology that positioned women as domestic sanitarians, responsible for the care and defense of the home and of the moral and physical well-being of the family. White middle-class women contrasted the ideal of healthy home life against the problematic sexuality and domestic habits of immigrant Chinese women. On the one hand, Dr. Mary Sawtelle, editor of a local medical advice journal, argued that all Chinese women were vicious prostitutes who conspired to inoculate American families with syphilis. On the other hand, Presbyterian women missionaries encouraged home visits in order to reform the hygienic conduct of married Chinese women to match the standards of Christian and "civilized" behavior. In both instances white, middle-class household culture was defined in opposition to perceptions of unreformed Chinese living conditions, behavior, and culture.

Women physicians and missionaries promoted female authority in enabling the healthy reproduction of the middle-class family. Medical concepts of health and cleanliness increasingly contributed to the definition of normative American identity. Despite their experiences with frequent epidemics and ineffectual therapeutics in the nineteenth century, middle-class Americans displayed a zealous confidence that knowledge about human physiology and hygiene could assure a healthy life, supplanting eighteenth-century fatalism about the inevitability of sickness. In the context of nation building, rapid industrialization, and urbanization, health became "a civic duty and the emblem of a responsible life."[1]

The infusion of moral and patriotic purpose in ensuring the health of the body amplified the scrutiny paid to the relations, habits, and environment of domestic life. The domestic implied the spatial arrangements that sustained biological and social reproduction. As such, domesticity was a key regulative norm of modernity that reconfigured the conception of the family from a "temporal organization of kinship" to a specific "spatial entity" that encompassed heterosexual marriage, children, and servants in a self-contained dwelling.[2] In the flourishing nineteenth-century advice literature, the viability and health of the middle-class family life depended on the attentive labor of middle-class women in caring for children, in guarding against threats to marriage, and in tending to the physical environment of the home. These gendered programs of care and cultivation in the domestic space also prepared persons for their critical roles of citizenship in the public sphere.[3]

In tying citizenship to the work of the domestic space, white middle-class women sought to address the problem of who belonged to the American nation, and to emphasize their abilities in training others in proper social conduct. They parlayed their expertise on moral virtue and fitness in the domestic sphere by provoking public debates concerning issues of health, sexual morality, and family life. At the edge of American empire in San Francisco, white women's projects of domestic reform in Chinatown mobilized the cultural practices of "imperial domesticity" to manage and reform the "foreign" within the nation. In the late nineteenth century and twentieth century, white American women engaged in Protestant missionary projects to civilize the "lower races" within the United States and abroad in China and India and, later, in the U.S. imperial territories of the Philippines and Puerto Rico. The imperial reach of American modernity depended on the success of white women in creating domestic space in foreign terrains that protected against the disorder and contagion of alien races.[4] Through the example of their domestic management and housekeeping advice, San Francisco Presbyterian missionaries and Dr. Sawtelle sought to tutor both Chinese and white women in the cultural practices of a healthy American home life that stood in sharp contrast to the lifestyles, standards, and norms of the Chinese race. Racial differences subtly permeated the emerging cultural standards and ideals of white, Protestant, middle-class families, which were increasingly depicted as the American norm.[5]

## RACIAL WAR AND THE CHINESE SYPHILITIC PROSTITUTE

In the 1870s and 1880s, San Francisco politicians, labor leaders, and public health officials had declared that Chinese immigrants imperiled the "white race" by undercutting wages, subverting government authority, and spreading vicious diseases. Sawtelle underscored the medical menace by speculating that the Chinese immigrants willfully distributed "germs of death to another better race."[6] In this racial war, the most pernicious weapon was the Chinese female prostitute, who, Sawtelle warned, was "infusing a poison into the Anglo-Saxon blood" and imperiling the "future of the American nation."[7] She claimed that the "almond-eyed, olive-brown courtezans [sic] of the Orient" transmitted virulent strains of syphilis because of their "filthy habits" and an unwillingness to use "preventive measures," unlike the more conscientious "white women" prostitutes. Sawtelle echoed the ominous predictions of San Francisco physicians and public health authorities who feared an epidemic of syphilis transmission from Chinese female prostitutes to white male clients and their families. Sawtelle characterized Chinese women as "saturated" with disease, dehumanizing them and reinforcing the perception that these women were the embodiment of syphilis and therefore uncommonly dangerous and expendable.

Since Chinese prostitutes embodied syphilis, Sawtelle was able both to ignore the female prostitutes of other nationalities who worked in San Francisco and to attribute a pandemic of syphilis on the Pacific Coast exclusively to the sexual labor of Chinese women.[8] She scolded the exclusively male Board of Health for its reluctance to confront syphilitic Chinese prostitutes. Sawtelle crusaded against the perils of Chinese female prostitution as part of her campaign for providing women with health education and care. In addition to operating a clinic for women and children, Sawtelle gave middle-class women "practical" advice on topics that ranged from diphtheria prevention to proper dress for infants, through the *Medico-Literary Journal*. With her publication she targeted the "daughters, wives and mothers" by couching her health advice in "plain and palatable language." Sawtelle anticipated that her audience would be young mothers with "unborn babies and infant children." She believed that men "care little for health until they have lost it," while women would intently apply their knowledge to "preserving health or preventing disease."[9] Although the middle-class advice literature of the time insisted that habits of personal hygiene reflected individual "enlightenment," morality, and self-discipline, the gender differences in prescriptive literature considered hygienic vigilance to be an intrinsic characteristic of feminine "nature" and the justification for women's domesticity.[10]

This gendered asymmetry, Sawtelle believed, was reflected in her own autobiography as a "medical pioneer" whose contributions were not readily recognized by the male-dominated medical profession. She had received her medical degree from the New York Women's Medical College in 1872 at the age of thirty-seven. She returned to Oregon, where she had grown up, to open a practice in Salem, awaiting the graduation of her husband, Cheston, from Willamette Medical College. After receiving certification to practice medicine in California in 1876, the Sawtelles had moved to San Francisco, where Mary Sawtelle operated a sanitarium for women and children at her home at 120 Capp Street. Shortly afterward, in 1878, she began publishing the *Medico-Literary Journal*. Professional physicians in California were reluctant to admit her into their fold; at first, in 1879, the California Medical Association denied Mary Sawtelle's application for membership but readily admitted her husband. When Sawtelle was admitted the following year she boasted that she was the first woman admitted to a professional medical association. She pursued her vision of medical and hygienic education for women through organizing the Women's Medical College of the Pacific Coast in 1881. However, both the college and the journal were short-lived ventures: the college closed in 1883 and the journal ceased publication two years later.[11]

Sawtelle advocated that government and society should extend the hygienic jurisdiction of middle-class mothers. As an advocate herself for hygienic conduct, Sawtelle urged mothers to become more vigilant of their sons' activities, "lest they become ruined in body and soul by contracting the foul contagion."[12] She implored "enlightened" women to dispense with propriety and force authorities to protect "white Christians" from the menace of Chinese syphilitic prostitutes.[13] In her rhetoric, she rarely vilified white men for their multiple sexual partners or for their infidelity to white women. Often she characterized these men as uncommonly young and innocent. Sawtelle narrated how men went by the "thousands nightly" to the "dens of Chinese women" and engaged in "beastly scenes." [14] The consequences of an individual man's immorality, however, would put the nation at risk by generating a syphilis plague that would "ultimately sink this nation into effeminacy and political death." [15]

For Sawtelle, the risks of effeminacy entailed grave upheavals of the political and social order. She criticized the race and gender treachery of the "effete statesmen" and the East Coast ministers who supported the continued Chinese immigration on the grounds of respecting the Burlingame Treaty and principles of nondiscrimination. The pernicious influence of abolitionists' promotion of racial coexistence had allegedly blinded East Coast elites to the necessity of keeping racial bloodstreams separate.[16] In Sawtelle's writing, the effete man was a particularly sinister figure. In both sexual scenarios and political debates, the effete man had lost his will and his moral compass, he was vulnerable to Chinese sexual and political seduction, and his activity jeopardized the vital interests of the race. Effete men demonstrated a careless disposition to race-mixing that undermined national strength and the perpetuation of a properly gendered social order.

For the men effeminized by their encounters with Chinese female prostitutes, the dual danger of their treachery was the contagious disease, which marked the contamination of men's bodies and souls, and their gender inversion, which made them disinterested in the social obligation and sexual bonds of heterosexual marriage. Because of male effeminacy, the magnetic bonds of feminine and masculine would no longer adhere, and therefore the white woman's intrinsic "purity," sensitivity, and "divinity" would no longer "inspire [man's] strong, rough, honest soul" to the masculine ideal.[17]

The Chinese prostitute threatened the integrity of marriage and the purity of reproduction. For Sawtelle, Christian marriage presented the "highest earthly tribunal before which white-souled purity is sublimated" and sex became sanctified in the service of procreation. However, venereal disease soiled and twisted these ideals of companionate marriage. Sawtelle bemoaned the fact that a woman's faith in the "marriage contract" could be destroyed by the failure of health authorities and police to suppress Chinese prostitution. A married woman must "bow her head in anguish when she learns that the law fosters a demon to destroy her husband by her side, to inoculate her pure blood with a poisonous virus[,] and [that she] must still continue to give life to polluted children."[18] This contamination of bloodstreams and the dangers of degenerated offspring demonstrated Sawtelle's astonishingly prescient efforts to bridge mid-nineteenth-century anxiety about race degeneration and twentieth-century programs for eugenics and racial fitness.[19]

Sawtelle advocated legal prohibitions to rid the nation of syphilis, demanding that the syphilis "victim" be "prohibited from contracting marriage."[20] Sawtelle proposed the creation of a federal bureaucracy that would employ public health's police powers to "track syphilis to its lair . . . whether in man or woman" and make it less likely for others to contract the disease. She recommended a system of compelling physicians to register all venereal disease cases, report the condition of victims to their sexual partners and families, and isolate them in locked hospitals. Sawtelle's proposal, which was aimed at both men and women, was far more aggressive than the western European and colonial system of mandatory inspection and treatment of female prostitutes. Through her advocacy of radical syphilis suppression, Sawtelle intended to secure health for future generations of the white race. This form of "racial hygiene" relied upon eugenic measures that prohibited the "diseased" from reproduction.[21] She viewed marriage as an arena for state intervention when racial health and national vitality were at stake.

In the decades that followed, male physicians and politicians would see syphilis as a cause of race depopulation and degeneration. Before and during World War I, San Francisco and other U.S. cities experimented with the medical regulation of prostitution. By then only a handful of Chinese women worked in the commercialized sex industry, and the official focus shifted to white and Latina women.[22] Proposals for public health registration of syphilis victims and medical testing of marriage applicants were entertained in legislatures and conferences.[23] In 1939 California joined other states in adopting serological testing for syphilis for marriage license applicants, and the courts later justified the state's interest in prohibiting those marriages in which perilous diseases could be transmitted to a spouse or the offspring.[24]

## NURTURING HOMES AND HOMEMAKERS IN CHINATOWN

In contrast to Sawtelle, who viewed Chinese women as a threat that required eradication, white women missionaries regarded Chinese women as instruments of social reform. Women missionaries believed that the cultivation of Chinese domesticity and respectable womanhood would transform Chinatown society. These white middle-class women boldly entered the arena of "sexual politics" to transform the reputation and lives of Chinese women.[25] Typical of the efforts of Protestant missionary organizations in the American West, in 1874 Presbyterian women established the Chinese Mission Home to "rescue" and "reform" Chinese female prostitutes. In an environment of intense racial hostility, and despite opposition from the church's male leadership, missionary women organized a controversial program to provide refuge for Chinese women.[26] The Chinese Mission Home enabled middle-class women simultaneously to promote female moral authority and to assist victimized women. Their reformation programs combined instruction in housekeeping with Christianity. Missionaries adopted the language and expectations of hygienic culture in their training programs for former Chinese prostitutes. By teaching Chinese women to emulate the gender and domestic roles of white middle-class culture, the missionaries hoped to train Chinese women for positions as domestic servants, seamstresses, and teachers, with the eventual goal of their becoming middle-class housewives.[27]

This training of Chinese women in middle-class domesticity simultaneously made "fallen" women "respectable" and served to transform Chinese society in the United States. Presbyterian missionaries envisioned the education of Chinese women as the centerpiece in a program of racial "uplift," believing that each Chinese immigrant woman they schooled might become "the keystone in the arch that will lift thousands of her race from misery and degradation."[28] Christian philanthropic work intervened to produce proper nuclear families for Chinatown society, perceived to be socially disordered and populated by social deviants and a handful of endangered families.

In their zeal to reform Chinese society, Presbyterian missionaries developed an outreach program of house-to-house visits to bring instruction in Christianity, civilized domesticity, and cleanliness to Chinese merchant wives. Mrs. I. M. Condit, a Presbyterian missionary fluent in Cantonese and whose husband was a prominent figure in Chinese missionary work in California, established the program of house visits. In 1879, Condit was replaced by her assistant, Emma Cable. Over a period of twelve years, Condit and Cable averaged fifty visits a month to a clientele of thirty households. They engaged in house-to-house visitations in Chinatown, concentrating on "respectable," often older, women who sewed or kept house for their husbands and families. Condit reasoned that in order to reach Chinese merchant wives who lived in seclusion, Christian missionaries must "carry the Gospel" to Chinese women in their homes. She added emphatically, "*It is the zenana work*

*of San Francisco.*"[29] By alluding to "zenanas," Condit invoked a series
of exotic images and evangelical narratives familiar to her readers of the
highly publicized British and American missionary activity in India,
where white women visited South Asian women secluded in so-called
harems, rather than in public spaces such as churches, schools, and medical clinics. She highlighted the sense of foreign adventure and mystery
and imparted to the missionary work in Chinatown the noble purpose
of female emancipation. Condit emphasized the vulnerability of heathen
women who, unlike middle-class American women, could not rely on the
strength of women's networks and associations for assistance. Chinese
women, despite evidence to the contrary, were portrayed as isolated,
helpless, and in dire need of the help of enlightened white women.[30]

Emma Cable frequently described the process of spiritual enlightenment in terms of changes in the hygienic habits and material culture of
the Chinese women she visited. In a typical narrative of Christian conversion, Cable began with a description of entry into a dark, decaying,
and putrid Chinatown tenement where "God's sunshine never enters."
In a style reminiscent of sensationalist journalists and public health
investigators, Cable detailed the precarious journey of conversion for
missionary-report readers. She visited a Chinese woman who lived in a
dark, cramped apartment that resembled a grave. Cable described her
heroic efforts to set aside "all feelings of loathsomeness" and repulsion
in the atmosphere of "filth and darkness" and begin the task of "illumi-
nating a soul of corresponding degradation."[31] The conscious mirroring
of environment and the soul became more pronounced as Cable charted
the spiritual and hygienic transformation of the Chinese woman. She
contrasted the Christian utopia of "God's love, pure air and sunshine"
with the Chinese woman's "present surroundings": "Each succeeding
visit found a growing appreciation of my words, 'till finally she became
as thoroughly nauseated with her surroundings as myself. To-day we
find her in a cheerful room at 822 Dupont Street, which she has thoroughly cleaned, whitewashed and papered."[32] Cable mobilized the metaphors of sanitation and health—"pure air" and "sunshine" to sharpen
the contrast between "heathen degradation" and Christian enlightenment. The moment of conversion was marked by the intolerance of the
Chinese woman for dirty habitations and signified by the cleansing and
redecoration of her apartment. In conversion narratives the movement
from "darkness" to "light" consciously mixed spiritual and medical
meanings. The success of the missionary conversion brought "air and
light" to the homes and swept away "the diseased parts." As Cable

described it, "Instead of darkness we have air, light, sunshine, birds and flowers. Rooms enlarged and beautifully furnished, walls papered, [and] floors carpeted." [33] Missionaries were insistent on training Chinese women to be "practical housewives" and encouraging them in "neatness of person and homes." [34] Ideas of cleanliness, sanitation, and middle-class white material culture were conflated as the indicators of Christian belief and "civilized" behavior. [35]

In several instances, Chinese husbands took the initiative to convert the material circumstances of their homes, and they instructed their "wives and children to appear in order and cleanliness." In one case a merchant told Cable, "By and by, I make you an office to teach my children; just now I know too dirty for an American lady." Cable was astonished with the renovation completed by her next visit: "Imagine our delight upon our next visit to find on the walls gilt paper, pictures, the wood work grained, a beautiful Brussels carpet, and in the center of the room a table on the cover of which lay the books, with chairs surrounding it—all ready for teaching." Ironically, the special room was "locked and only opened" for missionary visits. The room did not reflect changes to the everyday life of the Chinese family, but it demonstrated the commitment of this merchant to appear to assimilate to American material culture and social conduct. [36]

For the missionaries, what was significant was that the formerly "Christless people" were transformed, through the adept and persistent labor of the women missionaries, into "the resplendent material" necessary to build "a strong Christian nation." [37] Unlike Mary Sawtelle, the missionaries perceived American national identity as malleable, not necessarily restricted to any particular race. Yet the adoption of a particular material culture was absolutely necessary in securing participation in the nation and eventually in the Christian church. Although the women did not relinquish Chinese clothing, hair styles, or food preparation, reformed Chinese women adopted the decorative styles of middle-class American culture. Condit noted that, as exemplary evidence of reform, in the apartments "tidies are on the chairs, and pretty little ornaments are on the shelves. And what is better, our English and Chinese Bibles are on the tables, and we know they are read." [38] The reproduction of middle-class material culture signaled Chinese women's receptivity to Christian teaching. Cable boasted that with regular work among families, in five years she could "Americanize Chinatown, and in ten years it will be Christianized." [39] By converting a few exemplary families to middle-class Protestant culture, Cable believed, missionaries could effect the reform and eventual conversion of Chinese society. "Every home we gain access to," Cable explained, "becomes a separate and distinct congregation that must first be organized, disciplined and taught before we can hope to successfully reach the hearts and understandings of this strange and peculiar people."[40] The "congregation" was one of the organizational symbols that converted the privacy of religious faith into participation in a public society.

The politicians and public authorities rarely recognized that the labor of women missionaries had compelled Chinese families to join in the "march of civilization" and to embrace the Christian "Gospel of culture and comfort." Condit claimed that these conversions resulted in a growing "sentiment against untidy rooms, as well as untidy persons," well in advance of the highly publicized sanitation campaigns initiated by the Board of Health in the 1880s. These changes were not acknowledged by the public health authorities because they had not "had a look into any of our 'upper rooms,' where the birds sing and flowers bloom, while the soft-voiced Chinese mother sits sewing beside her children."[41] These private apartments, with their familiar maternal domesticity, were the antithesis of the bunkrooms and semipublic dens that horrified the authorities and the missionaries. In the "upper rooms," where converted Christians lived, the air was "Americanized by the perfume from the flowers in the windows, and the neat and cheerful furniture of the room."[42] The transition from disgusting and degrading Chineseness to "sweet" and "neat" Americanness was the result of the "power of Christianity to reach a Chinese woman's heart."[43] Condit was convinced it was unlikely that public health regulations alone could purify Chinatown. In her experience, only Christian teaching, from woman to woman, had the power to transform Chinese hygienic habits.

Even Condit realized, however, that the zeal to clean was not the exclusive trait of white Christian women. Chinese custom also promoted sanitary renewal during Chinese New Year, when Condit witnessed that "fresh paper on the wall, renewed paints, a lavish expenditure of soap and water . . . give promise of a coming millennium of cleanliness in these homes." Condit expected to convert this "latent" sanitary impulse into a daily habit. Missionary instruction and public health regulation could extend the spirited activity of "pagan" holidays into the realm of regular and orderly domesticity.[44]

When Cable stopped making house-to-house visitations in 1891, they became a less significant part of the Chinese Mission Home's work. The organization increasingly focused on rescue work and providing institutional care for Chinese single women and orphans. Emerging Chinese Protestant congregations and their ministers increasingly took over Christian conversion. At the turn of the century, house-to-house work continued to reach "shut-in" Chinese women but was undertaken by a committee of volunteers. One of the most effective missionaries was Mrs. Ngo Wing, a former resident of the Chinese Mission Home who went to school, married, and made a home for herself in Berkeley. After spending years as a Bible reader for the Sunday school, Ngo began work as a committee member by accompanying white women on visits. Her fluency in Cantonese and the trust she inspired in other Chinese women soon led Ngo to work independently.[45] Ngo reversed the procedures of home visits by asking Chinese women to visit her home in Berkeley. As a reformed Chinese woman, Ngo's example of domesticity and "housekeeping" were considered by the white missionaries to serve as an extraordinary "object lesson."[46] On one visit the women and children were delighted by everything in the house, "even the bathtub." As "entertainment" for the guests, the "children had a bath, for the first time in their lives, in a real bath tub." This entertainment brought about by the innovations of American material culture had profound residual effects, according to the white missionaries who relayed that the Chinese women were so overwhelmed by Ngo's domestic arrangements that they remarked, "We would like to have a home like this and we would not need to have idols."[47] As Chinese women from the Mission Home returned to their community as Christian women, their own conversion and the material effects of marriages arranged by the organization served as a spectacular advertisement for conversion to the civilized culture of middle-class hygiene and Christianity.

## NATION, CIVILIZATION, AND WHITENESS

The sharp contrasts between the material culture of "Christian homes" and "ordinary heathen homes" in Chinatown revealed the association of hygiene with civilization and whiteness in the materiality of furnishings, decoration, and odors. In an article for a national women's missionary publication, New Yorker Mary Field used these stereotypical contrasts to authenticate her description of a journey with a Presbyterian missionary on her rounds through Chinatown homes. The sensory details ensured the foreign nature of the journey: "As they descended the street the usual disgusting sights and malodorous smells of Chinatown assailed their senses. They turned in at a dingy entranceway and began to go up narrow stairs[,] . . . following the dark and devious hallway. Always the same ingrained, immemorial dirt above, below and on all sides; the same litter of ashes, parings and papers; the same vile blending of tobacco, opium and coal-oil smoke; the same shrill chatter of voices penetrating through thin partitions; the same scampering, miniature Chinese preceding and following the visitors."[48] Field's use of filth, darkness, pungent odors, and cacophonous noise highlighted the typical, reviled circumstances of "heathen" existence, circumstances readily intelligible to her readers as signs of decay, disorder, and disease. The journey to the apartment oriented the reader to the predictably dire circumstances of the family to be visited. The missionary and Field entered a tiny room and were "assaulted" by a "swarm of children" and a mother carrying a baby. The "assault" and lack of proper greeting from the mother emphasized the idea that unwholesome circumstances had bred uncivilized inhabitants. The room was dark, cramped, dirty, and in disarray: "The floor seemed to never have been cleaned, and the walls were cracked and stained and as dirty as the floor. The one little table was heaped with dishes and jars and sewing. . . . Not a ray of sunshine could creep into the one dingy window." Metaphors of dirt animated Field's evaluation of the visit: "The accumulated grime of years seemed to have incrusted [*sic*] itself on everything and everybody. She shuddered when a child leaned against her."[49]

By contrast, the missionary took Field to the house of Mrs. Wong Lee, one of the Chinese Mission Home's graduates, who lived on Prospect Place. The street was "pleasant," the house steps "exceedingly clean," and the visit "cordial" and humane, as they were greeted by a "bright little Chinese girl dressed in a neat American gingham frock." The girl showed them "through a clean hall into a cheerful living room with neat American furnishings" and left to retrieve her mother. The cleanliness of the home and its inhabitants and the adoption of American material culture were emblematic of Americanness. Wong arrived, gracious and smiling: "Her hair was glossy, smooth[,] and the clean blue sahm [*sic*] she had evidently taken time to slip on was a triumph of laundry work." When she proudly exhibited her baby boy, the last of seven children, Fields remarked that he was a "clean, wholesome, lovely manikin whom the ladies could hold without drawbacks." Wong displayed a home that was "the model of tidiness" with model children who were polite, eager, and mission-educated. Tidy housekeeping and "civilized" social behavior were perceived as the twin results of Presbyterian missionary training.

The interior of Mrs. Wong Lee's home reflected a cheerful confluence of cleanliness, whiteness, and Christianity: "The floor was white as scouring could make it; the windows shone, the curtains were snowy, and on the neatly papered walls were Scripture texts." [50] In Field's description the cultural practices of whiteness emerge. Since whiteness defined itself in opposition to other racial categories, it is not surprising that whiteness was revealed through the missionary work of assimilating Chinese women to white norms. Whiteness became an indicator of cleanliness and purity, as demonstrated in the contrasting descriptions between Mrs. Wong Lee's scoured "white" floors and the "dirty" ones in the "heathen home" of the unnamed Chinese woman.

In addition, white cleanliness accompanied a specific transformation of material culture: Mrs. Wong Lee's curtains were "snowy," while the other home had no curtains to frame the "dingy window." In the late nineteenth century, the conflation of whiteness and hygienic purity found its most salient cultural manifestation in the new indoor bathrooms of the middle class. With the growing emphasis on the medicinal advantages of regular bathing and the development of large-scale, municipal sewage systems at the turn of the century, the construction of indoor bathrooms became popular among the middle class. At midcentury, baths and water closets had often been located in dark rooms, but as whiteness and hygiene became inseparable, tubs, tiles, and toilets were painted a "hygienic" white. These white tubs "were placed in stark, white bathrooms hygienically covered with white tiles on walls and floors and topped by washable oil cloth wallpaper." The white tiles and tub easily alerted occupants to the presence or absence of dirt and made the bathrooms "cheerful and light." [51] The scrupulous absence of dirt, darkness, and gloom characterized the American vision of hygienic whiteness. The manifestation of "whiteness" in women's domestic culture demonstrated the ways in which white racial coding was articulated, often obliquely as a set of unmarked, unnamed, and seemingly normative cultural practices. [52]

Like all racial categories, "whiteness" displayed astonishing flexibility in late-nineteenth-century San Francisco. At one end, Mary Sawtelle perceived the boundaries of "whiteness" to be firm and nonnegotiable, allergic to the Chinese presence. On the other, Emma Cable believed that proper training in Christian hygienic culture could result in the erasure of Chinese difference and in Chinese assimilation to American norms. Although the Presbyterians contested medical recommendations for the expulsion of Chinese immigrants, their practices revealed that hygienist discourse became crucial to reforming Chinese women.

As domestic custodians, women were expected to be acutely sensitive to sanitary maintenance. Both Mary Sawtelle and Emma Cable considered the feminine gender to be naturally more inclined to household hygienic discipline than men. Middle-class women also articulated another dimension of the gendered preoccupation with whiteness: they identified moral purity as a definitive component in their conception of womanhood. This fixation with female purity provoked Mary Sawtelle to defend "white-souled" womanhood against the corrupting influences of Chinese prostitution. Concern with female purity also coaxed other middle-class white women to join the missionary crusade to "rescue" Chinese women from lives of prostitution and to reform the behavior and living styles of Chinese merchant wives and their families. Both Sawtelle and Cable reflected larger trends in American Protestant Christianity. Nineteenth-century Protestants developed an axiomatic "identification of the Christian way and the American" through a shared affiliation in whiteness.[53] The historian Wesley Woo has characterized the American Protestant vision of "America's destiny" as the exemplary Christian and civilized nation that was most threatened by Chinese and other immigrants who could pollute or corrupt "American institutions, morals, faith, and civil order."[54]

Sawtelle's crusade against the moral corruption and physical pollution generated by Chinese prostitution coincided with the American Protestant impulse to keep America pure. Her agenda was to expel the threat from the nation, whereas Presbyterian missionaries preferred to demonstrate the power of Christian civilization by engaging in active conversion of Chinese immigrants. The test of assimilation, nevertheless, placed the burden on the foreigners to adapt to American standards, styles, and norms. In 1911, Charles Nash, president of the Pacific Theological Seminary, argued that Asians must assimilate to "American standards" in physical and mental behavior in order to ensure the American quality of life and Christian civilization.[55] Nash echoed the concerns of the journalist Horace Greeley more than a half century before him. In 1854 Greeley had ranted against Chinese immigrants, arguing that the United States could not absorb the "flood of ignorant, filthy idolaters" and that only "Christian races" and "white races" were welcome to immigrate, since only they could "assimilate with Americans."[56]

Domestic society and domesticity frame the broad canvas of American empire. The ideas and projects of Sawtelle, Cable, and Condit demonstrate the permeable borders of public and private spheres. These projects disrupt easy assumptions about the gendered divide of the female home and the male civic world. However, as Amy Kaplan has so deftly argued, the "deconstruction of separate spheres" leads to a reconsideration of the common placement of "the domestic in intimate opposition to the foreign." In the borderlands of San Francisco's Chinatown, one of the preeminent contact zones of frontier and empire, the work of white middle-class women addressed the intimate proximity of the "foreign" and the domestic. In San Francisco an imperial domestic discourse emerged that contrasted white middle-class American modernity with the putatively alien and "backward" Asian cultures. Asian American critical histories demonstrate how the idea of Asians as perpetual foreigners shapes the ontology of the modern nation-state of the United States. Racial exclusion and respectable gender relations have culturally and politically turned the "imperial nation into a home," one that has continually dodged "specters of the foreign that lurk inside and outside its ever shifting borders." [57]

Standards of cleanliness and health, the categories produced by hygiene, were among emerging standards of American Christian civilization. In the nineteenth century, health reformers employed the language and sensibilities of religious commitment in their promotion of hygienic ideology. Christian missionaries seized the new hygienist discourse and adapted it to their older moral conceptions of cleanliness as intrinsic to spiritual regeneration. Health was perceived as goodness and purity, and sickness was identified with sin and corruption—even as the relationship between sickness and evil was being infused with medical theories of bacteriology, germs, and pathogens in the late nineteenth century.[58]

This domestic and hygienic ideology was malleable. In the 1920s and 1930s, Chinese American social workers took up the discourses of hygiene, domesticity, and gender and reworked them in their advocacy for access to municipal social services and for improved housing. They took statistics indicating the small but increasing number of childbirths as a sign that Chinatown was nurturing a "family society," and they held up the educated Chinese American housewives as most able to apply the norms of American middle-class domestic culture. Their intention was to position Chinese motherhood as a foil against the nineteenth-century image of a Chinese society composed of male bachelors and female prostitutes. This process of political purification through discourses of hygiene and nuclear family society ultimately enabled Chinese Americans to claim access to American civic polity and social resources.[59]

# CHAPTER 5

# Plague and Managing the Commercial City

On the night of March 6, 1900, the assistant city physician Dr. Frank P. Wilson arrived at the basement of the Globe Hotel in San Francisco's Chinatown to examine the dead body of Wing Chung Ging, a forty-one-year-old Chinese man who had worked in a wood yard on Pacific Street. A routine postmortem examination quickly led to a public health crisis when Wilson noticed swollen lymph nodes in the groin of the body and alerted the city bacteriologist Dr. Wilfred Kellogg, who took smears of the glands for further testing. After a preliminary microscopic study, Kellogg suspected that the man had died of bubonic plague. Kellogg immediately rushed the smears for further investigation to Dr. Joseph J. Kinyoun, who ran the bacteriological laboratory at the Angel Island Quarantine Station. Kinyoun inoculated two guinea pigs, a rat, and monkey with the glandular tissue, but it would be several days before conclusive results would be available. Later that night the Board of Health, at the insistence of the city health officer Dr. A. P. O'Brien, ordered an immediate quarantine of Chinatown. Early the next morning, the chief of police dispatched thirty-two officers to the Chinese quarter with orders to first remove all whites from the affected area, then to cordon it off and thereafter allow no one except white people to leave it and no one at all to enter it. By noon on March 7, the Chinese quarter was effectively sealed off from the rest of the city.[1]

Although the sequence of events appeared to the Board of Health to be natural and inevitable, controversy exploded almost immediately.

The Board of Health expected that their swift response to a suspected Chinese bubonic plague case would draw enthusiastic support from white politicians and the popular press. Instead, city health authorities and their federal colleagues faced searing criticism from politicians, clinical physicians, newspaper editors, and businesspeople. California's Governor Henry Gage rebuked both city and federal authorities for overreacting and provoking widespread national panic. Some business and political leaders accused public health officials of the rash and wanton destruction of the city's commercial reputation over the unverified suspicion of plague.

The very existence of bubonic plague and the public health tactics employed to combat it were questioned. Both white and Chinese critics contested the reliance on bacteriological verification and the blanket quarantine of Chinatown. In 1900, bacteriological knowledge was experimental, so both the microscopic diagnosis and the federal inoculations drew challenges from both Chinese and white critics. The order to remove all white people and seal off the Chinatown District faced claims by Chinese leaders of brazen racial discrimination, leaders who would take their case to federal courts. The method of quarantine itself, while acceptable for individual houses, was unprecedented in sequestering an entire district and all Chinese residents. For more than a year San Francisco's newspapers would vociferously debate the existence of bubonic plague and government containment measures; the debate exposed disputes in medical knowledge, and the newspapers readily solicited medical experts to substantiate their opposing positions.[2]

Throughout the crisis, municipal and federal health officials believed they could divide the contaminated from the uncontaminated along racial lines. Within the context of nearly five decades of medical concern and surveillance of Chinese immigrants in San Francisco, the quarantine of Chinatown was extraordinary but consistent with the logic of public health measures that routinely conflated deadly disease with Chinese race and residence. The leap from one Chinese suspect to suspicion of the entire Chinatown District was reasonable to health authorities; but they were unable to contain the crisis in terms of a clear binary arrangement in which protecting the white public meant isolating a Chinese threat. The assumption that all white and all Chinese residents would react like the other members of their own race also unraveled immediately. The splintering of white businesspeople, politicians, physicians, and newspaper editors at the announcement of a bubonic plague epidemic in San Francisco's Chinatown illustrates different positions regarding the tactics of governing Chinese residents in San Francisco, as well as a range of divergent economic and political interests at stake. Chinese residents gave spirited opposition to public health measures; however, Chinese diplomats, merchants, and laborers disagreed about how and when to protest or cooperate with health authorities.

Bubonic plague pandemics had a notorious history, and the public health authorities, white businesspeople, and Chinese residents had followed with great trepidation the news of the most recent pandemic that had hit major cities in China and India in the 1890s. Thriving ports in Hong Kong, Bombay, Honolulu, Sydney, and Cape Town had all halted trade when plague erupted; thousands had died in its wake. The terrible history of devastation drove San Francisco and U.S. public health authorities to take swift and extreme measures upon even the suspicion of bubonic plague. Businesspeople reacted at first with caution and skepticism because even the suspicion of plague in San Francisco would cut off commerce with the rest of the nation and the world. Health officials believed they had understood business worries by attempting to contain plague in Chinatown rather than by quarantining San Francisco's port; however, they had underestimated that the city's commercial elite would fear that any mention of bubonic plague's existence in San Francisco would drive officials across the United States to quarantine trade with San Francisco.

Because of the explosive oceanic commerce of European expansion, the use of quarantine had become widespread during the eighteenth and nineteenth centuries in all European ports and in European nations' colonial possessions in Africa, Asia, and the Americas.[3] In the late nineteenth century, as the United States became a rising commercial power, the federal government's involvement in the maintenance of quarantine and epidemic disease information systems attempted to allay fears that disease was transmitted through trade and migration. Production and dissemination of scientific knowledge were considered imperative in an era of imperial ambitions and global trade.[4] Shipping companies and merchants recognized the value of disease tracking and containment systems in inspiring an image of safe and regular transactions in an unpredictable environment, where epidemic disease, war, and natural disaster jeopardized commercial activity. Vast global and impersonal trade required insurance—not only financial guarantees but health guarantees as well. In practice, however, quarantine was an ambivalent strategy that both swelled hopes of containment and incited panic. By drawing a boundary that separated the contaminated from the noncontaminated, quarantine focused fear on the suspect ship, house, district, or person.[5]

In 1900, public debate about the existence of bubonic plague in San Francisco exposed the stark cleavages in scientific knowledge about epidemics and unease with government strategies for its suppression. Differences in the scientific epistemology of bubonic plague demonstrated the uneven and ambivalent transformation of both popular and professional medical understandings, from environmental theory to the germ theory. More broadly, the bubonic plague crisis revealed how scientific knowledge circulated in the public sphere and shaped public opinion and policy. Both federal and municipal public health agencies contested and attempted to discredit the concerns of white politicians, journalists, and physicians, as well as criticism from elite Chinese merchants, political leaders, and diplomats. The debate that occurred in elite daily newspapers, medical journals, government correspondence, and official reports also exposed positions that reflected different epistemes of the body and of epidemics and advocated different intervention strategies.

At this moment Chinese diplomatic and merchant elite leadership had become effective in petitioning the federal courts to register their protest and force local governments to desist from action. Their willingness to contest regulations and policy on grounds of discrimination, as well as to cooperate with city officials in order to negotiate more satisfactory outcomes, did not always please the Chinese laborers and small merchants they were supposed to represent. Through the courts, public hearings, and newspapers, the Chinese diplomats and merchant leaders of the Chinese Consolidated Benevolent Association (CCBA) could stake their positions in the dominant public sphere. However, Chinese laborers and petty merchants were disqualified from participation in either the dominant public sphere or the official Chinese opposition. Unlike physicians, journalists, and politicians, who could circulate their contrary opinions in a robust public-sphere debate in the print media, Chinese laborers had few arenas in which to speak. At best they were the collective authors of anonymous rumors. When their ideas did appear, their positions were distorted, ridiculed, and dismissed.[6]

The methodologies of subaltern studies, historical epistemology, and historical genealogy pay careful attention to rumors and discredited ideas in order to explore the historical formation of knowledge and power. Writing the history of the struggles between scientific bureaucracy and the socially marginalized raises several methodological problems. How does one analyze a history of incommensurate and unequal knowledge formations that entailed the discrediting and subjugation of one group of speakers and their ideas by another? How can one provide the texture and depths of the discredited ways of knowing that often appear fleetingly and fragmented in the dominant archival record produced by U.S. government officials, journalists, and politicians? One approach directly compares rumors with systematic science and, in doing so, exposes the competing categories that structure thought, pattern arguments, and certify the standards for explanation of reality without reinscribing science as the singular authoritative truth.[7]

The controversial events that surrounded the 1900 San Francisco bubonic plague crisis have prompted historians to analyze the mechanisms of power and authority. Many have connected the crisis to national transformations in public health administration, medical politics, and civil rights law. These studies have focused on public health authorities and their various critics. For historians of medicine and public health, the crisis was a pivotal moment in the establishment of public health power, demonstrating the value of nationally coordinated and managed policies under federal direction. The chronicle of events and the outcome have been frequently interpreted as a vindication of "objective" medical officials over paranoid and parochial politicians, businesspeople, and journalists.[8] More recent historical treatments of the crisis have recognized the racial antipathy that governed medical policies and media coverage and that made claims of objectivity suspect.[9] Finally, Charles McClain's exhaustive analysis of the legal proceedings in the first months of the crisis has focused attention on the role of the federal courts in circumscribing public health powers and in championing the rights of oppressed social groups.[10]

This chapter draws on these insights to examine contested social relations and knowledge formations that emerged as the state engaged in the medical management of society at a moment of epidemic crisis. The bubonic plague epidemic in San Francisco raised questions about the place of medical science and the authority of medical practitioners in the social order, and about the political and legal constraints on medical intervention. The development of the municipal public health infrastructure and the intervention of federal bacteriological expertise made the state management of epidemics at the cusp of the twentieth century substantively different from the measures taken in the smallpox epidemics of the 1870s and 1880s. The successful management of public health required the acceptance of scientific authority and the appearance of control. However, in San Francisco, health authorities were beset by sharp, political disputes and, frequently, public refusal. Although health authorities promoted bacteriological discoveries and public health therapies with unflappable confidence, the effects of disseminating medical knowledge were intensely ambivalent. The information about bubonic plague and its rapid spread both heightened anxiety and produced the assurances of control that were meant to assuage distress.[11] In San Francisco, public health management and medical knowledge inflamed prevailing fears of the menace of Chinese migration and Chinatown.

Concerns about the viability of commerce became a central issue in the debate over whether bubonic plague existed and how to contain its spread. White businesspeople and politicians worried that, on the one hand, rumors of contagion could cripple commerce and, on the other hand, the rapid spread of the disease on the U.S. mainland could devastate the economy. Anxiety over commercial viability also animated the class antagonism between the Chinese elite and the laborers and petty merchants that the crisis exacerbated. For Chinese elite and subaltern groups, commerce and property relations became key sites at which to register their disapproval and distress over the policies of health authorities. The suspicion of plague in Chinatown and policies of quarantine were likely to impoverish the livelihoods of merchants and force Chinese laborers into destitution because they could not travel to work on farms, in orchards, and at canneries across western North America. The commercial viability of the city and its inhabitants hung in the balance as health authorities and politicians attempted to manage the bubonic plague crisis and contain the epidemic in Chinatown.

ANTICIPATING EPIDEMIC

Although the diagnosis of bubonic plague cases in San Francisco was sudden, it was hardly unexpected. Public health authorities had anticipated bubonic plague's arrival for nearly four years, even predicting that one of the Pacific Coast's "Chinatowns" would be the most likely site of the epidemic's first strike on the continental United States. In 1894 the Public Health Service (PHS) had tracked the spread of the late-nineteenth-century bubonic plague pandemic from the interior of China to the ports of Canton and Hong Kong.[12] From southern China, plague spread rapidly to India, Egypt, South Africa, and seaports in France, Britain, and Australia.[13] The devastating death tolls in India, in particular, made public health authorities across the globe brace themselves for the "invasion" of this fatal pandemic.[14]

Revolutionary developments in bacteriology in the late nineteenth century had made the diagnosis of bubonic plague possible. Using the methods developed in 1870s by the German microbiologist Robert Koch, European and Japanese scientists had discovered the specific microbial causes of numerous human and animal diseases, such as typhoid, malaria, and diphtheria.[15] In the 1880s, Louis Pasteur began to experiment with the controlled injection of pathogenic microbes to produce immunity. Pasteur and other bacteriologists were able to identify the structure of antibodies and to artificially replicate their functions in order to create vaccines and serums for cholera, typhoid, and yellow fever.[16] These bacteriological developments revolutionized the scientific understanding of bubonic plague. In 1894, the Swiss bacteriologist Alexandre Yersin and the Japanese bacteriologist Shibasurburo Kitasato independently identified the bacillus responsible for causing plague. In 1897, the renowned Russian bacteriologist Waldemar Haffkine developed an experimental bubonic plague vaccine. It was first tested on Bombay prison inmates, but it was met with widespread resistance when colonial authorities suggested its general application.[17]

Although U.S. laboratories were not at the forefront of bacteriological discoveries, the PHS readily applied the new scientific knowledge to systematic procedures in an effort to arrest the entry of epidemics into the U.S. mainland. During his tenure as surgeon general, from 1891 to 1911, Walter Wyman developed a system of information exchange to track the spread of epidemic diseases at ports throughout the globe. Under Wyman's direction, the PHS grew from a small domestic agency of 54 medical officers in 1891, with a $600,000 budget, to an international bureaucracy employing 135 medical officers and more than 1,200 additional civilian employees by 1911, with a budget of $1,750,000. Wyman frequently rotated medical officers through intense tours of duty at domestic quarantine stations, in foreign ports, and in bacteriological laboratories. The quick relay of accurate microscopic verification of disease at any port across the globe became the goal of the PHS worldwide network.[18] Under the leadership of Dr. Joseph J. Kinyoun, the PHS set up the first bacteriological laboratory in the United States, at Staten Island. The laboratory moved to Washington, D.C., and became the Public Health Service Hygienic Laboratory, the center for developing therapeutic sera and antitoxins and training scientists from state and municipal health agencies.

Tracking bubonic plague and developing strategies to prevent its entry in the United States became one of the chief concerns of the PHS in the late 1890s.[19] PHS officers readily conflated the Chinese race and the spread of bubonic plague in their health policies along the Pacific Rim. In 1896 Wyman sent a trained bacteriologist to San Francisco and directed him to inspect and fumigate all Chinese and Japanese passengers and baggage because of the "prevalence of plague in southern China."[20] In the summer of 1899, PHS officers were under heightened alert when a thirteen-year-old Chinese boy died of bubonic plague on the San Francisco–bound *Nippon Maru* en route from Hong Kong to Yokohama. After disinfection in Yokohama the ship proceeded to San Francisco, and panic about the plague escalated.[21] The city bacteriologist hastily diagnosed bubonic plague in two stowaway Japanese passengers who had jumped ship at the harbor and drowned. The city health officer ordered the *Nippon Maru*'s passengers held in quarantine, but Dr. Kinyoun, the preeminent bacteriologist who was stationed at Angel Island Quarantine Station to track the bubonic plague, rejected the diagnosis and lifted the quarantine.[22] Kinyoun blasted the city bacteriologist's expertise and ill-equipped municipal facilities for mistaking pneumonia for bubonic plague.[23] The incident did not shake the PHS expectation that "vessels carrying Chinese" passengers from Hong Kong would continue to produce plague cases.[24] Later in the summer of 1899, after several "outbreaks of plague" aboard transpacific liners, steamship companies refused passage to lower-class Chinese steerage passengers. PHS officials endorsed the discriminatory practices as a necessary precaution to prevent an outbreak of plague in the United States.[25]

PHS officers based in China and in North American "Chinatowns" feared that the "filth" and "overcrowding" characteristic of all Chinese living environments incubated bubonic plague.[26] On December 12, 1899, officers of the Honolulu Board of Health examined the body of You Chong, a twenty-two-year-old Chinese bookkeeper, and concluded that Chong had died of bubonic plague. Within a few hours, four of his Chinese neighbors were diagnosed with plague, and they died soon afterward. The Honolulu Board of Health swung into action. U.S. military guards were called to secure the fourteen-block district, where ten thousand mostly Chinese and Japanese people lived, permitting no one other than medical officials and the police to leave or enter the district. A volunteer medical force joined the soldiers in ferreting out sick men and women for isolation and treatment. The Honolulu Board of Health proceeded to thoroughly disinfect and fumigate all streets and houses in the Chinatown District. The PHS ordered all shipping to cease and all steamships to remain in quarantine in the Honolulu harbor. After Honolulu authorities lifted the quarantine on December 19, new cases of plague infection appeared, prompting more aggressive action.[27]

The president of the Board of Health, Henry Cooper, ordered a systematic burning of buildings to rid the district of bubonic plague. On January 20, 1900, just after a controlled fire was set, the wind rose, carrying embers to nearby roofs. By afternoon, every block in Honolulu's Chinatown was ablaze. The fire burned for seventeen days, destroying thirty-eight acres and four thousand homes, and leaving forty-five hundred people homeless. By using extreme procedures of environmental sanitation—"destroying all known sources and centers of infection"—health authorities expected the epidemic to disappear.[28] However, this policy ignored the consequences of forcing humans and rodents to disperse. Within days two new cases of plague were reported in the business district and the PHS officer D. A. Carmichael concluded that "infection has been spread by rats or other vermin driven from Chinatown." After the burning of Chinatown, health officials diagnosed plague cases in other parts of Honolulu as well as in ports on other Hawaiian islands.[29]

As early as July 1897, PHS officers had associated rats with the transmission of plague and had employed special disinfection procedures to kill and remove rats from vessel cargo holds.[30] PHS officers observed that rats were the "chief means of conveying plague from port to port" and that "sick rats . . . about the wharf and Chinatown" in Honolulu were signs of plague.[31] In a widely disseminated pamphlet, Wyman argued that one could contract bubonic plague by contact with an infected wound, by inhaling the dust from infected houses, or by consuming infected food or liquids. Plague germs got in the dust or the air from spit, excrement, and the exhaled air of the infected person. Wyman suspected that filth and unsanitary conditions were responsible for breeding bubonic plague. In his account, rats were more readily infected only because of their snouts, which were an inch above the floor and therefore most likely to inhale plague-infested dust.[32] The PHS disregarded scientific evidence that rats were the primary conveyors of disease and instead focused their inspection and suppression efforts on Chinese and Japanese travelers.

The PHS anticipated that Chinese and Japanese passengers would transmit plague directly from Asia to "Chinatowns" along the Pacific Coast. Immediately after Honolulu's plague crisis, Wyman ordered his officers in Pacific Coast ports to conduct surveys of the sanitary conditions of local Chinatown districts. The surveys were intended to prepare the PHS to battle the potential epidemic. The survey and political mobilization conducted by the PHS officer Charles E. Decker in San Diego in January and February 1900 was typical of efforts to anticipate plague in Chinatown districts. Decker's initial drive through San Diego's Chinatown confirmed expectations of an unimaginably "filthy" district, populated by "exceeding unclean" Chinese inhabitants and filled with shanties and tenements, albeit "not as thickly crowded together as is usual in 'Chinatowns.'" Decker told San Diego's health officer that it would be difficult to find a "district more favorable to the lodgment and spread of plague" than San Diego's Chinatown.[33] Decker then used medical literature and popular pamphlets prepared by the PHS to convince the city's politicians and business elite that the "bad sanitary conditions . . . in Chinatown render[ed] the city . . . vulnerable to plague" and endangered the city's commercial future. Decker manipulated anxiety about a city's commercial future to solicit public and private funds in order to prevent plague strikes.[34] The PHS influenced local politicians and health officials in the Pacific Coast port cities to counter the threat of epidemic disease and to establish federal oversight.

The outbreak of plague in Honolulu's Chinatown prefigured the suspect status of every other Chinatown. Decker's immediate comparison of San Diego's Chinatown to an image of the general qualities of all "Chinatowns"—filthy, thickly crowded, vice ridden, immoral, unsanitary—indicated that "Chinatown" functioned as a generalized category that PHS officers used to predict the emergence of health problems. Since one of the fearful elements of epidemic disease was its transgression of boundaries, Chinatown, as the conflation of race and place, provided the illusion of impermeable boundaries. When national barriers failed, health authorities still believed that the boundaries of racial geography promised containment.

## RESPONSE AND RESISTANCE

San Francisco health authorities after nearly five decades of intensive scrutiny of Chinatown needed little encouragement to assume that the Chinese would be the first victims of bubonic plague in the city. Once the postmortem diagnosis of Wing Chung Ging on March 6, 1900, confirmed plague, the federal public health authorities swiftly intervened to provide expert advice and vaccine delivery. The day following the quarantine of Chinatown, Surgeon General Wyman wired instructions recommending that the local Board of Health undertake immediate sulfur disinfection of Chinatown, treatment with a therapeutic serum devel-

oped by Alexandre Yersin for the infected, and inoculation of all Chinatown residents with Haffkine's prophylactic vaccine.[35] The Board of
Health selectively followed federal guidance, opting initially for familiar
strategies of containment and environmental sanitation over experimental bacteriological therapeutic and preventive measures. Throughout the
spring, the Board of Health recalibrated its policies in relation to public
pressure and the discovery of new plague cases.

The deployment of standard public health procedures of fumigation,
disinfection, and quarantine on Chinese residences would have hardly
been considered unusual if the magnitude and extent of the measures
undertaken by the Board of Health had not been so severe. Public health
officials' ability to subject all of Chinatown to quarantine and conduct
thorough inspections and fumigation of its dwellings reflected the new
administrative capacity of the Public Health Department, which had
mushroomed in budget, personnel, and duties in the last years of the
nineteenth century. Deployment of public health technologies was no
longer inconsistent and haphazard as it had been during the smallpox
epidemics and political crises of the 1870s and 1880s. In the effort to
eradicate bubonic plague, local authorities were also aided by federal
expertise and staff.

However, what remained crucial to the systematic deployment of invasive public health practices was the preeminence of "epidemic logic."
As Linda Singer has observed, the specter of epidemic pushed "forms of
regulatory intervention into the lives of bodies and populations which
might, in other circumstances, appear excessive," and which could be
justified as necessary for "damage control and prophylactic protection-
ism." [36] This "epidemic logic" justified extraordinary intervention as well
as an astonishing mobilization of resources and the disruption of the cer-
tainties of everyday life.

The very intensity of medical intervention generated a rich array of
Chinese responses to the public health management of the epidemic.
White officials and writers have frequently represented the Chinese community as monolithic and have attributed homogenous responses to every social problem and official action. The dearth of Chinese-authored
sources in late-nineteenth-century San Francisco tended to permit that
representation in historical analyses. This is part of a general problem
scholars encounter in analyzing the discourses of marginalized social
groups. Historians rely on the written sources that are preserved, and
the fact that these tend to be official documents and elite newspapers frequently leads to analyses that are skewed toward the subjectivity of the

elite.[37] Historians can, however, interrogate those very elite sources for hints of the concerns and perspectives of people, such as Chinese laborers in San Francisco, who were socially marginal. Unlike previous epidemics, the bubonic plague crisis generated astonishingly detailed documentation in the popular press, in official correspondence, and in the Chinese-language newspapers, particularly the *Chung Sai Yat Po,* which reflected the editorial vision of the Chinese Christian Ng Poon Chew.[38] This array of sources exposed heterogeneity and conflict in Chinese responses to public health measures, revealing layers of resistance, accommodation, participation, and sharp political differences between the merchant elite, on one hand, and small shopkeepers and laborers, on the other. Although Chinese merchants, diplomats, and newspaper editors were racially excluded from the hub of political power, they connected Chinatown society with the wider world and participated in San Francisco political and economic life as commercial middlemen, community spokesmen, and court litigants. Although many of the elite readily spoke for all Chinese Americans, their responses more often reflected their own class concerns.

Since the late nineteenth century, the social and political hierarchy of Chinatown had been shaped by the pursuit of commercial wealth and the influence of powerful Chinese merchants. The major organization was the Chinese Consolidated Benevolent Association. The CCBA was a confederation of six district associations that coordinated efforts in 1882 to fight anti-Chinese discrimination. The presidents of the district associations rotated the position of CCBA president. The district association presidents were gentry-scholars from China on diplomatic passports and served as members of the Chinese consular staff. The other half of the CCBA board were major merchants who made fortunes in California. The CCBA and the district associations managed the immigration and financial life of many of the small merchants and laborers. The district associations and the individual merchants who ran them registered arriving immigrants, coordinated debts and labor recruitment, and provided exit permits necessary to secure passage back to China. The CCBA coordinated legal challenges and political responses to federal and local government and projected an image of protecting the welfare of Chinese Americans. As a mutual aid and benevolent protection association, the CCBA and its district associations took an active role in responding to the health authorities and in guiding Chinese American residents.[39]

The initial imposition of quarantine drew a swift and bitter response from Chinese residents. Consul Ho argued that the Board of Health had overstepped its authority in administering a "blockade of Chinatown," and appealed to the courts to dismiss the order. Consul Ho gathered information that cast doubt on the correctness of public health authorities' suspicion of bubonic plague. According to testimony by his brother, Wing Chung Ging had been ill for six months. On February 7 he had called on Dr. Chung Bu Bing and complained of fatigue, fever, headache, and pains in the chest, back, and bladder. Dr. Chung offered a diagnosis of inflammation of the bladder and prescribed an herbal remedy. By the time Wing consulted with Dr. Wong Wo a week later, his fever and pains had subsided, but he suffered from urethral discharges, swelling in his right groin, and a lame right leg. Wing feared that he had gonorrhea but refused an examination of his groin and genitals. He accepted further medicine to alleviate his painful urination but grew rapidly worse. After two weeks of severe vomiting and diarrhea, he collapsed and died. Some of Wing's symptoms—the fever, severe headache, extreme fatigue, muscular atrophy, and painful swelling of lymph glands in the groin— signaled bubonic plague. However, bubonic plague usually kills quickly and spreads rapidly. Many in San Francisco were doubtful that Wing Chung Ging had died of bubonic plague. Journalists at the *San Francisco Chronicle,* as well as Consul Ho, believed it was more likely that Wing had died of typhoid or venereal disease. The indeterminacy of the diagnosis fed doubts about the decision to quarantine Chinatown.[40] Ng Poon Chew, editor of *Chung Sai Yat Po,* expressed astonishment at the extent of the quarantine: "According to the epidemic prevention laws a yellow flag should be planted in the front of an epidemic-afflicted house, or the house should be encircled by tapes to warn people off. But never have we heard of blockading the whole town."[41] The CCBA did not dispute the limited use of quarantine; house quarantines had frequently been used in the late nineteenth century during smallpox epidemics and were widely considered to be a reasonable precaution. However, the "blockade of Chinatown" seemed to be an explicit act of racial discrimination against Chinese residents. Small shopkeepers protested in front of the offices of the CCBA. Chinese merchants, big and small, feared that the quarantine would bankrupt Chinese businesses.

The damage to commerce had much to do with the Board of Health's decision to lift the quarantine on the afternoon of March 9. The protests of Chinese leaders and merchants were echoed in the pages of the big city daily newspapers by white politicians and businesspeople worried that the plague reports would result in a national quarantine of San Francisco. Eager to scuttle plague rumors before they ruined Chinatown businesses, the Chinese consul and CCBA cooperated with public health orders of environmental sanitation once the quarantine had been called off. The Board of Health assembled a volunteer force to conduct a house-to-house inspection and fumigation of Chinatown. Sewers and dwellings were disinfected with sulfur dioxide and all the cellars were thoroughly whitewashed. The Chinese consul posted notices that Chinese residents should summon white physicians in cases of illness to assuage the authorities' worries that the Chinese hid potential plague victims. He also urged compliance with the Board of Health order that "every suspicious death" be certified by a "Caucasian physician" before burial.[42]

The inspection and disinfection of the Chinese quarter proceeded through the spring and provoked alternating moments of medical confidence and anxiety about the effectiveness of sanitary measures. Three additional plague cases were discovered at the end of March, and the Associated Press dispatched the news to East Coast newspapers, producing consternation in San Francisco commercial circles and prompting Mayor Phelan to telegraph assurances of the sanitary cleansing and control of Chinatown to fifty East Coast mayors.[43] The Board of Health's president John Williamson accused Chinese residents of concealing cases of plague from the health authorities. Nearly a month passed before another suspected case of plague appeared. By the end of April, health officials were confident that the plague crisis was under control. Their confidence was rudely shattered several weeks later in mid-May, when a cluster of four suspicious deaths in the Chinese quarter over three days stoked the anxiety of municipal and federal health authorities.[44]

On May 15 the PHS intervened to demand that San Francisco authorities take drastic measures. Wyman's chief recommendation was a mass inoculation of San Francisco's Chinese population. On the diplomatic front, Wyman urged the Chinese foreign minister in Washington, Wu Tingfang, to persuade his brother-in-law, Consul Ho, to "have the Chinese comply cheerfully" with the vaccination campaign. Three days later Wyman sent another telegram that extended the vaccination program to Japanese immigrants and ordered railroads to refuse passage out of San Francisco to any Chinese or Japanese who did not possess a certificate of inoculation.[45] Two days later the secretary of the treasury gave legal authority to restrict public travel of "Asiatics or other races particularly liable to the disease." The order confirmed that the putative racial susceptibility to bubonic plague would organize public health measures nationwide.[46]

Word of the mass vaccination campaign spread quickly through Chinatown. On May 17, the *Chung Sai Yat Po* reported that large crowds had gathered outside the offices of the CCBA, shouting their determination not to submit to inoculation. The CCBA leadership and the Chinese consul were caught off guard by the intensity of the opposition to the inoculations. One leader, in an attempt to disperse the crowd, took the floor and promised that the CCBA would pursue legal action against the health officials.[47] The following day an even larger crowd gathered at the association offices. Many could not squeeze into the association's premises and stood outside. Someone in the assembly pointed out that the proposed vaccination was quite different from a smallpox immunization: persons inoculated with the plague vaccine would run a fever for several days, and the inoculation would be devastating to a frail person. Another man proposed that all business establishments in the Chinese quarter be shut down in protest on the following day when the campaign was intended to begin. This proposal met with overwhelming approval from the crowd.[48]

That night the CCBA and Consul Ho both sent urgent telegrams to the Chinese foreign minister in Washington, D.C., informing him that "all Chinese object" to inoculation and insisted that there was no plague in San Francisco. The Chinese leaders warned that "if they inoculate by force there might be trouble and bloodshed." The Chinese foreign minister passed along these pleas to Wyman and urged PHS officers to "use more tact and discretion."[49] The health authorities refused to yield and threatened that Chinese who had not been inoculated would not be permitted to travel beyond the city limits.

On the eve of the mass vaccination campaign, a Chinese-language circular was posted across the Chinese quarter. It advocated the shutdown of commerce, both to register disapproval for public health policy and to threaten Chinese merchants who were willing to cooperate with the authorities:

> It is hard to go against an angry mass of people.
>     The doctors are about to compel our Chinese people to be inoculated. This action will involve the lives of us all who live in the City. Tomorrow . . . all business houses large or small must be closed and wait until this unjust action [is] settled before any one be allowed to resume their business. If any disobey this we will unite and put an everlasting boycott on them. Don't say that you have not been warned at first.[50]

The warning was meant to bend the will of the undecided merchants by warning them of the dangers of acting against the will of an "angry mass of people." The plea for participation in the commercial shutdown was supplemented by the not-so-subtle death threat of "everlasting boycott." The warning was so effective that when a force of physicians and municipal health workers descended upon Chinatown to administer the inoculation, they found businesses closed and few volunteers for vaccination. Many Chinese were frantically trying to leave the district. Circulars accused the Board of Health of seeking to "poison the Chinese by injecting drugs under the skin" and challenged the legitimacy of the Chinese consul and the CCBA to represent Chinese residents. "So bitter is the antagonism against the injection," Dr. Williamson claimed, "that the Chinese merchants who favored its use have been forced by the lawless element into closing their stores." The "everlasting boycott" threat had brought "all business . . . [to a] standstill." [51] Williamson overlooked the Board of Health's disruption of Chinese businesses and instead characterized resistance to state policy as a "lawless" protest and an implied death threat.

The distrust of health officials' activities extended to sanitary measures such as the procedure of killing rats, in which health inspectors "nailed dead fish on wooden boards and placed them in the sewers. The fishes' abdominal cavity was filled with arsenical (sic) paste to poison the rats." The practice incited rumors that the Board of Health was "inoculating the fish with bacilli of bubonic plague and feeding them to the rats so that these animals would contract the disease and carry it among the Chinese." Williamson was astonished by the rumors but refused to attribute them to the "Chinese brain." Instead he credited them to "some Caucasian, possibly a physician," who opposed the plague-suppression policies of the Board of Health and the PHS. [52]

These signs of Chinese resistance and refusal do not have to be understood exclusively within the frames of interpretation employed by public health authorities and journalists. A careful reading of Chinese rumors described in the official accounts and newspaper reports may provide some hints of the discursive contours of Chinese response. There are many difficulties in trying to interpret rumors as a type of popular discourse. The transition from oral to written form inevitably involved selection and distortion. Plague rumors were often printed in the dominant white press and official records in order to show the absurdity, the ignorance, and the irrationality of the masses. [53] Officials were likely to discount the agency and intellectual acuity of the Chinese, as Williamson demonstrated in his speculation that the source of subversive ideas was renegade white physicians rather than the Chinese shopkeepers and laborers.[54] Williamson's perception that the "cause" of protest was external to the Chinese consciousness was a way of ignoring and disparaging the subjectivity and agency of Chinese protesters.[55]

Chinese residents reacted to the public health declaration of bubonic plague in three sometimes conflicting, sometimes overlapping ways. First of all, some believed that there was no unusual disease affecting the San Francisco Chinese community. Second, others believed that there was disease but not bubonic plague. And third, many were convinced that bubonic plague was actually injected into Chinese bodies by public health authorities who were malevolently poisoning Chinese people. Chinese residents disputed the idea that they were the source of bubonic plague. Although they granted that some of their neighbors had been ill and died, the Chinese residents did not share the confidence of public health authorities who diagnosed bubonic plague. Instead, they preferred to believe that the illness was pneumonia or syphilis, a diagnosis shared by white politicians and medical skeptics as well. The bubonic plague epidemic had raged in southern China for six years, and many Chinese were familiar with the intensity of plague infection. Bubonic plague in China had spread like wildfire; it affected dozens of victims daily, rather than producing a half dozen cases spread over three months.[56] This competing folk knowledge undercut the claims of the health authorities, further exacerbating not only suspicions that the medical professionals had produced the hysteria of plague but also the belief that the PHS had either maliciously injected the disease into Chinese bodies or had ulterior motives in detaining and confining Chinese residents.

The rumors of poisoning indicated a deep suspicion about the source of bubonic plague. The Chinese challenged public health officials' purported role in extending life and instead became obsessed with their association with death. The health authorities carted dead bodies away and then diagnosed them with bubonic plague. Many of the rumors of poisoning focused on the experimental Haffkine vaccine and the invasive injection of pathogens into the body. The concern about inoculation perhaps demonstrated an astute awareness that the vaccine was prepared with the very pathogenic microbes that produced the plague. No matter how confident the health authorities were about their ability to calibrate the pathogens in order to manufacture a safe vaccine that would build immunity rather than induce death, the Chinese residents had enough experience with the health authorities to doubt their motives. And an assault on the body figured prominently in the general refusal to submit to inoculation. The concern of one merchant who refused vaccination on the grounds that he wanted to "protect his person" suggested an unwillingness to relinquish his body to suspect strangers who did not appear to exhibit concern about his well-being.[57] These protests rebuked health authorities for seeking the containment of the epidemic instead of the care of ill Chinese.

Rumors of the involvement of the consul and the CCBA leadership in the poisoning of Chinese laborers and petty merchants reflected the diminishing trust some Chinese had in the allegiances of their elite representatives. Some Chinese residents had a gnawing suspicion that their leadership's interests differed from their own. The distrust of Chinese laborers and petty merchants must have come as a rude shock to Consul Ho and the CCBA. Since his arrival in 1897, Ho had had extraordinary success in getting warring district associations to put aside their differences and restore the peace broken in the 1890s by internal assassinations and boycotts between secret societies. However, Consul Ho's tactics in threatening secret society members' relatives had also made him unpopular among many San Francisco Chinese residents.[58] Businesses had revived and Ho and the Chinese commercial elite were anxious for a quick resolution to the current crisis. They worried that quarantine would have financial consequences far more onerous than the consequences of inoculation. The leadership's initial efforts in cooperating with the public health authorities—their advice to the Chinese "not to argue with the health officers," and their frequent pleas for businesses to remain open despite the protests—fed a popular belief that the Chinese leaders had sided with the white authorities. The widely publicized protests of Chinese laborers and petty merchants against inoculation demonstrated a cleavage between the Chinese political elite and their constituents. Such challenges made public health officials and politicians rethink their belief that Chinese laborers offered unquestioned obedience and compliance to the orders of the CCBA and Chinese consul.

Actions taken by health officials did little to relieve tensions. Wyman advised his officers to use "tact and discretion in enforcing the Haffkine inoculation of the Chinese" and to persuade the reluctant Chinese by vaccinating "some whites."[59] The example of health authorities themselves being inoculated publicly, however, did little to loosen the resolve of most Chinese residents. A handful of Chinese merchants and leaders also submitted to vaccination. The Board of Health tried other tactics of persuasion, including posting notices stating that the government had spared no expense in preparing the medicine that was being used for vaccination and that the Chinese could be inoculated by their own doctors if they so chose. The notices also carried a cryptic warning of harsher measures if the Chinese continued to refuse vaccination.[60]

Showcase vaccinations of prominent Chinese individuals backfired, however, when reports of the health of those who had submitted to inoculation began to appear in the press. On May 22 the *Sacramento Record-Union* quoted the Chinese consul as saying that many of the Chinese who had been inoculated, his own clerk among them, were deathly ill and that this was well-known throughout the community.[61] The next day the *Chung Sai Yat Po* published a detailed account of two Chinese men who had submitted to the vaccination. According to the report, Zhao, a young man, had received an injection of the vaccine in the stomach and shortly afterward developed a fever and suffered excruciating pain. Soon after reaching home, he lost consciousness and his father had to summon a physician. Another man, Shen, had received an inoculation at the San Francisco wharf after returning to the city from the East Bay. Almost immediately he began to convulse in pain. He went to the offices of the CCBA to complain, collapsed there, and had to be revived by a doctor. News of his condition spread, and a crowd of several hundred gathered at the association offices.[62] These incidents reinforced notions of the toxicity of the vaccinations and heightened the apprehensions that health authorities were injecting the plague into unwitting Chinese. By May 23, the Board of Health had moved to desist from forcible inoculations and return to a familiar strategy of sanitary surveillance: house-to-house inspections.[63]

The travel restrictions drew legal challenges that were coordinated by the CCBA and Chinese consul. Over two decades the CCBA had become adept at using the federal court system to challenge both local and federal laws and policies that restricted Chinese immigration and trade. The CCBA secured the most prestigious legal counsel in San Francisco and strategized and coordinated test cases to serve primarily the interests of Chinese merchant classes. By the time of the 1900 bubonic plague crisis, the CCBA had become effective in presenting iron-clad legal challenges to discriminatory laws. Their lawyers were able to provide the most robust and persuasive challenges to laws that discriminated against Chinese Americans engaged in economic activities. These activities were most readily supported by the Supreme Court jurisprudence of the Fourteenth Amendment, which stated that "no one should be arbitrarily disadvantaged by government in the pursuit of economic advantage."[64] In May 1900, CCBA lawyers filed a lawsuit in the federal court on behalf of the San Francisco merchant Wong Wai, who had been denied by pub-

lic health officials the opportunity to travel for business purposes outside San Francisco. In his ruling Judge William Morrow acknowledged
the broad discretionary powers available in public health emergencies
but characterized the travel restrictions during the plague crisis as "arbitrary" and "discriminatory." These measures were "boldly directed
against the Asiatic or Mongolian race," Morrow argued, and demonstrated no scrutiny of individual "habits, exposure to disease, or residence" that would likely result in infection. Morrow rejected any policy
that presumed a racial susceptibility to plague, and he invalidated the
travel restrictions.[65]

When the courts lifted the travel restrictions, Texas and New Orleans
public health authorities considered unilateral quarantine of San Francisco freight to contain the epidemic. Under heavy political pressure,
San Francisco authorities again ordered the quarantine of Chinatown.
The Board of Health imposed this second quarantine of Chinatown at
its borders of Kearny, Broadway, Stockton, and California Streets. These
borderlines did not guarantee racial homogeneity, since some Chinese
lived outside these borders and a handful of whites lived within the
boundaries. This reality encouraged the board to leave the exact boundaries to the discretion of the police and public health authorities. The
deft selection of quarantine lines was not lost on the *San Francisco
Chronicle* correspondent who remarked that by a "careful discrimination in fixing the line of embargo, not one Caucasian doing business on
the outer rim of the alleged infected district is affected. . . . Their Asiatic
neighbors, however, are imprisoned within the lines." The only Chinese
and Japanese residents allowed to leave the quarantine zone had to carry
certification that they had received the Haffkine vaccination. The restrictions based on race were still upheld in the new quarantine policy.[66]

The CCBA and Consul Ho again accommodated the quarantine and
cooperated with sanitary measures. However, Consul Ho accused city
authorities of ignoring the health and welfare needs of the Chinese and
urged them to employ the more effective house quarantines in order to
safeguard healthy Chinese from disease, and to develop programs to
feed and care for the thousands of destitute Chinese effectively "imprisoned" in the quarantined district.[67] In order to head off economic disaster, an alliance based on shared commercial interests developed between
Chinese and white business groups. In response, the San Francisco Board
of Trade organized a mass meeting of white city merchants to raise funds
for the Board of Health's program to inspect, fumigate, and cleanse Chinatown; to remove residents to a detention camp; and to feed indigent

Chinese. In a matter of hours, the white "merchant princes" formed the Citizen's Relief Committee and raised $28,200 in contributions to pay for the work of the Board of Health.[68] Most of the money pledged was used to finance the Board of Health's sanitary measures, but some was allocated to feed indigent Chinese. Although the *San Francisco Examiner* acknowledged the city's responsibility to feed the quarantined Chinese, it rebuked the "arrogant" and "threatening" tone of Consul Ho's request, reminding him that, humanitarian considerations aside, the Chinese were "unwelcome guests" who through "their unsanitary habits" had given plague a "foothold" in San Francisco.[69]

The Board of Trade's intervention demonstrated one of the varying commercial interests at stake during the bubonic plague crisis. Businesses that prospered through manufacturing and shipping goods across the nation feared that the suspicion of uncontrolled bubonic plague would damage San Francisco's commercial reputation and ruin their businesses. Many of these large manufacturing and shipping businesses, as well as bankers and insurers, were represented on the Board of Trade. They shared with the CCBA, Consul Ho, and Chinese merchants an interest in supporting quarantine if it would quickly restore trade and assuage the concerns of public health agencies across the country. The Board of Trade and its white "merchant prince" members eagerly supported efforts to quarantine Chinatown alone, instead of allowing San Francisco and its commercial goods to be quarantined by others. Many of the white property-holders who leased their buildings to Chinatown businesses and residents had other property, manufacturing, and financial interests in the city. This group of white businesspeople had a greater interest in regulating and managing Chinatown and retaining the lucrative rentals from Chinese tenants than in destroying the district. Moreover, they were not ignorant of the rapid spread of bubonic plague throughout the Hawaiian Islands after the accidental burning of Honolulu's Chinatown. In order to contain the bubonic plague in Chinatown, in both perception and reality, many white businesspeople were willing to contribute financially to feeding quarantined Chinese residents.[70]

The Board of Trade's food distribution could not meet the vast daily needs of the nearly four thousand destitute Chinese within the quarantine borders.[71] Chinese men made desperate by hunger were accused of a dozen burglaries that occurred in Chinatown during the quarantine's first week. These break-ins can be interpreted as attempts to both satisfy hunger and register resistance to the quarantine. Chinese stole from wealthier Chinese as well as from white groceries, claiming the resources

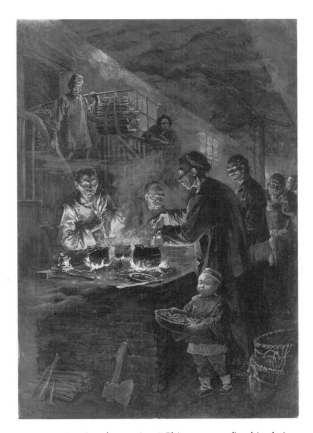

Figure 6. Bearing the caption "Chinamen confined in their quarters, cooking their meals," this drawing by Roger Williams Allen illustrated the article "The Bubonic Plague in San Francisco," published in *Harper's Weekly* 44 (June 2, 1900): 505. Reproduced from the Collections of the Library of Congress, 808321 262–120792.

from both within and beyond the quarantine boundaries. Other angry Chinese laborers and merchants protested the quarantine by refusing to pay bills and rent owed to white landlords until the quarantine was lifted.[72] (See Figure 6.)

During the second quarantine, Chinese laborers continued to harbor fears of poisoning. Rumors circulated that the Board of Health had sent out "emissaries to scatter disease germs throughout Chinatown." Chinese watchmen vigilantly guarded water and food supplies. One night, a Chinese watchman noticed a strange white man coming from a passageway that led to a water tank and sounded the alarm. Chinese men came from all the surrounding houses and the "word was passed about that the white man had been caught in the act of poisoning a tank." A crowd gathered around the watchman and shouted, "Kill him! Beat him! Make him eat his own poison." When police officers arrived who were familiar to the neighborhood, they tried to calm down the crowd by persuading them that the accused man was a newly assigned police guard and "not connected with the Board of Health." [73] The incident revealed not only the depth of Chinese anxiety about poisoning but also the extent of their suspicions about Board of Health representatives. The mob could "trust" police officers but not health officers. This incident and other altercations between health officers and Chinese residents convinced Dr. Chalmers, the head of the sanitary department, to order the corps of medical inspectors to work in pairs and be "extremely careful not to incur the enmity of the Chinese." [74]

The fears of health department poisoning were aggravated by the introduction of Dr. Kinyoun's street and sewer fumigator. The Citizen's Relief Committee had funded the operation of the new gadget, which began working on June 11. The fumigator pumped sulfur fumes through all the sewers in the district. Many were dismayed by the acrid smoke rising from the manholes and refused to have their rooms fumigated. After some Chinese threatened to destroy the fumigator, a guard was posted to protect it. [75] The state of alarm grew two days later when a crowd of Chinese threatened to wreck the butcher shop of Long Wo and Company at 849 Dupont Street, "because a silver dollar, cooked with a piece of pork, turned black." A CCBA representative offered the disquieting explanation that the "sulfur fumes" had produced the discoloration. Apprehensions about the toxicity of the fumigating machine were already high, and this incident made even more Chinese residents convinced that their food supply was poisoned. A volunteer ate the food, but even his apparent good health afterward did little to dissuade an anxious Chinese public. [76]

Rumors of foul play fomented fears of race betrayal and threw suspicion on anyone who had contact with white people. In one instance, a street-corner seer declared that a Chinese woman who had married a white man and who lived on Waverly Place had contrived with the public health authorities to scatter plague "germs" throughout the district. A crowd assembled outside her house, and when they did not find her at home, they searched the district in an unsuccessful attempt to locate her. [77] In this case, the treasonous connotations of interracial marriage dovetailed with already prevalent fears that people were working from the outside to destroy and betray the Chinese community.

Professional contact with white physicians drew the ire of Chinese crowds as well. A crowd gathered after news spread that a white woman physician was permitted to cross the quarantine lines and attend a Chinese infant. The crowd gathered outside the building and angrily called on the mother of the infant to explain her conduct in allowing a "white devil doctor" in her home. They threatened to wreck her home. CCBA representatives arrived and persuaded the crowd to disperse. But later in the evening, an anonymous circular was distributed that warned the Chinese residents against allowing white doctors to attend the sick in their homes. These protests signaled both a distrust of white physicians and a threat of mob violence to those residents who would seek their services.[78]

Chinese residents treated violently those among their fellows who sought white physicians or who took the plague vaccine. A handful of merchants submitted to inoculation in hopes of being allowed free access out of the quarantined district. For example, in a tent in Portsmouth Square, Dr. Frank Fitzgibbon inoculated a Chinese merchant. An angry crowd gathered and threatened the merchant with assault. Many members of the crowd considered the inoculation to be an act of submission to the "right of the Health Board to insist upon" mandatory vaccination. Several public health inspectors rescued the merchant and escorted him home.[79] Two days later, Quong Chong, a leading merchant, submitted to inoculation and was attacked by a mob and chased through the district, before seeking refuge in the rooms of the CCBA.[80] These incidents clearly demonstrated a breach between Chinese laborers who protested the health regulations and Chinese merchants who were willing to obey them for their own personal interests.

Court cases filed by a number of Chinese complainants challenged the maintenance of the quarantine. On June 13 Judge John De Haven of the U.S. District Court permitted Chun Ah Sing to walk out of quarantine and return to his work as a cook at Mrs. Davis's boardinghouse on Bush Street. De Haven ruled against Chun's enforced residence in Chinatown. Chun did not suffer from bubonic plague, nor did he live at or near any house where plague existed. The lack of proximity or contact with bubonic plague made the quarantine policy suspect. Although De Haven remarked that the quarantine represented "unjust discrimination against [Chun] and his race," the ruling did not invalidate the quarantine.[81]

Several days later the U.S. District Court ruled upon the case of Jew

Ho, a grocer who complained that the quarantine was enforced selectively upon the Chinese. On the block of Stockton Street were Jew Ho
lived and conducted business, every other business and residence was
occupied by whites and was free of quarantine restrictions. Jew Ho's attorneys supplemented their case with eighteen affidavits from licensed
San Francisco physicians disputing either the Board of Health's diagnosis of plague or the methods the agency had used to combat the epidemic.
The attorneys were also able to supplement medical findings with Governor Henry T. Gage's conclusions that no plague existed in the city.[82]

On June 15 Judge Morrow invalidated the quarantine. He argued
that there were limits to the "police powers" invested in public health
authorities and that the exercise of that power was "subject to the supervision of the courts." Putting an entire district and race under quarantine far exceeded the legal authority of the agency in preventing the
spread of disease. Morrow admonished the health authorities for making Chinese residents more vulnerable by not strenuously isolating the
houses of plague victims within the quarantined district. He ordered the
Board of Health to desist from the general quarantine of Chinatown and
to return to the more localized use of quarantine on individual buildings
where a known plague victim had lived. For a second time the courts
had forced the Board of Health to lift the quarantine, and the health
authorities returned to fumigation and sanitary measures in Chinatown
buildings and sewers.[83]

The Chinese press responded to the court victory with satirical ven-
geance. *Chung Sai Yat Po* published a large front-page cartoon showing
a Chinese man injecting a large dose of Haffkine prophylactic directly
into the top of Dr. Kinyoun's head, while Judge Morrow looked on with
approval. In a reversal and displacement of perceived roles, a guinea pig
also observed the forcible inoculation with satisfaction.[84] The Chinese
were no longer the "guinea pigs" subject to federal bacteriologists of
medical experimentation; Morrow's ruling had vindicated those Chinese
who defied the invasive power public health officials had exerted or attempted to exert over their bodies and movements. In an inversion of
power dynamics the cartoon artist employed the vilified instruments of
medical power against public health authorities in a fantasy of revenge.

In San Francisco's courtrooms and newspapers, lawyers, reporters,
and physicians debated what constituted "medical expertise." The court
records reveal deep fissures within the medical and scientific establishment in the city and state. The medical affidavits summoned for the Jew
Ho case demonstrated how sharply divided physicians and medical sci-

entists were about the existence of bubonic plague. Several licensed physicians who had firsthand experience with the alleged cases, sharply contested the bubonic plague diagnosis made by public health officials.[85]

One source of division was between clinical and bacteriological methods of diagnosis among professional medical practitioners. Many clinical practitioners were uneasy with the new bacteriology's emphasis on understanding the body's ailments by means of microscopic slides and germ cultures. No scientific medical consensus existed, though the partisan practitioners confidently claimed the superiority of their respective diagnoses and therapeutics. Bacteriological knowledge conceptualized the human body as plague's source and vehicle. Plague detection required intense physical scrutiny of the groin to detect the glandular swellings; however, the diagnosis was not straightforward. In clinical diagnosis, early symptoms of bubonic plague, such as prostration and high fever, resembled those of typhoid and typhus fever, and painful swollen lymph nodes in the groin readily suggested venereal disease.[86] The indeterminacy of physical examination made microscopic imaging attractive. Many bacteriology experts claimed that postmortem testing could offer the only reliable confirmation. The discovery of the plague bacilli and the ensuing production of therapeutic sera and prophylactics contributed to the medical perception that only invasive procedures on the human body could detect, protect one from, and cure bubonic plague.[87]

The U.S. secretary of the treasury intervened in the controversy in January 1901 and established a national commission to investigate the existence of bubonic plague in San Francisco.[88] The commission spent two weeks in San Francisco. They conducted bacteriological examinations on the body tissues of thirteen dead Chinese men and women and confirmed that six of these had died of bubonic plague. California's Governor Gage refused to accept the study and ordered a state commission to refute the national commission's findings. Fearful that the national commission's report would devastate San Francisco's commerce and tourist trade, Gage dispatched publishers from the city's newspapers and officials from the Southern Pacific Railroad to Washington, D.C., in early March 1901. The California delegation lobbied President McKinley and Surgeon General Wyman to suppress publication of the commission's report and future plague reports nationwide and remove Dr. Kinyoun from San Francisco. Under intense political pressure, Wyman agreed to a news embargo in exchange for California state authorities' cooperation with the PHS and San Francisco Board of Health to eradicate the disease from Chinatown. Shortly afterward, Washington officials abruptly transferred Kinyoun to Detroit.[89] Under the direction of the California state health inspectors, the San Francisco Board of Health and the PHS arranged for inspection of all sick and dead Chinese, cleaning and fumigation of all Chinatown buildings, and quarantine facilities in the Tung Wah Dispensary, which they commandeered for the purpose. The PHS surgeon M. J. White suspected that not all sick or dead Chinese individuals were made available for PHS inspection. Although White believed the state officials willfully deceived federal and local health authorities by concealing bubonic plague cases, his fury was aimed at Chinese residents and the CCBA leadership: White concluded that the Chinese were "the most incorrigible and utterly conscienceless liars on the face of the earth."[90]

Nearly sixty days of joint federal and state inspection yielded no new cases of plague. On June 1, 1901, Wyman and Gage called an end to the operation, with only half of the Chinatown buildings inspected. The lull in bubonic plague cases lasted until July 5, when a severely ill Chinese man arrived from the Sacramento River region and died immediately afterward. A Chinese undertaker reported the death to a man whom he thought was a state official, but who was in reality a PHS officer, Dr. Rupert Blue, who had replaced Kinyoun. After both a physical and a bacteriological inspection, Blue pronounced the case to be bubonic plague. Three days later, on July 8, four more cases of plague were discovered in a single Japanese household. It was impossible for state officials to continue to suppress news about the bubonic plague. Plague cases mounted over the summer—more than twenty-five new cases were confirmed by October. PHS officers hired Chinese interpreters to bolster detective efforts to find plague victims who had been secretly carted off to nearby cities or who were concealed in Chinatown.[91] Despite the resurgence of plague cases confirmed by the PHS and a death toll of nearly ninety, Governor Gage and his allies remained skeptical, believing that the deaths were due to acute syphilis, not bubonic plague. In November 1902, a physician, Dr. George Pardee, was elected governor. His election lifted the hopes of health authorities nationwide that this signaled an end to the impasse between California state officials, on the one side, and local and federal public health officers, on the other, in responding to bubonic plague.

In an attempt to sway Governor Pardee, two dozen state boards of health petitioned Wyman for an emergency plague conference. The conference was held in Washington, D.C., on January 19, 1903, during the last days of Gage's term. Health authorities from twenty-one states attended and passed a resolution criticizing the "gross neglect" of the California State Board of Health and the "obstructive influence" of Governor Gage. They threatened a massive quarantine of all commercial and passenger traffic from California if California state authorities did not cooperate with the PHS in suppressing bubonic plague.

## THE TRIUMPH OF SANITARY MANAGEMENT

Following the election of Governor Pardee, state, local, and federal authorities developed a coordinated program to suppress bubonic plague. Under the guidance of the PHS, an alliance of California business leaders developed a vehicle for reconciliation of the quarreling health agencies. Recognizing the likelihood of commercial quarantine, a nervous local business leadership acted quickly to assuage nationwide concerns about the spread of bubonic plague. Through the formation of a Joint Mercantile Committee, the business elite of the city and state coordinated and led a thorough inspection and cleansing of Chinatown. The Joint Mercantile Committee included representatives from the California State Board of Trade, San Francisco Board of Trade, San Francisco Chamber of Commerce, Merchants' Association of San Francisco, Merchants' Exchange of San Francisco, Manufacturers' and Producers' Association of California, and California Promotion League. These associations represented the white businesspeople who ran the large transportation, manufacturing, agricultural, and financial businesses in San Francisco. Many of them lived in Pacific Heights and had led campaigns for civic improvement, civil service government, and centralized municipal services that brought James Phelan into the mayoral office in 1896 and led to the successful approval of a new city charter in 1898. These white businesspeople intently supported the program of sanitary management of Chinatown in order to eradicate bubonic plague from the city and restore the city's commercial and civic reputation. The Joint Mercantile Committee's strategy of fiscally supporting direct improvements, instead of increasing the salaried staff of the Board of Health, suited the fiscal policy of the white business establishment constituencies in both the James Phelan (1897–1901) and the Eugene Schmitz (1901–07) mayoral administrations. Their economic interests also dovetailed with those of Chinese and Japanese merchants who contracted Chinese and Japanese laborers for work on farms, in canneries, and in factories throughout the West Coast. Wealthy white and Asian businesspeople both had an interest in eradicating bubonic plague, managing its perceived epicenter in Chinatown, and maintaining the mobility of Asian workers and merchants.[92]

The sanitary management supported by the white Joint Mercantile Committee and the CCBA offered intensive surveillance and medical monitoring of Chinatown residents and a variety of measures to eradicate sanitary nuisances and destroy rats. When the "systematic inspection" began on February 10, 1903, the CCBA offered to assist with the sanitary investigations and help obtain access to the "sick people of the Chinese race of the city." Public health authorities created a new surveillance plan that divided Chinatown into five sanitary districts, each assigned to a permanent medical inspector. Each medical inspector, by conducting daily rounds, was expected to gain familiarity with the district's sanitary problems and win the trust of Chinese residents. The inspection went through several phases, including police raids of lodging houses suspected of being overcrowded, intensive rat poisoning and trapping efforts, and medical identification of all sick Chinese residents.

The process of regulating and sanitizing Chinatown had made both public health officials and their white business supporters recognize that Chinese laborers were particularly suspicious and resistant to the authority of both health officials and the Chinese diplomatic and merchant-elite leadership. The objective of winning the trust of Chinese residents entailed not only a kind of strenuous surveillance of recalcitrant Chinese but also an awareness that public health authorities needed to cultivate hygienic consciousness and tutor sanitary conduct among a wider range of Chinese residents, not just the merchant elite.

The surveillance program was accompanied by the targeted destruction of condemned buildings. On March 30 the Board of Health began a demolition campaign against the profusion of small, "unsanitary" wooden structures built on the sides of houses, which "choked" Chinatown alleys and backyards. These board shacks, which served as "water-closets, kitchens and sleeping bunks," lacked adequate plumbing and collected debris and garbage. Labor gangs demolished the structures, unless spared by court orders, and then washed the existing walls with lime. By mid-October, the inspectors had razed 160 buildings, vacated 70 more, and made 400 plumbing repairs.[93] The emphasis on demolition of targeted unsanitary structures and on improvement of plumbing systems followed the instruction of nuisance law and the policy of requiring sewer connections to all buildings, both developed in late-nineteenth-century San Francisco municipal regulations.

Using information gleaned from the systematic inspection of Chinatown, federal and local authorities developed a census and directory of Chinese residents. The directory was culled from registration books used for the residential inspections, which listed names, occupation of head of household, and a brief description of living conditions at each address.[94] This "fairly accurate directory of permanent Chinese residents" was intended to provide a "useful check" on the movements of the "Chinese from place to place in the city" and specifically to trace the "abode" of any sick person who had been removed by "friends." This directory made the official surveillance easier and house quarantine more reliable.[95] The public health authorities began to find identification of Chinese individuals much more helpful in surveillance than the broad, undifferentiated categories that had commonly been used before. Individual specificity did not erase the potency of the racial category: as with the use of individual case files in immigration regulation, the intensity of individual detail that officials could amass made racial surveillance stricter.[96]

The sanitary surveillance of the San Francisco Chinese extended to those traveling to other cities in California and in other western states. The Joint Mercantile Committee advised local health officers statewide to keep "their Chinese quarter . . . under close surveillance, especially for Chinese arriving from San Francisco." This effort specifically tracked Chinese traders and migrant laborers who were contracted to harvest crops. The suspicious public health authorities employed these surveillance measures to trace "sick Chinese" that had been surreptitiously sent away to other Chinese communities in California. This system improved the PHS's covert strategy of seeking intelligence reports on sanitary conditions in "Chinatowns," and on Chinese death records, in California cities when they had to circumvent the California State Board of Health's interference in bubonic plague suppression from 1900 to 1902.[97]

The prevalent model of sanitary management continued to presume that Chinese bodies and locales would be the foci of bubonic plague infection. In the handful of cases in which white men and women contracted bubonic plague, public health authorities tried to find a "Chinese connection"; the two most popular were proximity to Chinatown and physical contact with the Chinese.[98] For instance, in July 1903, plague was diagnosed in two members of an Italian family—a thirty-six-year-old railroad laborer and his mother. The PHS officer directly in charge of plague suppression, Dr. Rupert Blue, immediately attempted to fix a Chinatown cause for the infection. Blue speculated that since the son, Pietro Spadafora, often walked through Chinatown on his way home and purchased produce and other goods there, he might have "accidentally" brought the infection home. The family lived north of Chinatown in the Latin Quarter, where predominately Portuguese and Italian immigrants lived. After a door-to-door inspection of the district, Blue remarked that the inhabitants were "cosmopolitan" and therefore did not oppose public health procedures such as disease reporting, house quarantine, and fumigation. Blue acclaimed European immigrants for their compliance with public health regulations, which attested to their "modern" sensibility as citizen-subjects. In the months that followed, no other human cases of plague were found in the Latin Quarter, but infected rats were discovered, aggravating public health concerns that the focus of plague infection had spread. The thorough sanitary management imposed on Chinatown was extended to the Latin Quarter for the duration of the summer.[99]

In February 1904 the Joint Mercantile Committee redoubled its efforts to bring the bubonic plague epidemic to an end. They ordered property owners in Chinatown to cement all basements and cellars as an essential "rat-proofing" measure. The PHS manufactured and distributed Danysz's virus to poison the rats, first in the sewers of Chinatown and then, by October 1904, in the Latin Quarter and so-called Japantown.[100] Plague cases, however, increased across the city and in the Bay Area. In the first three months of 1904, out of 10 plague cases only 4 were Chinese and 6 were white. The spread of bubonic plague infection was drifting away from Chinatown; 2 of the white cases lived and worked in the far western Richmond District, and 1 white death occurred in the East Bay town of Concord. When the San Francisco Board of Health declared the end of the plague in February 1904, the final figures for those afflicted by bubonic plague in San Francisco were 121 cases and 113 deaths. Of those deaths, 4 were identified as Japanese, 2 as white, and 107 as Chinese.[101]

Such statistics of overwhelming Chinese mortality from the 1900–04 bubonic plague epidemic could serve as a striking affirmation of public health officials' efforts to contain plague in Chinatown. It would seem logical to insist that since bubonic plague struck almost exclusively Chinese residents, aggressive measures targeting the Chinese were necessary to halt the spread of the epidemic. However, the history of the struggle to know and fight bubonic plague in San Francisco reveals the deep political and cultural dimensions of public health policies. These health policies and epidemiological statistics were not value-neutral. Both individual diagnoses and health policy were shaped by the conflation of the Chinese race and Chinatown with bubonic plague. Plague diagnosis was controversial, and physicians across San Francisco differed sharply about diagnostic methods and interpretations. It took several years for bacteriology to gain widespread authority in diagnosing bubonic plague among white physicians alone. Especially in the first year of the epidemic, when the PHS paid closest attention to death certifications of Chinatown residents, many white physicians may have diagnosed clinical symptoms such as glandular swellings, prostration, and fever in their white patients as acute syphilis or pneumonia rather than bubonic plague.

The statistics confirmed the popular perception that Chinese race, place, and behavior could explain the source, severity, and extent of San Francisco epidemics. It reinforced the knowledge that "being Chinese" created an environment that fostered disease. Did the predominance of Chinese victims of bubonic plague mean, however, that plague was peculiarly Chinese, as many San Franciscans presumed? A study by the historian William Deverell has adroitly demonstrated that it is necessary to untangle and understand how race, place, and culture became fused into an essential triangle to explain the predominance of Mexican plague victims during the 1924 bubonic plague epidemic in Los Angeles. It is apparent in both cases that bubonic plague struck individuals living in certain localities. Race, place, and culture were neither mutually exclusive categories nor inevitable linkages to explain epidemics. To think of bubonic plague as an essentially Chinese or Mexican affliction was to overlook then-contemporary medical understandings of how healthy people came into contact with plague-infected people or rat fleas. The containment and segregation strategies employed by public health officials in both San Francisco in 1900 and Los Angeles in 1924 may have shaped the circumstances in which the dead were nearly all of one ethnicity. The insistence that the fusion of race, place, and cultural behavior were key epidemiological factors was part of the "perceptual practices of dominant culture to view and explain plague epidemic" along lines of familiar racial stereotypes.[102]

Despite the freight of racial stereotype in health policy and explanation, the federal courts and Chinese protests restrained the most excessive public health initiatives and redirected health officials to undertake sanitary management to stamp out bubonic plague. Although the fear of Chinese aliens as epidemic menace circulated widely in both popular and medical discourse, public health officials did not excise Chinatown but, rather, sought to regulate and manage it. Health officials used prac-

tices of selective nuisance abatement, destruction of unsanitary buildings, and demands that plumbing be connected to sewer systems in order to rehabilitate Chinatown neighborhoods. In 1903, bond measures
designed to extend sewer and waste disposal infrastructure incorporated
Chinatown in the city system rather than ignoring it. Ironically, the destruction of San Francisco's Chinatown was achieved soon after—not
by state design but by natural catastrophe.[103]

THE AFTERMATH OF DESTRUCTION

In the early morning of April 18, 1906, a violent earthquake roared
through San Francisco, rocking and toppling buildings. Smashed gas
pipes set off dozens of fires throughout the city. Ruptured water mains
cut off the water supply, and firefighters relied on explosives to contain
the blazes. The strategy backfired, igniting fresh fires and hurtling them
out of control. The fires raged for nearly two days, destroying the South
of Market area, Chinatown, Hayes Valley, and most of the business district. Medical journals and newspapers hailed the destruction of Chinatown as the purification of San Francisco.[104] In the disaster's aftermath,
white politicians led by former mayor Phelan floated plans to relocate
the Chinese to the city's outskirts and replace the Chinatown vice district with an expanded business district and parks. Chinese merchants
and white property-owners, however, rallied to rebuild the old Chinatown District. Chinese institutions and a handful of Chinese property-
owners borrowed from Hong Kong banks to rebuild on their properties.
White landlords, fearful of losing Chinese tenants who paid premium
rents, organized the Dupont Street Improvement Club and pledged to reconstruct Chinatown following a "sanitary plan." Faced with mounting
opposition and the resolve of white landlords to lease their buildings to
Chinese tenants, city officials relented and dropped plans to drive the Chinese out. Mayoral advisor Abraham Ruef and newspaper editorials scut-
tled plans for the relocation of Chinatown as an affirmation of property
rights of white landlords and their freedom to lease to Chinese tenants.[105]

During the reconstruction, city officials, white landlords, and Chinese
merchants worked together to establish Chinatown as a safe and sanitary tourist attraction. City planners widened streets and connected
them with other main streets in the downtown area, and eliminated
"blind alleys" to create "easily policed" thoroughfares. By removing the
"succession of ratholes and lurking places," they engineered a transformation from a topography of darkness and villainy to the transparent

and open layout characteristic of the rest of the city.[106] Sanitary precepts governed the city's more stringent regulations requiring tenement houses to have "sufficient air and light spaces for tenants" in order to avoid the "bad features of the old Chinatown." Dr. Winslow Anderson, editor of the *Pacific Medical Journal,* advised builders to incorporate "scientific plumbing and concrete basements" and link Chinatown buildings with the city's sewer system.[107]

The process of incorporating Chinatown, however, resulted in building styles and ornamentation that created a visual architectural difference. The San Francisco Real Estate Board met with Chinese merchants and white landowners at the Chamber of Commerce to suggest that all Chinatown buildings be constructed in "imitation oriental" style. The landowners gave ten- and twenty-year land leases to Chinese merchants and allowed them full latitude in building three- and four-story buildings. White architects designed buildings with a hybrid architectural style unique to San Francisco, referred to as "Chinese Renaissance." To attract tourist business, building facades featured tiered pagoda towers, Mission-style fringe-tile roofs, curving eaves, and dragon decorations. Tourist literature carefully distinguished between the vice and filth of the past and the "sanitary" exoticism of the rebuilt picturesque streets and stores.[108] Ervin Will heralded the "cleaner" Chinatown's appeal to tourists and encouraged Chinese residents to adopt "modern ways of life and health" necessary for their survival in the United States.[109]

Despite the improvements, Chinatown and Chinese immigrants continued to be linked to the dissemination of epidemic. An article in a national magazine, *Collier's Weekly,* claimed that at first bubonic plague had been "confined" to Chinatown, but that the earthquake had scattered "infected rats" and "human cases developed in other districts. . . . Whites are now attacked, whereas before it was almost entirely Chinese and Japanese." The article, widely appreciated by anti-Asian immigration organizations, indicted "Asiatic Immigration" and "infected" Asians as the "direct source of the bubonic plague—the most terrible and swift of fatal scourges known to modern science. It is a human disease, and the rodent family against which the war is now being carried on, is really the victim of human agencies."[110]

In the wake of the disaster, a second epidemic of bubonic plague broke out in San Francisco. This time when a bubonic plague case was diagnosed a year after the 1906 earthquake and fire, neither Chinese immigrants nor Chinatown was implicated as the source of disease. The first reported deaths in the second epidemic were those of a "white

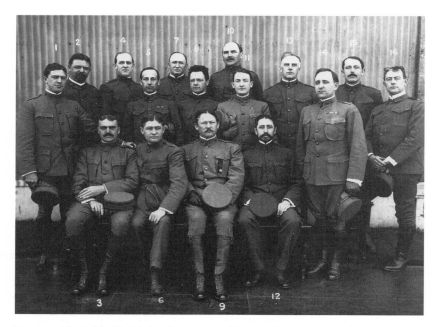

Figure 7. The Public Health Service sanitary officers on duty during the San Francisco plague epidemic of 1908 included Dr. Rupert Blue (seated third from left). Courtesy National Archives, College Park, RG 090–139–8.

sailor" on May 27, 1907, and an "Italian boy" on August 12, 1907. In September, twenty-two additional cases of plague were reported from throughout the San Francisco Bay Area.[111] The Board of Health did not recommend measures of quarantine or mass inoculation to combat the plague outbreak. The PHS officer Rupert Blue was sent back to San Francisco to take command of the plague suppression campaign, and the Board of Health immediately accepted offers of PHS financial and tactical support. (See Figure 7.) The program of systematic sanitary management they adopted divided the city into twelve administrative sections, each with a corps of inspectors, assistants, and rat catchers. Buildings throughout the city were rat proofed, procedures for catching and poisoning rats were initiated, and all incoming and outgoing ships were quarantined. Local residents were enlisted to help authorities by trapping and burning dead rats, burning daily refuse, and keeping their houses sanitary and dust-free.[112] During this second epidemic, scientific medicine readily identified the rat flea as the source of transmission of the disease from rats to humans. The San Francisco medical press endorsed the "rat crusade" as the most effective means to eradicate bubonic plague.[113] The plague outbreak lasted approximately a year and a half, resulting in 160 cases and 78 deaths. This time virtually all the victims were white.[114]

During the second plague epidemic, the bacteriological revolution identified the human body and its social conduct as the greatest agent of disease dissemination and the bearer of its essential diagnostic signs, but it also incorporated a focus on the extermination of rodents in the physical environment. The germ theory of disease renewed concerns about the environment but held humans responsible for cultivating the proper sanitary condition of their surroundings. Dorothy Porter has argued that "public health officials no longer viewed the individual simply as an isolated health unit; he or she was seen rather as the bearer of social relations of health and illness." In San Francisco, the cleansing of cellars and streets and the eradication of filth and refuse that would harbor rodents amplified the responsibility of individual conduct for the health of the community. Bacteriology produced new knowledge about the specific cause of disease, which sharpened the drive to implement preventive measures.[115] Bacteriological examination continued to stand as the authoritative proof of plague's presence in human and rodent bodies. And bacteriological technology was employed in the treatment of human plague through serum and as an instrument of biological warfare in rat poisons. However, sanitary management had succeeded as the principal strategy of plague eradication and prevention.

Despite the different mortality statistics and impact of the two epidemics, bubonic plague continued to have a tenacious association with the "Oriental" race and racial geography. In 1900, Walter Wyman wrote that the bubonic plague was an "Oriental disease, peculiar to rice eaters."[116] Seven years later when the majority of bubonic plague victims were white, Dr. Anderson referred to the disease as "Oriental plague" and California State Board of Health officials continued to monitor the "Chinatowns" and "Japantowns" in both San Francisco and Oakland for evidence of the plague's spread.[117] Frank Todd, in his report of the 1907 plague epidemic, explained how bubonic plague persisted in the popular imagination as an "Oriental" disease: "Plague no longer [was] a typically Oriental disease, nor wholly a filth disease. . . . Yet it was curious how hard these ideas were to dispel, even in the face of evidence furnished by white men's funerals."[118] The culmination of the successful suppression of the second bubonic plague epidemic could, therefore, find no more fitting venue for celebration than on the hill

above Chinatown, where a group called the Citizen's Health Committee honored the PHS officer Dr. Rupert Blue for eradicating the second
plague. The March 31, 1909, banquet attended by some three hundred
California luminaries was held at Nob Hill's Fairmont Hotel. In his
speech Blue declared, "We have vanquished the foes of the Orient, and
we are proud of the victory gained." The conflation of plague, the Orient, and Orientals provided the popular vocabulary to communicate the
nature of the threat and the urgency of sanitary reform.

The PHS program of rat eradication and sanitary reform comple-
mented the rebuilding of San Francisco after the 1906 earthquake and
fire. Dr. T. W. Huntington of the San Francisco Board of Health credited
Blue's sanitary campaign for wiping out the danger of typhoid, diphtheria, and other infectious diseases. Walter Macarthur credited the effectiveness of accurate information and the fact that people were persuaded
to disinfect their homes, streets, and sewers and to poison rats.[119]

During the bubonic plague epidemic, public health officials had confronted anew the problem and danger of Chinatown and how to rid San
Francisco of the perceived unsanitary conditions there that fomented
epidemic disease. At different moments in the crisis, three strategies
were entertained to deal with both Chinatown and bubonic plague. Frequently during the first epidemic and in the post-1906 rebuilding of San
Francisco, several civic and public health leaders revived a nineteenth-
century proposal to excise Chinatown from the central city. The proposal shaped the rhetoric and city beautification plans of land developers and city planners, but it did not win the interest of Chinatown's white
landlords and it underestimated the tenacity of Chinese merchants; both
of the latter profited from the concentration of Chinese businesses and
residences in the central city. The second strategy was to contain the disease within Chinatown. The early measures of quarantine and the racial travel restrictions followed this approach. However, both Chinese
residents and federal judges questioned whether disease could be pinpointed to a specific racial source that could then be contained by a
stringent racial boundary. Both the judges and Chinese residents suspected that the strategy was intended to kill off those expendable people
caught within the quarantine boundaries, rather than provide the most
effective means to suppress the plague irrespective of the race of the victims. The final strategy involved the public health management of Chinatown and its residents. This strategy had the support of the city's
white commercial and political establishment, federal judges, and the
Chinese diplomatic and commercial leadership. The aim was to improve

living conditions to the level of the norm and to incorporate Chinatown into the city system. The project of sanitary management entailed instructing citizen-subjects in the repertoire of caring for their immediate living environments and bodies as well as persuading them to follow extraordinary procedures necessitated during a epidemic crisis. The emerging consensus of public health management allowed for the delicate use of police powers within the constraints of civil rights to manage the city and its inhabitants in times of epidemic crisis. The aim was not to provoke fear but to inspire confidence and maintain the city's disease-free commercial reputation and to ensure the continuation of trade transactions even in times of upheaval.

The question remained, though, after the incorporation of Chinatown in the city's sanitary and sewer system, how could the Chinese residents, who were viewed as dangerous aliens, be drawn into the fold of society? The project of sanitary management already set the grounds for how public health officials might consider the Chinese to be citizen-subjects: they would have to exhibit hygienic consciousness and cultivate healthy conduct. Otherwise, city officials would continue to perceive Chinese residents as aliens who must be strenuously and rigorously regulated. During the bubonic plague epidemics, however, Chinese residents became effective in their ability to contest public health regulations. The Chinese merchant elite and the CCBA effectively used the federal courts, and Chinese laborers used public demonstrations, to challenge public health powers and the governance of their lives. Chinese residents of all classes demonstrated a variety of different visions of mobility, justice, and bodily autonomy. The racialization of disease did not disappear in either public health or popular representations. Chinatown and Chinese residents continued to figure as the typical and expected sites of disease and, by necessity, the targets of more forceful efforts of containment. But increasingly there was the possibility that if Chinese residents abided by the hygienic and sanitary standards of self-governance, they could be incorporated into city system and population.

# CHAPTER 6

# White Labor and the American Standard of Living

San Francisco labor politics in the late nineteenth and early twentieth centuries fixated on the threat posed by Chinese laborers to white jobs, health, and way of life. The imagery of a Chinese medical menace was a crucial element in the elaboration of the alleged threat to white households and livelihoods. Nineteenth-century labor and medical rhetoric had been generously laced with speculations about Chinese-manufactured cigars and slippers spreading epidemic disease.[1] Labor leaders, in particular, identified the Chinese production of consumer goods that whites purchased for their homes as the menacing *source* of such incurable diseases as leprosy and tuberculosis.

The terrifying combination of disease, "alien" invasion, and the contamination of white homes shaped labor politics in the late nineteenth and early twentieth centuries. In San Francisco and nationwide, union leaders in 1874 adopted the buy-the-union-label campaigns first popularized by the San Francisco cigar makers to discourage consumption of Chinese-made cigars. These consumer campaigns linked the presumed security of workplace with that of the domestic space. The revival of the campaigns in the twentieth century explicitly made the spread of disease a key consequence of consuming non-union products. By equating union production with sanitary workplaces, union leaders sought to bolster public support for the newly established norms of unionized factories, including well-ventilated work environments, worker safety, eight-hour workdays, the regulation of industrial home-work, and the repudiation of child labor. These new working conditions, produced through turn-of-the-century trade union and progressive reform activism, served as both the moral imperative and political vision of the future prosperity of white American working families.

This agenda of protecting the working families' livelihood, home, and health coalesced in the popular twentieth-century U.S. labor union creed of maintaining the "American standard of living." Unionization promised workers shorter workdays, good pay, and safe and sanitary working conditions—all elements considered crucial for the pursuit of a comfortable living standard for the American working family. The struggle to maintain the American standard of living demanded worker vigilance on the shop floor but also intervention in the practices of consumption. Union leaders feared that the merchandise produced under union conditions was undercut in the marketplace by goods made more cheaply under supposedly aberrant labor regimes, typically systems that hired racial minorities, prisoners, and recent immigrants. Rather than bring these underpaid workers into the organized-labor fold, union leaders attempted to squeeze out the competition by politicizing and policing consumption decisions. They developed a working-class consciousness about consumption practices that sustained the organized exclusion of Asians from unionization and the American public sphere.[2]

The American standard of living became freighted with discourses of racial danger, family security, and national vitality. By charting the rhetorical and activist strategies of the buy-the-union-label campaigns from the 1870s to the second decade of the twentieth century, this chapter explores how racial and national identities ordered the politics of production and consumption in white working-class consciousness, and the fact that the presumed threat posed by Chinese immigration reverberated for decades beyond the most intensive immigration to the United States in the 1870s and the greatest competition in manufacturing in San Francisco.

## RACIAL STANDARDS AND SANITARY SOCIETY

In nineteenth-century California, the consolidation of the labor movement had been based on anxieties about the "ruinous competition" from Chinese labor that fueled vigorous campaigns against Chinese employment and immigration.[3] In San Francisco, cigar making presented one of the first and most aggressive arenas for trade-union organizing against Chinese employment. As early as 1859 skilled cigar makers first

orchestrated boycotts of Chinese-made goods and demanded that employers fire Chinese workers. At first the Cigar Makers Association, a
group of white proprietors and journeymen, expelled one of its members for employing Chinese apprentices. With this breach, there was
no longer a racial boundary around the skilled trades that "insure[d]
the American white industrial classes immunity from the dangers" of
"enslaved Chinese labor." Along with other white tradesmen, the cigar
makers launched the People's Protective Union to fight Chinese competition, which they feared would retard "civilization" and destroy the
"country's prosperity," thereby bringing "want and suffering into the
homes of our people." The People's Protective Union tried to pressure
employers in order to keep them from hiring Chinese workers. Despite
the successful mobilization of trade union solidarity, Chinese workers
increasingly dominated the cigar-making industry; by 1866, 90 percent
of the two thousand cigar makers and nearly half the factory owners
were Chinese.[4]

Interest in combating Chinese labor competition resurfaced in 1874,
when white cigar makers and shoemakers both adopted a product label
in an effort to discourage consumers from buying goods made by the
Chinese.[5] The white Cigar Makers Association marked their products
with a white label that served as an explicit racial declaration that the
cigars had been made by "white men." The union appealed directly to
white consumers in order to create "a demand for white men's cigars"
and compel "manufacturers to employ white labor only."[6] The white label bluntly contributed to the emerging formation of white identity that
had exclusively defined trade union membership and generated racial
solidarity in order to ease potential conflicts among different European
immigrant nationalities and religious groups.[7] The label's initial use as
a means of distinguishing the race of producers developed into an appeal to sustain the living standards of white skilled labor when William
Woltz, the leader of the San Francisco cigar makers union, declared that
white cigar makers should not "live like coolies."[8] Labor leaders erro-
neously identified Chinese workers as "coolies," a racially coded term
that referred to indentured Asian Indian and Chinese workers who had
replaced slave labor on sugar plantations in the Caribbean. The image
of the "coolie" obligated to work under multiyear contracts at subsis-
tence wages amplified worries that a new form of racialized slavery
would replace recently emancipated black slaves.[9] Woltz and other
labor leaders worried not at all about living conditions of "colonized

classes" except as a foreboding scenario of the future of independent white workers forced to compete with "coolies."[10]

The union label not only highlighted racial differences in production and living but also underscored them with tales of medical menace. During this period the transmission of both syphilis and leprosy inflamed political rhetoric and medical concern about the dangers of contact between Chinese and white races.[11] A San Francisco delegate to the 1878 California Constitutional Convention and practicing physician, Dr. Charles C. O'Donnell argued that "Chinese leper[s]" were engaged in manufacturing throughout California. O'Donnell said that he personally had witnessed "three lepers making cigars" in a Chinatown hovel, and that he feared they could contaminate the rest of the city's population.[12] Labor leaders accused Chinese cigar workers of depositing "infectious germs" of leprosy and syphilis when they rolled the tobacco and moistened the tips of cigars by inserting the cigars in their mouths. The image of infection focused on the Chinese cigar workers illicit oral contact with the cigar. The dried saliva on the cigar was feared to be the conduit of disfiguring disease. The scenario of contagion traveling from the orifices of Chinese cigar makers to white consumers emphasized how careless oversight of workplaces imperiled consumer culture.[13]

The medical menace of Chinese production not only informed labor's nascent consumer campaigns, but it also provided a potent and putatively scientific alibi to the white labor political mobilization in San Francisco in the 1870s. The rhetoric of disease had its most direct expression in the political agenda of the 1879 municipal election, when Issac Kalloch, candidate of the Workingmen's Party of California, was elected mayor. One of Mayor Kalloch's first initiatives was to spearhead an investigation into the public health conditions of Chinatown. When the Board of Health declared Chinatown a public health nuisance and recommended its demolition, the Workingmen's Party readily published the report and amended it with its own controversial investigation. The Workingmen's Party report gave a striking assessment of the itinerary and consequence of "infected" products that linked the presumed security of the domestic space with the conditions of the workplace. The Workingmen's Party warned against purchasing Chinese-manufactured "cigars, clothing, even articles of food" because they were produced in the "filthiest holes imaginable" and exposed in such dens to the "impregnation of germs of diseases." The careless consumption of those goods would introduce sickness into the "fold of private families."[14]

In this formulation the reproduction of germs and disease occurred in the marginal spaces of production—the "filthy dens of Chinatown"— which were at odds with the supposedly sanitary union work floor. And transmission of disease suggested sexual reproduction and feminization as the consumer goods were "impregnated" by disease germs in these "dens" and then transferred into the feminized, domestic spaces of "private families."

By pinpointing the Chinese worker and the Chinatown den as the imagined source of domestic infection, the Workingmen's Party infused consumer culture with political and social consequences. Tracing the conditions of the product's manufacture and its itinerary from the hands of the producers to its entry into the home both revealed the workings of commercial capitalism and shaded the process with potent racial and national meanings. The notion that impure products could infiltrate the home of the white worker carried disturbing undercurrents of sexual danger and the sense of insidious and indirect assault on "private families." During this era, the vitality of the family and its successful reproduction had been vigorously associated with conceptions of the purity of race and the strength of the nation.[15] Thus the relation of Chinese producers to a commodity for domestic consumption intensified the potential peril of the white home, the white race, and the American nation. The exposure of the production and distribution processes served white trade unions to emphasize how Chinese labor not only undercut the system of white labor production but was also responsible for the ruin of the seemingly pure material culture and health of the nation.

The publication of the report came after a month of white-worker protests and anti-Chinese violence. Thousands of unemployed men gathered in the sandlots and marched to businesses, demanding that they immediately discharge Chinese workers. White men assaulted Chinese men on the streets and torched Chinese laundries at night. In February, the Board of Health's proclamation that the "Chinatown nuisance" must be abated fortified the white workers' conviction that they must drive the Chinese from San Francisco. Members of the Workingmen's Party gathered weapons and formed "military companies" to protect themselves from hostile police and to amass the firepower needed to carry out the removal of the Chinese. The merchants and property holders organized the Citizen's Protective Union in order to quell the labor protests and reestablish "order and protect property." In an effort to head off the showdown between angry workers and anxious merchants, the opposing forces reached a compromise that established the independent status of public health action. The Citizen's Protective Union gave assurances to the Workingmen's Party that there would be "no illegitimate interference" with enforcing the Board of Health's order to abate the Chinatown nuisance.[16] Although the Workingmen's militias disbanded, an unsympathetic Board of Supervisors and police force made it impossible for public health authorities to do more to Chinatown property than enforce building codes in the case of individual violations.[17]

The violent street protests and the rapid but short-lived rise of the Workingmen's Party were the most visible political manifestations of widespread desperation and dissatisfaction among white workers. The 1870s had been punctuated with severe economic depressions that had made steady employment nonexistent. Although the 1873 national economic collapse did not initially punish California as severely as the East Coast states, the influx of unemployed workers to the West Coast and an 1876 drought pushed California to economic depression in 1877. Poor business conditions and a large labor pool delayed recovery until 1880.[18] The acute competition for work could have pitted skilled against unskilled workers, recent arrivals to California against old-timers, and European immigrants against the native born. However, the sandlot protesters that gave public and electoral support to the Workingmen's Party developed a white workingman's coalition that refocused competitive anxieties on Chinese immigrants. Even after the Workingmen's Party lost power, white skilled workers continued to protest against Chinese labor competition.

The hysteria of a racialized threat also masked the dramatic structural changes that had made skilled artisans economically vulnerable. For instance, in the cigar-making industry, factory owners had begun to use cigar molds, imported from Germany, which increased the pace and scale of production dramatically and required less skillful labor. This change in the production process made artisans who were skilled in hand-rolling cigars increasingly obsolete, as employers found it more profitable to hire less-skilled Chinese, eastern European, and Latin American immigrant workers.[19] The struggle to maintain skilled artisan production inspired the Cigar Maker's International Union (CMIU) to adopt the union label in 1880. The CMIU broadened the label's legend, so that it highlighted issues of skilled workmanship and sanitary conditions and folded them into the structural differences of production and labor markets. Their light blue label guaranteed "first class workmanship" and served as a "positive Detective to help separate and weed out filthy, inferior tenement house, Prison, Chinese and rat-shop workmanship."[20]

The national union replaced the explicit mention of the producer's white racial identity with an inventory of unsanitary and abject alternatives to the quality of workmanship ensured by its "skilled mechanics." The union highlighted the site of non-union production and the race of the non-union producer as markers of filth and inferiority. Other local unions could then widen the union label's effectiveness as a weapon in struggles against an assortment of less skilled workers across the country, whether the competitive "menace" was prisoners; Chinese, eastern European, or southern European immigrants; African Americans; or Cubans.[21]

The union label grew in popularity in the United States in the 1890s and was rapidly adopted by dozens of national trade unions. By 1908, 68 of the 117 national trade unions affiliated with the American Federation of Labor (AFL) were using the label. The membership of these label-using unions was 724,200, representing 47 percent of the aggregate membership of the AFL. At the turn of the century, trade unions in England, Australia, and France successfully adopted the label in their labor and consumer campaigns.[22]

The versatility of the union label did not undermine its malleability to local conditions. In San Francisco, the union label could continue to serve a narrower agenda that honored its local history of labor solidarity and trade union protest. In 1886, when the local city trade unions banded together to form the Council for Federated Trades of the Pacific Coast, the coalition affirmed the roots of its solidarity with the politics of "union label agitation" in the service of "Chinese Exclusion." This combined agenda of consumer campaigns and the anti-Chinese crusades sustained the federation when it became the San Francisco Labor Council in 1892. Although the explicit racial markers were deleted from the union label, racial exclusion persisted and informed the programs of organized labor. In the first third of the twentieth century, the consumer campaigns spearheaded by the San Francisco Labor Council elaborated on the racial meanings of labor solidarity.

In the first decade of the twentieth century, *Labor Clarion*, the Labor Council's official weekly publication, periodically presented organizational reports and persuasive essays that developed the conceptual and practical agenda of buy-the-union-label efforts. The discussion of racial and national identities critically informed label campaign rhetoric. The *Clarion* maintained an anti-Asian-immigration stance throughout the first third of the twentieth century. The politics of anti-Asian immigration dominated its pages in the form of frequent reports about restrictive legislation, immigration statistics, and the different Asian nationalities arriving in California in the early twentieth century. Although the first Chinese Exclusion Act in 1882 had stemmed the tide of incoming Chinese laborers, Japanese, Asian Indians, Koreans, and Filipinos began to freely immigrate to the United States at the turn of the century. The *Clarion*'s inaugural issue in February 1902 featured the Labor Council's efforts to lobby Congress for the passage of a more stringent Chinese exclusion act. The *Clarion* published Labor Council resolutions that accused "unfair" Chinese competition of depressing "the standard of wages, living and morals" and destroying the "national prosperity" upon which American citizenship and democracy relied.

San Francisco's Mayor Eugene Schmitz was one of a dozen local and national political leaders featured in the newspaper's first issue who endorsed the Labor Council's position on Chinese exclusion. Mayor Schmitz employed the rhetorical strategy of the eyewitness Chinatown excursion to blend medical and labor critiques of Chinese manufacturing. He recounted that an "ordinary living room will be crowded to suffocation with coolie slaves (many of them afflicted with cancerous and loathsome hereditary diseases) busy eighteen hours a day, making cigars, or clothing, or shoes, or a hundred other products." Schmitz seamlessly incorporated worries about the hygienic status of unventilated, improper work spaces and diseased workers into labor critiques of enslaved workers and unrelenting working conditions. Schmitz argued that the mode of production in Chinatown's "countless sweatshops" damaged both unsuspecting American consumers and American workers. Unlike these "coolies," Schmitz argued, "American labor" could not "live on a few cents a day," and American living standards required "nourishing food and suitable clothing, as well as good air to breathe and reasonable hours to work." He doubted that greedy manufacturers and retailers would relent in patronizing Chinese labor, and so advocated that federal intervention restrict immigration and that labor activism sustain a humanitarian ethics of consumption.[23] Schmitz's commentary echoed the Labor Council's continued efforts to call for a general boycott of all Chinese-made goods and of all Chinese establishments. The Labor Council leadership reasoned that the boycott would "convince the employers of Chinese labor that there is no sale for the products of such labor" and influence "the Chinese coolies to stay in China."[24]

Boycott pressure seemed unnecessary to dissuade Chinese immigration after nearly two decades of restrictions on the immigration of Chinese laborers, which had forced the rapid decline in the number of Chinese workers in San Francisco and throughout the United States.

However, labor leaders maintained that the Chinese "coolie" was a pervasive and viable racial threat to white American workers. The political struggle to prevent Chinese immigration and the symbolic appeal of the Chinese as a scapegoat reconfirmed the boundaries of race and national difference that were crucial for union solidarity.

When invoking the history of the union label's origins, the label promotion articles appreciatively highlighted the anti-Chinese stance of the white San Francisco cigar makers.[25] A 1902 Fourth of July speech in the *Clarion* provided a fairly typical assessment of the enduring significance of the nineteenth-century anti-Chinese stance. Consumption of union-made goods was observed as a patriotic American duty performed in the interests of skilled labor. Honoring the union label was all the more important in an age of tremendous immigration that had brought a "horde of cheap and unskilled labor" to American shores. Attention to the eastern and southern European origins of the turn-of-century "hordes" was skillfully deflected by focusing on the Chinese as the most abject and unassimilable immigrant.[26] The American standard of living could be sustained only through the careful distinction between the assimilable immigrant who came to "be among us, share our liberties, adopt our customs and laws[,] and advance and progress with us" and the "Chinese coolie, sweatshop and colonized classes, which represented a far too low standard of living for our citizens to adopt."[27] The invocation of the anti-Chinese history of the label buttressed the recognition among union members that perceptions of "unfair" racial competition had shaped labor organization and influenced the possibilities of labor solidarity. John Graham Brooks, a social reformer and president of the National Consumer's League, considered immigration's effect on labor to be a "question of race." The need to preserve an "American" standard of living overrode the ideal of a brotherhood of universal workers and of political equality. For Brooks, the choice of cigar consumption became a decision to "maintain the white as against the coolie standard of life and work."[28]

In U.S. labor politics at the turn of the century, the living-standard rhetoric was characterized by interchangeable codes of race and nationality; the so-called American standard of living, or more bluntly "the white man's standard," was defined in resolute opposition to the "Asiatic" or the "coolie" standard of living.[29] The AFL, founded in 1881, engaged in a persistent political crusade to deny Chinese and other Asian workers entry into trade union ranks and into the nation. Samuel Gompers, a longtime president of the AFL, and Herman Gutstadt, a San

Francisco–based official of the Cigar Makers International Union, coauthored a nationally distributed essay that telescoped five decades of anti-Chinese politics into an explanation of how Chinese living standards were incompatible with and destructive to the political and cultural fabric of U.S. society.[30] They argued that "you cannot work a man who must have beef and bread alongside a man who can live on rice. In all such conflicts, and in all such struggles, the result is not to bring up the man who lives on rice to the beef-and-bread standard, but it is to bring down the beef-and-bread man to the rice standard."[31] They predicted that sharp wage differences between the putative Chinese rice-eaters and white beef-eaters would precipitate the collapse of white wage levels, depleting white confidence in the political order and fomenting white discontent and sedition.

In a bid to ensure the renewal of Chinese-immigration-restriction legislation in 1902, Gompers and Gutstadt developed an argument for national stability based on racialized living standards and masculine self-preservation. The contrasted food consumption patterns of the workingman formed a shorthand code that harbored anxieties about downward social mobility and the loss of masculine privilege and the status of manhood. During the nineteenth century the structural assault on artisan production made it increasingly difficult for a skilled workingman to be the sole provider for a wife and children—a key element of the working-class ideal of manhood. The assertion of independence and respectable masculinity for working-class men was structured around the ability to have and sustain dependents.[32] Since Chinese workers were perceived as bachelors without family obligations, the notion of the "coolie" standard was invested with fears about a socially disordered world of unemployed men, women prostitutes, and working families ripped apart by vice, poverty, and disease. The vigorous diatribes against "Chinese coolies" emphasized the irreconcilable differences between putatively unfree, racially inferior, and alien Chinese workers and the free, independent, white producer-citizens. In labor rhetoric the presence of the Chinese antagonized American workers and contaminated their aspirations for prosperity, democratic citizenship, and family life.

In the union propaganda on boycotts and immigration controls, the mapping of race difference in terms of opposing living standards and styles seized upon the dramatic transformations of the social and economic order. The caricature of the "Oriental standard" functioned to shore up moral support and political leverage for organized labor's program to both regulate industry and dampen the effects of rapid industrialization. The sanitation references became increasingly significant in the definition of living standards because of the intensity of public health reform in trade union initiatives. Turn-of-the-century social reform and labor campaigns for sanitary and safe work conditions in factories, crusades for spacious housing and urban park space, and campaigns to secure eight-hour workdays and to ban child labor were premised upon protecting the health and safety of workers and their families.[33] Since these reforms were insecure and uneven, labor activists were extremely sensitive to any perceived threats to hard-won gains. The racial contrast served to establish the new conditions as normative and necessary to ensuring the humanity of working families, to preserving the white race, and to maintaining civic stability.

The meanings attributed to "sanitary" workplaces often relied upon late-nineteenth-century visions of a separation of living and working environments. The "promiscuous" combination of leisure and work had, in preceding decades, alarmed public health authorities, who feared that the ill and immoral would "infect" consumer goods with disease. The possibilities of careless "infection" were observed in an illustration entitled "Scene in a Chinese Broom Factory," which accompanied an article that equated convict labor and Chinese labor as the twin threats of white union broom makers.[34] The drawing highlighted the questionable mixture of activities—eating, opium smoking, and sleeping—in a cluttered and crowded workshop where only a few Chinese men were actually making brooms. The image drew together typical images of Chinese vice and disorder with more general insinuations of laziness and poor productivity, which were not usually ascribed to Chinese workers. The racialization of the broom factory developed its significance from the use of images of "crowding," opium smoking, and the general mixing of work and leisure that had aggravated health inspectors in San Francisco laundries and cigar factories in the late nineteenth century, and that had then readily been blamed for disease transmission to consumers.

Hygienic practices and the achievement of sanitary norms gave a scientific patina to labor's goal of improving the "standards" of work and life for working-class families. The production of norms and standards in industry entailed the use of hygienic practices to make heterogeneous production systems uniform. There were many types of unhygienic environments but a singular norm of hygiene. The American standard of living served as the uniform standard for different, particularistic labor and living systems. It was a process that paralleled the consolidation and systematization of capitalist production as well as the transformation of varieties of European ethnicity into white American citizens.

In consumer campaigns in the early twentieth century, union label promoters explicitly made the connection between sanitary standards, working conditions, and health. Label promoters contrasted non-union goods made in "poorly ventilated, over-crowded, disease-propagating tenements by the overworked, poorly-paid slaves of grasping employers" with the union goods made in sanitary workplaces by well-paid workers.[35] The union label was promoted as a health "safeguard" against the "vile, disease-breeding sweatshop" that scattered "the seeds of disease and death over the entire country as long as [the sweatshops'] products can be sold."[36] Narratives of potential disease transmission connected the producer and consumer by emphasizing that the "unwholesome conditions for the worker . . . mean sorrow, disease and death to the consumer."[37] Union cigar makers claimed that union-made products were the "enemies of dirt and disease" and sought the endorsement of physicians certifying that the union-made cigars were hygienically manufactured and thereby "positively prevented germ transmission."[38] By "insuring" the consumer against "filth and contagion," the union label established the reorganization of "purchasing power" that coupled the "health and morality of the producer" and the "well-being of the purchaser."[39]

Most of the direct commercial advertising regarding the union label "insurance" played upon fears of diseases that could be spread. In a series of United Garment Workers Union (UGWU) advertisements for men's suits, the caption for one advertisement informed the reader, "Clothing with this label *insures* the buyer against contagion. *Guarantees* that it came from a Clean Modern Shop. *Was Made* by Skilled Union Tailors."[40] Other advertisements associated cleanliness and health with union production, and the antithesis with the products of sweatshop manufacturing. One advertisement advised the consumer to "Discriminate against inferior unclean sweat-shop clothing."[41] (See Figure 8.) Another advertisement, featuring the Miller-Made brand of clothing embossed with the UGWU label, included the pledge that the "clothes [were] made by the most skilled workmen in absolutely sanitary, well-lighted, airy and clean shops."[42]

The guarantees of sanitary standards and skilled workmanship were framed by a racially exclusive union membership. For more than half a

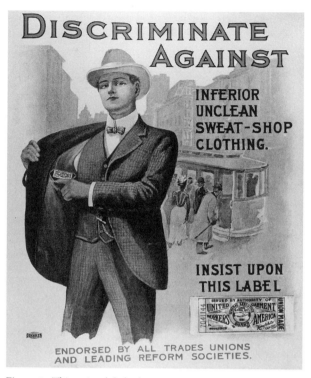

Figure 8. This union label advertisement, sponsored by the
United Garment Workers of America, appeared in the *Labor
Clarion* 1, no. 25 (August 15, 1902): 13. Courtesy San Fran-
cisco Labor Archive, San Francisco State University.

century white worker solidarity on the West Coast was premised on the
perceived fears of Asian worker competition. The garment workers'
unions in San Francisco had prohibited the inclusion of Asian workers and any attempts to organize Asian workers.[43] When the UGWU
formed its first local in San Francisco, in December 1900, the leadership
vowed to defend white women workers from the "demoralizing competition of Chinese and sweatshop workers." These scenarios of "demor-
alization" suggested that white women would be thrown out of work
because their wage rates could not compete with Chinese wages. Forced
out of "honest" labor, these women were likely to take up street prostitution to survive. The UGWU transposed this protection of women's integrity and virtue in the workplace to the more general protection of the
purity of the domestic sphere from dangerous consumption. They prom-

ised that clothing produced under the UGWU label was made not only by "persons free from disease" but also that "no child under sixteen years of age has worked upon the garment" and that "no Asiatic has touched the garment." [44] This inventory of protections suggested several forms of contamination. On the one hand, the UGWU label guarded against the physical threat of infection and, on the other hand, it relieved the consumer of the moral danger of supporting exploitative child labor practices. However, the declaration of freedom from the "Asiatic" touch suggested how physical and moral taint were combined in the racial danger of Asian labor infiltrating the white home. The defense of the home from disease, aberrant labor, and racial difference was crucial to the home's success as the purified site of social reproduction.

## GENDERED APPEALS AND THE DEFENSE OF THE HOME

The imagery of the home under siege was a key trope in the consumer campaigns and made the labor issues all the more compelling and immediate. The perception of threat to social stability and family security paralleled contemporaneous public health and moral policing campaigns combating venereal disease, which focused on men bringing disease from the outside to the home and imperiling family reproduction.[45] Physical threats to domestic space resurrected conventional expectations of women's role as domestic sanitarians, entrusted with the care and defense of the home and of the moral and physical well-being of the family.[46]

At the turn of the century, labor union leaders attempted to reorder and elaborate on gender in their crusade for union-label consumption. In an essay that took first prize in a 1904 AFL contest related to the union label, Walter MacArthur, editor of the *Coast Seaman's Report* of San Francisco, formulated a constellation of distinctively gendered values and duties for men and women in promoting the union label. For men, the union label represented the bridging of citizenship between industry and individual life and the application of codes of integrity such as "cleanliness, morality, honesty, chivalry toward woman." The responsibilities and significance of the union label for women were less political and more "instinctual." MacArthur argued that union consumption would appeal to women's domestic virtues of "cleanliness, morality, the care of the young, [and] the sanctity of the home." By consuming union-made goods, the "mistress of the household" could wield her "purchasing power" for the union cause: "By demanding the union label the wife of the trade unionist becomes truly the helpmeet of the breadwinner, her powerful influence being thus extended from the home to the workshop, from which she is otherwise totally excluded."[47]

Women in trade union families organized the Woman's International Union Label League (WIULL) and developed branches across the United States and Canada, including an active organization in San Francisco.[48] Many members sought to widen the definitions of working-class women's domesticity to encompass the union's political struggle. In 1905 Mamie Brettel, the president and general organizer of the WIULL, claimed that the organization existed to "teach women" the altruistic mission of the "betterment of humanity" through their "everyday work."[49] Her successor, Annie Fitzgerald, argued that women's education concerning the union label must recognize a woman's power as the family "purchasing agent" and then guide that power with an enlightened understanding of political and economic interest: if a woman "buys a garment, for herself or her child, which does not bear a label, then she is working against the best interests of her husband whose trade may be represented by a union label."[50]

The member trade unions of the San Francisco Labor Council and the local chapter of the Women's International Union Label League developed publicity programs to target women consumers. They disbursed leaflets, union label calendars, and picture postcards to encourage women to buy union products and ensure the economic prosperity of union men.[51] The Labor Council sponsored variety shows that promoted label consumption through vaudeville acts and public speeches.[52]

In the campaigns, women were constantly described as upholding the "home and family" and as the "custodians of family income" and the "purchasing agents of the home." Women were perceived in relation to union men as their wives, sisters, mothers, and daughters. MacArthur's and Fitzgerald's presumptions of strict gender role divisions in the working class were widely shared among their trade union colleagues. Images of working-class women's domesticity mimicked the existence of separate spheres within the middle-class and disavowed the existence of women as workers in factories, sweatshops, and their own homes.[53] This definition of proper gender roles—which consigned women to the sphere of domestic, unpaid labor—also dovetailed conveniently with the agendas of labor reform and public health reform, which sought to close down sweatshops and curtail industrial homework, effectively removing many women and children from the labor market.

By rearticulating women's domestic roles, union label promoters sought to impart working-class consciousness to women despite their presumed "indifference" to trade unionism. This condescension belied the policies of several AFL trade unions that opened membership to women and the eagerness of many eligible women to join.[54] In order to maintain gender differentiation in the wake of organizational transformations, labor leaders targeted their appeals to housewives who did not work outside the home. Therefore, the rhetoric aimed at women emphasized the improvements to home and family that would accrue from women's conscientious consumption: better wages and shorter hours for the "breadwinner" would translate into increased household "comforts" and improvements in the family's health and less work for the housewives. Although working-class women were often employed outside the home, in union propaganda they were relentlessly characterized as housewives.[55] This both reinforced the pervasive persuasion campaigns for the white working class to adopt middle-class gender roles and denied the possibility that through paid labor women might have access to arenas for developing political consciousness other than the domestic sphere. And, not least, it also reiterated the idea that a female relative working for pay represented a man's moral and financial failure. That she might "prostitute" herself in this way suggested that a woman could not rely on a man for security and prosperity.[56]

The union label campaigns promoted a vision of the citizenship of white working-class women that was distinguished by styles of dependence. In her political participation, an union woman was expected to enable her man, accede to his agenda, and not be in conflict with him or stand independently of him. Some women leaders began to reevaluate the content of their own citizenship and their ability to make rather than influence legislation. By 1909, the wives of union men were organizing for greater political participation in order to undertake duties of municipal housekeeping and promoting trade unionists' interest in ensuring union sovereignty in factories and sanitary workplace conditions.[57] In 1912 after the suffrage amendment had been passed in California, the San Francisco Labor Council financed the electoral mobilization of "working women and the wives, daughters, and female relatives of workingmen." Shortly afterward, the activist Alice Park offered a "women's agenda" that supported legislation for an eight-hour workday for women and children, as well as advocated feminist causes, including red-light district abatement, pay equity, and greater rights in property and child custody.[58] The alliance of white working-class women with white middle-class women reformers arrayed itself against, on the one hand, the business elite and, on the other hand, the disenfranchised and non-union workers (racial minorities, recent European immigrants, and prisoners). The alliance's interest in improving white women's political and social rights as well as white working and living conditions dovetailed with their stake in maintaining racial hierarchies and exclusions in the social order and general economy.

## RACE, HEALTH, AND LABOR

Union leaders juxtaposed the supposed affinity of white people and health with Asians and disease, drawing statistical and anecdotal substantiation from the layers of popularized public health knowledge. The emergence of bacteriological knowledge and its application as an incontestable bar for immigration particularly fascinated and influenced labor activists. Soon after news of the bacteriological detection of parasite diseases broke in the news media in 1910, the Asiatic Exclusion League endorsed the mandatory use of the PHS examinations of Asian immigrants to detect "germs of disease . . . endemic in Oriental countries, such as uncinariasis and filariasis." [59] Noting the PHS statistics on hookworm prevalence in Asian Indians and the trachoma incidence in Japanese, various white labor advocates concluded that any and all Asian immigration was an "invitation" to epidemic disease and "among the graver perils to American health." The differences between Asian immigrants were perceived by their opponents to be superficial, and labor writers argued that all "Orientals" should be treated to the same strict immigration barriers as had been placed in front of Chinese arrivals.[60]

The rank and file of the trade unions had already been primed for the message of public health reform and vigilance. In the first decades of the twentieth century, public-education campaigns, local and national government organizations, and private foundations and social-reform organizations had taken the message of public health reform to the working class and immigrants in the cities.[61] Like many of its counterparts across the country, the *Labor Clarion* regularly reported on public health programs, disseminated public health advice for the prevention of diseases such as typhoid and diphtheria, and reported medical profession debates on the issues of vaccination, fumigation, and quarantine. The health coverage emphasized the necessity of assiduously tending to personal hygiene and the consistent control of environmental sanitation.[62] In addition to supporting public health programs and broadcasting health advice, the *Clarion* and labor leaders became involved in the production of health expertise. Labor leaders nationwide organized sanitary committees to evaluate the effectiveness of municipal and state health laws, offered expertise in issues of industrial hygiene, and served on municipal health boards.[63] In their participation in the dissemination of health advice and in the creation of health policy, union leaders emphasized the threat to life and livelihood posed by disease.

Labor and medical concern about the influx of Asian immigration and the manufacture of Asian immigrant goods in the United States logically developed into an insistent concern about the dangers of imported products. A cigar maker and former soldier, William Backner of Springfield, Massachusetts, feared the dangers of "Manila cigars" imported by the unscrupulous "Tobacco Trust." In an open letter to George Perkins, president of the CMIU, Backner opposed congressional legislation to reduce tariffs on goods from the Philippines, a newly acquired colony of the United States. The contents of the letter were printed in labor publications across the country, including the *Labor Clarion*. Backner's impressions revealed an astonishing manipulation of racially coded languages of health and hygiene and their promiscuous application to any racialized population:

> Now every soldier knows the uncleanliness of the average Philippino, and if you ask him he will tell you that many a poor fellow came home in a box by too close association with them, as they are poison to the white man. They are all affected with a skin disease and a large majority are covered with open sores and scars. Leprosy, beri-beri, cholera, bubonic plague and other infectious disease, are, as everyone knows, prevalent there. They sit half naked and work and scratch, while the air is rank with the smell of decayed fish and coconut oil, which the women use on their hair. Now imagine one of these natives, whose teeth have rotted black by the constant chewing of the betelnut, biting out [cigar] heads, which I took particular notice to see if they did, and using their spittle to help paste the heads on their work, you form some idea of what the American smoker will get when the [tobacco] trust dumps these far-famed Manila cigars on the market. The United States government spends thousands of dollars to quarantine against these Asiatic diseases, and when one leaves the island for this country, himself and effects are thoroughly disinfected, and in the face of all this our law makers propose to put their seal of approval on this bill which will put into the mouths of thousands of our citizens a most prolific means of contagion, and if as I firmly believe, it will be the means of infecting those filthy Asiatic diseases into the blood of the American people, the present administration can thank itself for it.[64]

Backner's fears of an alien invasion of epidemic diseases and his ascription of endemic disease to Asian races presented a new version of the "yellow peril" that had preoccupied nineteenth-century public health officials and labor leaders. His descriptions and characterizations of the "repulsive habits" of Manila cigar workers reproduced both the detail and the narrative emphasis that had been employed in exposés of sweatshop labor in New York's East Side and San Francisco's Chinatown in the late nineteenth century as well as in colonial narratives of labor in Asia. His description highlighted the disfigured bodies oozing with contagion and the lack of separation of living arrangements from the workplace.

These patterns revealed far more than Backner's familiarity with the rhetoric of contemporary urban reformers and public health physicians. They demonstrated the extent to which union men had adapted the concerns and conclusions of national public health vigilance to their own interests for a secure and safe livelihood. The preoccupation with good health as precarious and difficult to maintain must have resonated with their own life experiences, where illness and disability frequently threatened economic survival.[65] The repeated attribution of vicious epidemics and debilitating diseases to immigrants in both medical and labor discourses through the nineteenth century had accrued in a domain of uncontested "common sense."

The sanitary consumption campaigns of the early twentieth century had renewed the infamous melding of racial danger, insidious health catastrophe, and unfair labor. The crosscutting discourses of race, nation, health, and gender that had shaped the campaigns for sanitary consumption would have an enduring legacy in labor and national politics. The discursive elements that had preoccupied nineteenth-century white labor leaders in relation to Chinese workers in the United States translated well into the dire, doomsday scenarios that animated twentieth-century labor rhetoric about foreign (usually Asian and Latin American) competition, particularly in the post–World War II period. Although union labor workers recognized themselves as the grateful subjects of public health reform of their own work sites and the improvement of their living circumstances, they remained vulnerable to any aberrant labor regime—a system characteristically identified by inhumanely low wages, unsanitary and unsafe working conditions, and the labor of the disenfranchised ("sweatshop" workers, prisoners, "colonized classes," and racial minorities). Labor union rhetoric about the potentially perilous decline of American workers in the wake of "foreign" competition mirrored public health reformers' concerns that "aberrant" behavior endangered the "normal" population or environment.

The progressive reform struggles to ensure sanitary factories and to discontinue practices such as child labor had tragically been caught in a vortex of racial fears and phobias endemic in the American experience. Rather than extend the struggle for public health reforms to vulnerable and disenfranchised populations, the labor unions maintained a racial limit to the definition of "public" in its application to practices of health and welfare—the very same limit the unions secured in the delineation of union membership. The visionary and noble fights for universal standards of health, labor, and livelihood were stymied by this racial limit. The restriction of progressive reform to true racial and national boundaries crippled the possibilities of labor solidarity as well as guaranteed the vulnerability of union workers and their families.

The labor movement's health consciousness had combined fears of alien Asian presence and production with the ever-threatened pursuit of "progress" and "improvement." Reformers, labor activists, and union men and women increasingly recognized that public health reform had made the vision of the American standard of living a plausible reality for a growing number of white working families. The management of three kinds of reproduction were at stake in reproducing the American standard of living. First, union leaders sought to ensure the reproduction of labor power. They struggled to preserve hard-won union improvements in working conditions and wage levels that ensured the capacity of white workingmen to secure the livelihoods of their dependent women and children. Second, labor advocates sought to advance the social reproduction of the home. Ensuring financial security for male wage earners would facilitate the removal of working women and children from factory and industrial home-work and therefore guarantee an idealized system of strictly separated gender roles and responsibilities for male breadwinners and female housewives. Male authority within the nuclear family would be maintained through this division of workplace and domestic space. And third, the embrace of the American standard of living would curtail the reproduction of germs and disease in the work site and in the home. Union demands for higher wages, shorter workdays, and sanitary work conditions maintained the health of the worker, enabled the improvement of living conditions for the worker's family, and assured the consumer of the hygienic purity of goods and production processes. The agenda of the American standard then tied the reproduction of labor, gender, and health to the pursuit of national progress and prosperity for American workingmen in their interrelated roles as producers, consumers, and citizens.

However, at any moment this "progress" could be undercut. The prospect of the invasion of contaminated consumer goods would not only infect an individual family but result in a horrid reversal of the reformist vision of social "progress" for the working class, the white race, and the American nation. "Progress," because of its inherent comparison to "aberration," sustained xenophobic fears. The specter of racialized threats would invariably haunt the American working class in its pursuit of the American standard of living. If the American standard of living was heralded as the achievement of the promise of "progress," then it was a precarious promise that was always under siege and liable to reversal.

# CHAPTER 7

# Making Medical Borders
# at Angel Island

It is indeed pitiable the harsh treatment of our fellow countrymen.
The doctor extracting blood caused us the greatest anguish.
Our stomachs are full of grievances, but to whom can we tell them?
We can but pace to and fro, scratch our heads, and question the blue sky.

Poem number 50 in *Island: Poetry and History of
Chinese Immigrants on Angel Island, 1910–1940*

From the turn of the century until 1940, the ordeal of immigration for
Chinese and other Asian migrants to San Francisco began with medical
inspection at Angel Island. The poem above, a translation of one of the
hundreds of poems carved on the walls of the Chinese detention barrack,
expresses the distress and helplessness that many Chinese immigrants
faced. On arrival, they confronted military-style examinations that were
commanded by uniformed white public health inspectors who barked
orders in English, with terse translations offered by Chinese subordi-
nates. Many immigrants found the often unexplained procedures painful and bewildering. Although the exact requirements of medical examination shifted over the period of Angel Island's operation, the required
submission to nude physical exams and the inspection of body parts,
and the demands to supply bodily substances, were remarkably consistent features throughout the period 1910 to 1940. There was no opportunity to object or withdraw one's body from scrutiny.

These medical examinations were part of an emerging worldwide network of quarantine and health inspection that served as the "imperial
defence" against the potential invasion of epidemic diseases into metropolitan ports in North America and Europe.[1] Along with the European
imperial powers, U.S. health authorities created information relays to
track the spread of epidemic diseases at ports throughout the globe from

Hong Kong to Rio de Janeiro. Public health officers sought to allay fears
that disease traveled with trade and migration. Responding to the widespread fears that immigrants carried disease into the American nation,
the federal government established measures to detect diseased aliens and
to deny them entry.[2] As quarantine intensified and immigration medical
exams developed, health became a crucial gauge in the management of
national borders.

Chinese immigrants experienced the most strenuous hurdles to legal
entry into the United States. The passage of and amendments to the Chinese Exclusion Acts (1882–1902) prohibited the immigration of Chinese
laborers, required registration and extensive documentation for Chinese
settlers, and denied them the opportunity of naturalized citizenship.[3]
The health-screening process presented further obstacles to settlement
in the United States. In the early twentieth century, immigration restrictions were extended to impede other Asian nationalities. Since San Francisco served as the principal Pacific Coast gateway for Asian commerce
and migration into the United States, Angel Island became the site of
special medical and immigration hurdles for Chinese, Japanese, Korean,
Filipino, and Asian Indian migrants.[4]

In the twentieth century, health-screening practices moved from quarantining epidemic diseases to screening for the fitness of future citizens.
PHS officers developed a range of techniques to coax "truth" from the
recalcitrant body and to interpret that truth. These techniques, loosely
gathered under the umbrella of medical purpose, can be analyzed as
three stages in the development of medical inspection practices. They
reveal different layers of medical sight and interpretation of the body.
The first technique involved the inspection of the naked body for suspect
symptoms that were visible on the skin or in the swelling of the glands.
Inspectors paid particular attention to swellings and lesions that indicated epidemic diseases such as bubonic plague or "loathsome" conditions such as leprosy. The second set of techniques scrutinized specific
organs to detect infections and defects. During the first decade of the
twentieth century, PHS officers carefully inspected eyes for ailments that
could impair sight and therefore lead to disability. The PHS's third set
involved examination of the body beneath the skin through the microscopic inspection of internal fluids or waste products to detect traces of
internal parasites. Parasites caused fatigue and declining productivity,
yet the sufferer displayed no visible sign of ailment.

Each new layer of visual scrutiny revealed hidden threats, which, the
PHS confidently asserted, only their specialized expertise could deci-

pher. With their increasingly specialized expertise, the PHS projected an image of unequivocal confidence in scientific diagnosis to both the detainees and the American public. The PHS used science's claims of objectivity and disinterested inquiry to place its policies above politics. Scientific forms of knowledge dominated the often heated medical debates and even mainstream political criticisms of disease screening.[5]

As the truth of the immigrant's health shifted away from the physical examination of the body and toward the bacteriological examination of the body's fluids and wastes, PHS officers developed a scientific knowledge of race that became increasingly enmeshed in a framework of bodily norms and aberrations. Scientists and administrators of the time and historians of the period have proclaimed that bacteriology's focus on germs, "the most democratic creatures in the word," would overthrow a parochial reliance on invidious distinctions of race and class.[6] How was it that, far from making race irrelevant, the PHS's use of bacteriology made racial assumptions crucial to its own system of border control? Why did the pursuit of "invisible germs" produce new thresholds for the visibility of social difference? How did the PHS's system of inspection produce an understanding of bodily norms that ignited exceptional vigilance against aberration that was interpreted in racial and class terms? And how was it possible that the anomalous procedures imposed on Chinese, Asian Indian, and Japanese migrants at Angel Island became justified in PHS explanations as part of a system of universally applied border controls?

Through the process of medical inspection on Angel Island, other forms of knowing were also produced about bodies in transit. The power struggles over naming and defining a body and its excludable defects and diseases produced a range of different epistemic positions. In Guangdong villages, onboard the ships, on Angel Island, and in Chinese communities in the United States, Chinese men and women exchanged knowledge about the experience of invasive examination that countered PHS claims about their bodies and the necessity of inspection. The traces of this immensely varied subaltern public sphere persist in a textual historical record found in the poetry Chinese men wrote on the Angel Island barrack walls; in the satirical editorials published in Chinese newspapers in San Francisco; in the coaching papers that offered prospective immigrants strategies by which to negotiate border obstacles; and in the oral histories that suggest the stories, gossip, and advice that Chinese women and men shared. These forms of knowledge, which disputed the official, scientific positions, were often ridiculed or ignored in the dominant record of policy debates. Since PHS medical officers and U.S. politicians perceived the Chinese and other arriving Asians as "alien" and unlikely to ever become American citizen-subjects, the American elite ignored the subjectivity and the agency of the Chinese "aliens."

Chinese detainees insisted on explaining their reality and seizing a position from which to speak. Many of the Chinese who were detained left behind poems, either written in ink or carved on the walls of the barracks, that tell tales of the suffering caused by detention on Angel Island. They sought to impart their experiences to those who followed them from Guangdong province. The poetry came to public attention thirty-five years after the government closed its Angel Island immigration station. In the late 1970s, San Francisco Chinese American activists and community historians fought successfully to halt destruction of the Chinese detention barracks and preserve the poems. Chinese American community historians translated and compiled the poetry. In all they collected 135 poems. The poems followed classical style and form, and the majority of the poems were undated and unsigned. The poems that have been preserved were written by literate men. Most immigrants did not have formal schooling beyond the primary grades, and often the poems violate rules of rhyme and tone required in Chinese poetry. Community historians have supplemented these poems with extensive interviews with the detainees who successful entered the United States. The oral histories were supplied by both Chinese women and men during the late 1970s and 1980s. Although the poems offer the more immediate expressions of anger, frustration, and depression at being in detention, the oral histories provide remarkable details about the everyday experience of detention and reflect the continued impact of the experience after decades of life in the United States. The poems, along with the oral histories, offer rare insight into the subjectivity and perspective of the detainees.[7]

Throughout this chapter, I have included barrack-wall poetry and satirical Chinese American press reports in order to emphasize the dramatic and often irreconcilable contests in the politics of bodies and their well-being during their forced encounter with the U.S. state. The PHS officials and scientists grudgingly acknowledged but dismissed the satire by Chinese journalists as well as the official representations of Chinese elite commercial interests by Chinese diplomats. However, Chinese barrack-wall poetry was ignored by the PHS officials, who had already disqualified any knowledge produced by the alien, the patient, or the ill-person as naive and beneath the required level of detached cognition or scientificness. Although denied, these Chinese insisted on explaining their reality and seizing a position from which to speak. Yet even with these re-markable recoveries there are limits to a historian's ability to assess the full dimensions of the subjectivity of Chinese detainees on Angel Island, since all of those who could write the poetry and the newspaper satires were literate men. It is even less possible to know the stories of those who were not male or not of the literate classes, or, in the case of oral histories, of those who failed to surmount immigration hurdles.

## ROUTINES OF INSPECTION

Inspecting travelers for signs of illness had its origins in nineteenth-century quarantine procedures. In San Francisco, quarantine in the 1870s targeted ships from Asia in order to prevent "invoices of small-pox" from China.[8] Quarantine was a low-threshold filter intended to thwart the spread of acute, contagious infections such as cholera, yellow fever, and bubonic plague. The target of investigation could involve per-sons, animals, commercial goods, or the ship's hull.[9] At many U.S. sea-ports, local authorities handled quarantine procedures until the last decade of the nineteenth century and applied general principles of in-spection, isolation, and fumigation in order to neutralize contagion.[10]

When the federal government consolidated quarantine responsibili-ties, it built permanent quarantine facilities at the busiest ports, includ-ing the Angel Island facility at the mouth of San Francisco's harbor. In 1890, two decades before permanent immigration facilities were con-structed, the Angel Island Quarantine Station boasted a hospital, fumi-gation building, and separate bathing facilities and barracks for all cabin-class and Chinese steerage passengers. Under the direction of the PHS, medical officers developed systematic procedures for disinfecting cargo, people, and ships to screen out contagious diseases such as smallpox, cholera, and typhoid.[11] In 1891, following a U.S. legislature mandate, PHS officers began to conduct health inspections of all arriving immi-grants and travelers.[12] Different stations developed specific procedures to respond to the call for mandatory exams. At Angel Island, when steerage passengers arrived for disinfection the PHS officers used the op-portunity to scrutinize the bodies of Chinese and Japanese immigrants by sending them to bathe. In the 1890s the medical gaze focused on the signs of epidemic diseases, particularly bubonic plague and cholera, which were believed to be infiltrating the United States from East Asia.[13] The PHS employed bathing not only for the disinfection advantages of "using soap liberally and vigorously" but also for the unparalleled opportunity to "discover glandular swellings and eruptions" that were the diagnostic signs of bubonic plague.[14] Hugh Cummings, the chief quarantine officer, valued any procedure that required the disrobing of arriving immigrants because it enabled the "careful examination of the individual."[15] The exam of the naked body could reap unexpected revelations, such as evidence of leprosy or hernia.[16]

Steerage and cabin passengers experienced different levels of scrutiny at the San Francisco quarantine station. Onboard the ship, a medical officer would examine all steerage passengers on the deck for quarantinable diseases such as smallpox and cholera. He would also make preliminary assessments of visible "physical defects and deformities" that would be more thoroughly investigated on Angel Island.[17] Then, the upper-class cabin passengers would be examined in the privacy of the passengers' rooms and without the kind of invasive physical contact and public examination that was routinely applied to steerage passengers. Cabin passengers were less susceptible to disease, PHS officers believed, because they could afford better sanitary conditions and nourishment on ship, and because cabin passengers supposedly possessed "higher intelligence to exercise a certain amount of self-care."[18] Medical inspectors also took special care to protect the health of cabin passengers and protect them from any transfer of disease in the medical inspection process. They guaranteed cabin passengers that the thermometers they used were "thoroughly disinfected" between uses.[19] PHS officers treated upper-class passengers with "discretion," providing them with the illusion of privacy. The classes of accommodation also masked racial distinctions. At Angel Island, the steerage passengers were most likely to be Asian immigrants, while cabin passengers were most likely to be white, usually U.S. citizens or European visitors.[20]

During the medical exam on Angel Island, steerage passengers received more intensive individual and physical scrutiny than those that arrived at Ellis Island in New York, where 70 percent of all immigrants to the United States arrived.[21] Upon arrival on Angel Island, Chinese men and women were led to sex-segregated barracks, where they deposited their luggage. Unlike at Ellis Island, men and women were examined separately at Angel Island because of the intrusive nature of the physical examination. In the examination of Chinese men, a PHS officer would command the detainees to line up and strip to the waist for the physical exam. Mr. Leung, a twenty-four-year-old at the time of his detention on Angel Island in 1936, recalled that "a whole bunch of us had to take off all our clothes like marching soldiers." The PHS officers in-

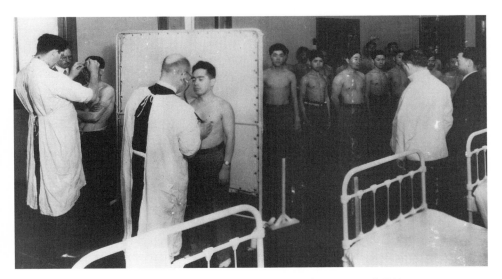

Figure 9. Public Health Service officers conduct a medical inspection of Chinese men at Angel Island Immigration Station, 1923. Courtesy National Archives at College Park, RG 090-G-152–2039.

spected the men's "teeth, ears, and nose" and conducted a stethoscope examination of the chest, and then took them "individually behind a ward screen," where each man was "completely stripped" in order to reveal any "abnormalities" below the waist. Chinese women underwent a less rigorous physical exam: PHS officers did not ask women to disrobe unless they detected specific signs of disease. In the twentieth century, two new procedures were added to the medical exam. First, all arriving immigrants had their eyelids everted for signs of trachoma infection. Second, after 1910, the detainees were sent to line up at the toilets and handed tin basins. Both men and women were required to "furnish a specimen of feces for hookworm examination." Afterward, the attendants offered the detainees denim uniforms to wear while their clothes were sent to be disinfected.[22] (See Figure 9.)

The medical examination of immigrants developed in tandem with other early twentieth-century systems of mass screening of healthy persons for disease and defects, such as the medical examination of applicants for life insurance, industrial employment, primary school education, and military service. Rather than addressing specific symptoms of illness in an individual patient, physicians developed new procedures for the new technique of examining healthy people. The immigration medical exam, like the exams instituted for insurance and the military conscription, sought to measure fitness and detect defects in a broad spectrum of the population. These large-scale health-screening processes were instrumental in identifying the norms of health and in applying the eugenic criteria of fitness.[23]

Although both quarantine and immigrant health exams ostensibly erected barriers to "contagion," the focus of medical scrutiny diverged. Unlike quarantine's focus on acute infectious disease, health exams of immigrants began to develop criteria of fitness and identified endemic illnesses that might have long-term consequences for the productive capacity of the arriving immigrant. Politicians and immigration authorities increasingly turned to physicians to arbitrate the grounds of immigrant exclusion. Although deportation never exceeded 3 percent annually from 1890 to 1924, medical certification became the increasingly dominant reason for deportation. In 1898 less than 2 percent of total deportations were for medical reasons, but by 1913 medical reasons accounted for 57 percent of deportations and reached 69 percent in 1916. Medical exclusion overshadowed the formerly "subjective" deportation criteria, such as subversive and anarchical political activities, criminality, and prostitution. Public health officials and politicians perceived medical screening as unfettered by politics and subjective judgments, even though they frequently designated specific races and ethnic groups to be "unfit" for entry.[24]

Despite the increasingly decisive role of medical certification, PHS medical inspectors positioned themselves as detached and objective, valued qualities in the creation of a scientific bureaucracy. The aura of objectivity insulated PHS physicians from accusations of political bias and prejudice. Although PHS officials refused to serve on the U.S. Immigration Service Boards of Special Inquiry where final appeals were reviewed, the PHS medical inspectors were comfortably ensconced in the formal machinery of medical exclusion.[25] Immigration and PHS officers were aware of the need for swift, scientific, and unassailable medical diagnosis and the necessity to adjust diagnoses to conform to administrative categories of exclusion.[26] The considerable confusion about, and variation in, the diagnostic interpretation of eye and parasite diseases in the first quarter of the century were a vexing problem for both immigration and medical authorities eager to put political judgments under the cloak of scientific objectivity.

## OPTICAL ILLUSIONS AND THE DIAGNOSIS OF TRACHOMA

In the first decade of the twentieth century, trachoma was the signature disease of medical exclusion. Trachoma as a proportion of medical deportations rose rapidly and paralleled the rise in medical deportations generally. Its swift dominance and sudden decline in medical certifications demonstrated how "epidemic" phenomena can be produced through the development of diagnostic methods and medical definition. In 1900 most of the trachoma certifications occurred at Ellis Island in New York, but within five years the diagnostic techniques and interpretation were applied at the other immigration stations, from Galveston to San Francisco. In 1900, only 1 in 1,631 immigrant arrivals had trachoma, but by 1908 it was nearly 1 in 300. In 1900 eye exams were administered only to those migrants with visible symptoms such as granules and inflammation around the eye. Medical deportations rose sharply after 1903, when excludable diseases were systematized and trachoma became one of two "contagious diseases" that would result in immediate exclusion.[27] Medical opinion considered trachoma a contagious disease that could in extreme cases result in blindness. In 1905 all immigrants at Ellis Island were subjected to eye exams; officers used buttonhooks or fingers to evert eyelids and discover the sores that were trachoma's telltale sign. In 1908 there were over 2,900 medical deportations, and nearly 90 percent of those deported were certified as having trachoma.[28]

PHS supervisors insisted that its officers fold various diagnoses into the official administrative definitions of disease in order to ensure ample numbers of trachoma certifications and deportations.[29] Officers at Angel Island were instructed to refrain from making diagnoses such as "granular eyelids," "granular conjunctivitis," or "folliclosis," no matter how accurate or medically sound. Similar inflammatory eye diseases generated unwelcome ambiguity for administrators, eager to distinguish trachoma from other unhealthy eye conditions that were not grounds for exclusion. The regulatory power of the trachoma diagnosis made PHS supervisors all the more suspicious of diagnoses that approximated trachoma.[30]

Heated debates about trachoma's symptoms and contagiousness within the PHS and the medical profession nationwide bedeviled the quest for uniform diagnosis.[31] In 1905 the PHS was embarrassed by contradictory diagnoses of the same immigrant by PHS inspectors in San Francisco and a PHS inspector stationed to certify U.S.–bound passengers in Victoria, British Columbia. The inconsistency gave critics within both the medical profession and the public grounds to question the PHS's definition of trachoma.[32] The clinical expertise of PHS officers was enlisted to account for the discrepancies in trachoma certification. Many officers, faced with symptoms that ran counter to textbook cases, developed explanations for the peculiarities of the "Oriental" race. Dr. Victor G. Geiser, chief quarantine officer in the Philippine Islands, argued that the "poor physical state of the average Oriental" was responsible for all kinds of inflammatory eye conditions. Trachoma in "Orientals" was endemic and impervious to the treatment that would successfully heal "another race."[33] Putative racial differences also influenced ideas about immunity. Dr. Carl Remeus, who had inspected immigrants in Honolulu and at Ellis Island, explained that "white races" suffered from "dangerous complications" from trachoma infection, but that "Asiatics" had relatively mild cases of trachoma because of their alleged hereditary immunity developed through thousands of years of contact with the disease.[34] These theories of the peculiar Asian susceptibility and inheritance instantiated a racial hierarchy in the medical knowledge of trachoma. Despite differences in their conclusions, all of the scientists measured trachoma in Asians as abnormal against the typical experiences of eastern and southern Europeans and against the norms of vulnerable health in western Europeans.

The theories about racial susceptibility and immunity underscored the insistence on racial measurement during this period. In this era, the sciences of phrenology and eugenics were not alone in assiduously tabulating the relationship between physical differences and race.[35] Despite claims that Europeans were more vulnerable to acute trachoma infection than Asians, PHS statistics revealed that Asian and Middle Eastern immigrants were far more frequently diagnosed with trachoma and deported than the European immigrants. In a study of trachoma diagnosis at all immigration stations from 1908 to 1910 in the United States, the PHS officer Victor Safford concluded that Chinese, Japanese, Syrian, and Asian Indian immigrants were more likely to be certified for trachoma than the most "susceptible" southern and eastern European "races." Among eastern and southern European groups, less than 1 percent of all immigrant arrivals were certified for trachoma. However, Asians experienced sharply higher ratios of trachoma detection, with as many as 8 percent and 11 percent of immigrant arrivals from China and India, respectively, being deported for trachoma.[36] These statistics revealed the increased vulnerability of Japanese, Asian Indian, Syrian, and Korean immigrants to medical deportations.

Among PHS officers there was a "wide divergence of views on trachoma," and diagnoses depended on the "personal equation of the observer."[37] However, PHS officers were confident that the discovery of a "specific microbe of trachoma" would provide an incontrovertible standard for diagnosis and systematize immigration health controls.[38] The hunt for such a microbe proved elusive. Physical observation and description, with the attendant dependence on the vagaries of "personal" interpretation, prevailed. However, PHS officers continued to rely on characteristics such as racial bodies and racial geographies to arrest the perceived external traffic in trachoma infection. When new, bacteriologically detected, parasite diseases emerged in 1910 at Angel Island, the proportion of deportations for trachoma detection dropped off sharply. In 1909 the proportion of trachoma certification of all medical exclusions hovered at 60 percent. Two years later, in 1911, the proportion had plummeted to 8 percent. Despite this severe drop in trachoma certifications, the overall number of medical deportations remained steady because hookworm had replaced trachoma as the leading cause of medical exclusion.[39]

## DETECTING "PARASITES"

The rapid proliferation of hookworm diagnoses ushered in a new era in immigration health exams. Prior to the establishment of a full-scale bacteriological laboratory on Angel Island in 1910, PHS officers relied upon the techniques of physical observation to interpret the health of immigrants. The new bacteriology, with its reliance on microscopic slides and germ cultures, provided a new means of visualizing the body beneath the skin. PHS officers drew blood and feces samples from the immigrants and, under the microscope, isolated the traces of intestinal parasites.

In the twentieth century, bacteriological examinations became a unique but vital technique in the health screening of Asian immigrants. In the late nineteenth century, bacteriological exams were a precautionary measure that supplemented the physical exams, particularly to address suspicions of bubonic plague and cholera. During the era of bubonic plague epidemics, from 1900 to 1908, bacteriological testing became a ritual of scientific confirmation and buttressed the PHS's authority in plague detection within San Francisco.[40] During the plague epidemics the PHS bacteriological laboratory had been located in the city, which limited its use for immigration inspection. In 1910, with the consolidation of the Angel Island Quarantine Station with the new Angel Island Immigration Station, PHS officers were able to pursue bacteriological testing of Asian immigrants who were already detained for other illnesses or who awaited immigration interviews.

The testing for hookworm in Asian immigrants developed from just such detention practices. In September 1910, after inspections onboard an incoming steamer, the PHS inspector M. W. Glover detained six Asian Indian men at the Angel Island Hospital with an initial diagnosis of anemia. After conducting tests of their feces, Glover determined that they had hookworm. What was visible under the microscope were the eggs of the hookworm parasite. Glover extrapolated that these eggs indicated that the parasite lived within the individual's stomach and intestine.[41] Glover ordered feces examinations of all Asian Indian men already in the hospital and found the hookworm ova present in over 70 percent of the Asian Indian patients.[42]

Bacteriological examination's success in providing visible evidence of infection prompted Glover to extend mandatory examinations to all Asian Indian and Chinese passengers. The investigations merged the two groups into the category of "Asian" and confirmed suspicions that all Asian immigrants were liable to be infected by "parasites," even when they demonstrated no visible signs of suffering or incapacitation. These apparently healthy "carriers" harbored a variety of dangerous portable pathogens in their bodies—hookworm, whipworm, and roundworm. These pathogens left the host unaffected but, Glover feared, would have devastating effects on unsuspecting white Americans.[43] Bacteriology opened a new visual layer to medical interpretation, and, with the discovery of the hookworm parasite in the "healthy carrier," microscopic examination supplanted physical observation of the epidermal body.[44]

At the turn of the century, medical scientists had identified hookworm as a disease condition with symptoms of anemia, diarrhea, and slight fever. The parasite caused those afflicted to suffer from lethargy and to experience diminished mental and physical development. It was not considered fatal, but the parasite was expected to remain in the human host for ten years.[45] Hookworm was often referred to the as the "germ of laziness," and it explained both the poverty of its sufferers, given the body's diminished physical capacity, and their disinterest in low-wage labor. PHS officers and the Rockefeller Foundation medical researchers developed campaigns to eradicate hookworm in the rural South and the newly colonized territories of Puerto Rico and the Philippines.[46]

The use of hookworm diagnosis to bar Asian Indian migrants reinvigorated campaigns on the Pacific Coast by labor organizations and sympathetic newspapers to limit Asian Indian immigration. Nearly seven thousand Punjabi men immigrated to the United States during the peak immigration years of 1907–11 before immigration restrictions were imposed. Many Punjabis worked on railway construction, at lumber mills, and on farms. The *San Francisco Bulletin* hailed Dr. Glover's discovery as "an effective dam to the torrent of Hindu immigration which has been surging the shores of the Pacific Coast at a speed of 5,000 of India's riff-raff a year." [47] Although many of these men followed the Sikh faith, the migrants were both matter of factly and derisively referred to as "Hindus." [48] The use of bacteriological knowledge to bar immigration particularly fascinated white labor leaders, who perceived Asian Indian immigrants as the new "Asiatic menace" for the white labor market. [49] Soon after news of the bacteriological detection of hookworm broke in the news media in 1910, the Asiatic Exclusion League endorsed the mandatory bacteriological examination of Asian immigrants to detect hookworm and other parasite diseases. [50] White labor leaders concluded that all "Orientals" should be subject to the same strict immigration barriers that had been erected against Chinese arrivals, since any Asian immigration was an "invitation" to epidemic disease and presented "grave perils to American health." [51]

Prior to Dr. Glover's discovery of hookworm, the PHS officers at Angel Island had been acutely aware of the controversy surrounding Asian Indian immigrants. The bacteriological testing of anemic Asian Indian immigrants in September 1910 had been spurred by an internal crisis over medical exclusion procedures. In May 1910 an Immigration Service (IS) officer had accused the Angel Island immigration commissioner Hart H. North of corruption and negligence in medical exclusion procedures. One of the complaints lodged was that many Asian Indian migrants with "poor physique" were allowed entry even though they had been designated as likely to become public charges. During the investigation, Glover testified that IS officers were not qualified to make judgments about the "physical capability" of the immigrant to earn a living without conducting a full medical exam. [52] In a move calculated to bolster the PHS's authority to determine physical fitness, Glover employed bacteriological tests to provide specialized knowledge of an immigrant's capabilities and the precise cause of an immigrant's disability. Popular anti-Hindu politics and the IS controversy emboldened Glover to demand time-consuming bacteriological exams of all Asian Indian immigrants. [53] Glover was fully conscious of the political effect of this power when he boasted in his annual report that the hookworm exam "was a large factor in stopping the influx of East Indians into this country." [54]

Glover enthusiastically championed Angel Island's capabilities in bacteriological examination for the unparalleled PHS research and training facilities it would provide in the field of tropical medicine. The volume and variety of immigration from Asia, he claimed, provided an "excellent opportunity for study of intestinal parasites as the supply of material is large and constantly new." [55] Glover freely used hospital patients as laboratory specimens, in one case administering an anthelmintic drug to extract "a hundred or more of the worms themselves" from one Asian Indian patient.[56] This use of detainees for medical experimentation without their consent was a standard practice in the formation of medical disciplines and demonstrated how bodies were made instrumental for medical data prior to the advent of patient's rights.[57]

Glover's desire to make Angel Island a laboratory for tropical disease research spurred sarcastic commentary from Chinese activists and journalists in San Francisco. The *Chinese Defender* satirized the inventiveness of the PHS: "So the arriving immigrants are now to have hookworm. Somebody must have stayed awake nights to think that out; it surely was a stroke of genius!" The *Defender* editorial characterized hookworm diagnosis as an arbitrary and petulant act that relied on inventing fictions comparable to the fantastic stories of Grimm's fairy tales.[58] The PHS's explanation of hookworm as a parasite that slowly consumed and incapacitated the human body from within but often manifested no immediate symptoms heightened suspicions about the fictive character of hookworm infection.

Despite protests to the contrary, PHS officers did target Asian groups for mandatory bacteriological exams. In hookworm investigations, they singled out Chinese steerage and second-class cabin passengers who were already detained, awaiting immigration hearings. In 1913, Chinese were examined for hookworm prior to embarkation in Hong Kong. Asian Indian male laborers and Japanese "picture brides" were also considered suspect, and mandatory hookworm exams were ordered for them as well. The latter two groups constituted high-risk groups because of their rural and agricultural origins, where parasites were presumed to be endemic.[59]

Bacteriological inquiry into the immigrants made new layers of the body available to medical sight. Through the examination of fluids such as blood and of waste products such as feces, bacteriology generated visible knowledge of new pathogens and multiplied the number of medical conditions that barred immigrant entry. In 1910 the PHS classified hookworm and threadworm (filariasis), and in 1917 added liver fluke (clonor-chiasis), as excludable diseases that were likely to make the sufferer be-come a public charge. These disease conditions linked disability with an immigrant's potential fitness for employment. The legislators and PHS officers feared that the parasite diseases could produce future disability and dependency that would strain community charity and state coffers.

Like the examination of feces to observe hookworm, the drawing of blood to test for filariasis drew suspicion from journalists and Chinese American leaders. The curious procedures became the subject of protest and ridicule when the *San Francisco Chronicle* reported on the theatrical strategies employed by the PHS to defend its diagnosis of threadworm in Chinese immigrants. The *Chronicle* reported that at midnight on Angel Island a group of attorneys, officials, physicians, and Chinese diplomats surrounded Lin Shee, a Chinese boy who had been brought unwillingly into the circle. Dr. Glover, "the immigration surgeon who discovered hookworm in the Hindus," cut Lin Shee's "right ear . . . until the blood dripped, while they gazed in rapt attention at the ruddy gore." The scene was reminiscent of the arcane sacrifice rituals of a cult or the initiation theatrics of an elite male club but was conducted in the "interest of sci-ence and immigration laws." The *Chronicle* writer mocked Glover's pro-cedures and the "scientific" purpose of the test's "peculiar" timing: "the filaria circulate only at midnight, and to catch them it is necessary to get the suspect's blood at that hour of the night."[60] The *Chinese Defender* ridiculed the demonstration of "midnight examinations" and the "shed-ding of blood" as evidence of the intimidation and terror experienced by Chinese immigrants. The skeptical journalists emphasized the scene of extraction of blood and ignored the scene of the laboratory identifi-cation of filaria residues from the blood. This perspective supported the position of the Chinese consul and attorneys who protested that the ter-ror produced in the scene of contact between arriving immigrant and physician could not be justified in the laboratory results of filaria infec-tion. Both the protesters and the journalists expressed extreme ambiva-lence in redirecting authoritative medical diagnosis away from the phys-ical encounter of physician and immigrant and in making the laboratory a privileged site of medical knowledge. Their skepticism was shared by many physicians, who doubted the diagnosis furnished through the new bacteriological world of germ cultures and microscopes.[61]

Federal immigration authorities dismissed protests about the "humil-iating or mutilating practices" and earnestly defended the procedures in innocuous clinical language. The exam for threadworm, for instance, re-

quired the "pricking of the alien's finger or ear lobe with a sterilized surgeon's needle, and the drawing of a drop of blood." The blood sample
could provide invaluable results for the officials in their mandate to
identify "infected" bodies. These tests were "incidentally" valuable to
the arriving immigrants, since those who could know the true "nature
of their affliction can take proper measures to cure themselves."[62]

The bacteriological examination only further distanced the arriving
immigrant from possessing control over the "true nature" of their bodies and heightened the adversarial character of the medical inspection
process. Since the diagnosis of parasites had only a "incidental" relationship to treatment, the "infected" immigrant was even more vulnerable to the systems of immigration and medical control. In certain instances, when the PHS did offer treatment options, the procedures and
their impact on the body were rarely explained. At the PHS hospital,
hookworm was treated with thymol, which loosened the worms from
the intestinal wall, allowing them to be expelled.[63] Mrs. Chin, who was
detained for two weeks at Angel Island in 1913, described the disori-
enting experience of the medical therapy required to "flush" hookworm
out of her system. She took the medicine three times a day and had to
refrain from eating. She recalled the effect of the medicine: "Your body
started feeling as weak as a snake's. You would walk to the hillside and
lay down like a drunkard." The following day the attendants gave Mrs.
Chin a pan for another feces examination. "Even if you didn't have any-
thing to go, you forced it out. After they examined it, overnight, they
would give you a little something to eat. Then you had to be examined
again. If you were cleared, you could go."[64] Once the hookworm parasite was flushed out of the body, one could enter the United States. However, the Chinese detainees perceived that the hookworm diagnosis
made them subject to medical authority and practices they did not understand. They did not perceive themselves to be under benevolent medical care. The willingness to accept the medical treatment, even by those
who were bewildered, was perceived by PHS officers as an acceptance of
their diagnosis and a willingness to accept modern health instruction.

Although they were obliged to submit to examination and treatment,
many Chinese were skeptical about the validity of the medical diagnosis:
One poet rejected the idea that his diagnosis, which he called the "the
shadow of hookworm," was serious enough to warrant his detention
and questioned why the cost of the hospitalization was borne by the immigrant. Another poet wrote of his hatred for white "barbarians" who
"continually promulgate harsh laws to show off their prowess" and char-

acterized hookworm exams as evidence of their "hundreds of despotic acts."[65] This poet refused to grant the medical officials any scientific legitimacy in the pursuit of their inspection for disease but rather perceived it as an arrogant abuse of power. Others considered the test results to be fraudulent. Mr. Tong, who at the age of seventeen was detained for two months in 1921, shared a story popular among former Angel Island detainees: "Before I came to Angel Island, I knew of a friend who shared his feces with another immigrant who couldn't eliminate at the moment. It was the same feces, but do you know, one was found to have hookworms and other didn't!" This story circulated as a grim joke to lessen the pain of seemingly arbitrary diagnosis. The PHS procedures of impersonal testing, forced treatment, payment demands, and indefinite detention heightened the arriving immigrant's sense of humiliating dependency. One poet wished to escape the "humiliation and oppression by the devils." He refused to perceive himself as ill, revealing his resistance to the PHS's quest to know his body and make its care dependent on their expertise.[66] The PHS championed scientific logic and the police practices of detention not to enable social and health change in an arriving immigrant but to neutralize a potential health hazard.[67]

The special scrutiny of Asians at Angel Island became apparent when Chinese began arriving at Atlantic Coast ports. In 1923 the immigration station in Boston was unprepared to conduct "satisfactory examination of Chinese aliens" when the Canadian Pacific Railroad began regularly transporting Chinese from St. John, New Brunswick, Canada, to Boston. Although Boston PHS officers were aware of intestinal parasites, they never had occasion to conduct full-scale, routine bacteriological examinations before the arrival of Chinese immigrants.[68] Following the racialized expectation that they were infected with hookworms, Chinese immigrants were also singled out for testing for filariasis and other parasites. The Boston station lacked the laboratory equipment to conduct a large number of bacteriological exams, but ordered more equipment once Chinese immigration became a regular facet of their work. The bacteriological protocol developed at Angel Island followed Chinese immigrants throughout the PHS system.[69]

Chinese American community organizations and Chinese diplomats mounted challenges to the PHS testing practices. In November 1910, the Chinese consulate and the Chinese Consolidated Benevolent Association had hired local physicians and professors of tropical medicine to testify that filaria was not directly communicable in North American conditions. One expert argued that a person infected with filaria could

"live in this community without being a menace to its health," was unlikely to become a public charge, and would benefit from a change in
climate.[70] Dr. King Kwan claimed that one could be a parasite carrier
without being a threat, in his challenge to federal officials to subject
themselves to a test for the "filaria germ," insinuating that they too were
probable disease carriers.[71] Kwan's challenge called into question several key assumptions in PHS social policy on parasites. The first is the
perception that a healthy body must be a pure body, independent of the
existence of any other organisms. In order for the body to be pure, it had
to be bound within its own flesh, closed off from its ecological context.
The very process of transmission of the parasite was alarming in the
ways in which it made vulnerable the pure, bounded body of the middle-
class ideal.[72] Parasites were considered to be foreign entities that poisoned and contaminated the body. The idea of the human carrier who
was able to transport pathogens but remain unaffected by the presence
of foreign organisms was deeply alarming to PHS officers, who feared
the possible harm to unsuspecting Americans and the potential financial
burden to the community. The judgment collapsed the identification of
a parasite organism within the body with the status of being a social parasite and dependent.

The conflation of the internal parasite and the social parasite had been
amplified in the political discourse on the health dangers of Asian immigration to the productive capacity of white Americans. Charles T. Nesbitt, health director of Wilmington, North Carolina, who testified before
the U.S. House of Representatives, claimed that Asia was the "fountain"
of the "most destructive pestilence" in recorded history and that Asians
have consequently "acquired such a high state of immunity to [its] effects that they have been unconscious carriers." In Nesbitt's mind, immunity produced stronger, more dangerous bodies that became carriers
that could destroy the health of a putatively parasite-free "white race."
He perceived Asian immigrants as likely to "introduce among whites on
the Pacific Slope insidious chronic diseases which will subject them to
physical deterioration." He feared that these "parasitic diseases, just as
capable of destroying the efficiency of the white race (as the hookworm
disease)," but with fatal consequences, were likely to infiltrate from
China, Japan, and India.[73] Nesbitt's fears of future infection drew from
the recent experience of hookworm in the South, where the PHS had
demonstrated that hookworm infection affected substantial portions of
the poor, agricultural black and white populations and was increasingly
found to disrupt the productivity of white factory workers in the South.[74]

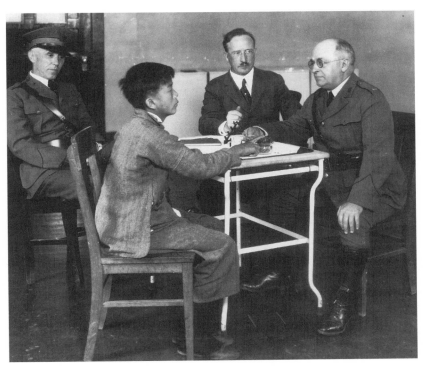

Figure 10. Public Health Service and Immigration Service officers interrogate a Chinese immigrant at a meeting of the Board of Special Medical Inquiry, Angel Island, 1923. Photo by the commercial photographer P. E. Brooks. Courtesy National Archives at College Park, RG 090-G-124–479.

Unlike immigration interrogations that required oral verifications of "authentic" life narratives and relied upon the subjective judgment of officers, medical investigation provided seemingly incontrovertible evidence of an individual's fitness for entry based on a normative notion of good health. Medical officers believed that immigrants could not be "coached" in health as they could be in the nuances of village geography and family relationships. The medical criteria, U.S. authorities believed, provided universal and objective criteria for entrance. They refused to acknowledge that special immigration procedures faced by the Chinese and, later, other Asian immigrant groups provided the PHS with a special opportunity to conduct bacteriological tests even when physical appearance gave no grounds for suspicion, and that the racialized expectations of disease were justified by the results of the examinations. (See Figure 10.)

## RESISTING MEDICAL PREROGATIVES

During the era of bacteriological examinations for the detection of parasite diseases, the PHS insulated itself within the arena of science. Through
the relentless championing of science as the only legitimate language for
dispute, the PHS foreclosed the exchange of crucial information among
the objects of medical scrutiny. Both the *Chinese Defender* and the CCBA
in two separate challenges to PHS policy employed medical expertise in
varying degrees to legitimate their opposition, complying with and mo-
bilizing the prevailing scientific logic of the regulatory structures. Thus,
not only were Chinese community organizations and periodicals forced
to employ medical expertise in their protests, but they had already ac-
ceded to the PHS philosophy that disease and ill-health were foreign conditions that justified strenuous border screening and exclusion policies.

The singling out of certain groups for intensive investigation drew legal challenges. In 1921 two Chinese merchants, Pang Hing and Hee Fuk
Yuen, filed federal lawsuits questioning the administration of immigration medical inspections. Both men had been denied reentry to the United
States after being certified at Angel Island as having liver fluke. People
afflicted with clonorchiasis have enlarged livers, bloody diarrhea, and
symptomatic jaundice. Their lawyer, Jackson Ralston, argued that the
targeting of Chinese immigrants reflected an "unequal administration
of the law," comparable to the San Francisco laundry regulations successfully challenged in *Yick Wo v. Hopkins* (1885). Ralston argued that
"Caucasian passengers no matter what class or nationality are exempt
from the microscopic test of their feces, only the Oriental alien traveling
in other than first class accommodations . . . is required to submit to a
specimen for microscopic tests." [75] The PHS had linked liver fluke infection to the Chinese and Japanese diet of raw fish and used this cultural
specificity to justify special racial hurdles for immigrant entry. The federal appeals courts and the Supreme Court affirmed that the cultural susceptibility could be a criteria for special investigation and that the practice of not testing all white and Asian first-class passengers could not be
interpreted as discriminatory or as "withholding of the rights of Chinese
persons." [76]

The Pang Hing case also challenged the administrative authority of
the surgeon general to designate a disease "loathsome and contagious"
without any opportunity for external review. The attorneys raised questions about the contagiousness of liver fluke and brought to the courts

the testimony of experts in parasite diseases who cast doubt on the threat the disease posed to others in the United States. The federal courts, however, were unwilling to intervene in the administrative authority of the surgeon general. On appeal, the attorneys for Pang Hing emphasized the dangers of allowing the surgeon general's dubious classifications to remain unaccountable and "invulnerable to judicial attack." They attacked the classification of liver fluke, describing it as an "abuse" of the surgeon general's authority since internal PHS studies indicated that not a single Chinese death had been attributable to liver fluke and that in North America there existed no intermediate hosts to transmit the disease to other humans. The Ninth Circuit Court of Appeals affirmed the authority of the surgeon general to classify dangerous contagious diseases and concluded that PHS officers were warranted in narrowing their investigation to "second-class Oriental passengers only," since the source of the disease was "supposed to be a diet of raw fish." [77]

The federal courts limited the grounds for challenges to the policy to persuading the PHS to change disease classifications. In its campaign against clonorchiasis certification, the CCBA hired attorneys to gather medical evidence that liver fluke was not contagious and to lobby the PHS to develop clinical cures for the disease.[78] They proposed to equip a research hospital with PHS personnel who would test experimental therapies on infected Chinese arrivals.[79] The politics of reclassification of excludable diseases was complicated. The PHS insulated itself from political challenges and maintained a reputation for professional independence. Surgeon General Hugh Cummings directed the PHS officer N. E. Wayson, who had served as chief medical officer at the Angel Island Quarantine Station, to conduct epidemiological and bacteriological investigations into the contagiousness of clonorchiasis.[80] After five years of study, Wayson came to the same conclusion that had been reached in earlier scientific public health and tropical medicine studies: that North America lacked the species of fish and snails that served as hosts to the fluke's larva, and therefore it was impossible for the parasite to spread to other humans. Finally, in 1927, clonorchiasis was reclassified from an excludable disease to a class "C" disease condition, which, at the discretion of the medical inspector, could be considered a class "B" condition if it was deemed to inhibit the sufferer's ability to earn a living.[81] Similarly, hookworm had been demoted in 1917 to a class "B" disease that might debar an immigrant only if the disease was deemed likely to make the individual a public charge.[82]

Surgeon General Cummings warned a jubilant Chinese community in San Francisco that the reclassification occurred despite political pressure and "solely as a result of scientific and epidemiological investigation" under PHS direction. The PHS had an interest in characterizing the reclassification as a "purely" internal matter. Cummings pointedly dismissed the idea that the findings of a non-PHS physician such as Dr. Fred K. Lam of Honolulu, whom Cummings had met, had any influence in the matter. Cummings disdained the credit Lam received in Chinese publications like the San Francisco–based *Chinese World*.[83] Since the CCBA had challenged the PHS within the parameters of medical decision-making, the CCBA eagerly credited PHS personnel for their scientific research. Nevertheless, they did take an opportunity to acknowledge "other scientific investigators" and "noted statesmen" for their "deep interest" in the reclassification. In the listing of acknowledgments, however, Fong did not include the names of any Chinese physicians or activists who had labored to change the policy, but rather took the opportunity to pay tribute to a plethora of white officials, physicians, statesmen, and attorneys.[84] Fong could declare victory only within the parameters of public health definitions. Clonorchiasis had been reclassified, but the ideological apparatus that adjudicated the exclusion policies of disease had not been dislodged. The Chinese American activists accepted that the PHS could and should police the entry of immigrants on the basis of their health status. The *Chinese Defender*, with its ridiculing and dismissive temperament, had, a decade and half later, been replaced by a more pliant coalition that was willing to comply with the regulatory structure if this meant it could gain certain adjustments to, and force official reconsideration of, policy. The CCBA's success demonstrated the unequivocal power of "scientific logic" to shape the contours of debate and to reinforce the prevailing regulatory structures.

The oral histories and barrack-wall poetry, however, expressed little tolerance for such a political philosophy shrouded in scientific logic. The frequent mention of assault, "humiliation," and unjustified oppression in the verses and testimonies recognized the PHS practices as a kind of despotic military oppression. The poetry, in particular, unequivocally refused such prerogatives, calling them "unjust" and highlighting the political intentions and psychic effects of such scientifically endorsed measures.

Many Chinese immigrants fundamentally doubted that they carried sickness in their bodies and instead presumed that the process of detention produced illness. In a long poem published anonymously in *Chinese World* in March 1910, an Angel Island detainee wrote:

> In this newly opened wild land, the environment is not agreeable.
> Drinking water, many developed coughs.
> Sipping it, not so few developed sore throats.
> A hundred symptoms of sickness developed; it is difficult to put our misery into words.[85]

The paradox of the PHS's detection and treatment of disease in Chinese and other Asian immigrants was that it forced these immigrants into detention in what was regarded by the PHS officers themselves as unsanitary and unhealthy conditions. In their pleas for appropriations for basic improvements, the PHS officers described the Chinese barracks as filthy, crowded, and rat-infested.[86]

The question remains, why didn't bacteriology, with its interest in the microbial pathogen, interrupt the medical obsession with racializing disease? The microscopic detection processes were intended to provide the "truth" of an individual's health condition independent of clinical signs or symptoms. Despite the PHS's unwavering justification of its policies as scientifically guided health measures, unaffected by politics or prejudice, the practices of bacteriological examination necessitated a selection strategy. The PHS had neither the facilities nor the political will to detain all incoming passengers for full bacteriological exams. Universal application would require that white first-class passengers be treated the same as most Asian steerage passengers. It would unsettle the health authorities' underlying insistence that disease was exclusively un-American and nonwhite.

The very means of identification and the statistical tabulation employed by the PHS both relied upon and reproduced categories of nationality and race. The naming of racial and national groups did not simply specify origins. They strategically influenced policies, expectations, and treatment while masquerading as objective, scientific findings. Throughout the bacteriological revolution, the ability to conduct individual diagnosis had been enfolded into group expectations. And the "truth" of national difference inexorably invoked race so that the expectation of Chinese health and illness served to define the characteristics of "Asiatics" or "Orientals" and affected the immigration treatment and health concerns of Asian Indians, Japanese, Koreans, and Filipinos.

The history of immigrant exclusion as a result of trachoma, hookworm, threadworm, and liver fluke at the San Francisco quarantine sta-

tion reinforces Charles Rosenberg's observation that medical knowledge
has been framed, in part, by a "socially constructed and determined belief system, a reflection of arbitrary social arrangements, social need and
the distribution of power." Medical knowledge, however, is neither arbitrary nor compulsively functionalist. The developments in microbiol-
ogy shaped the choices available to societies in developing institutional
responses to disease.[87] These choices operated within a political world
that had conflated fears of immigrants, particularly from Asia, and anxiety about disease. It was possible in managing national borders to mobilize bacteriological expertise to screen particular migrants. The bacteriological revolution did not disrupt racial formation of medical knowledge;
its techniques and insights meshed with prevailing policies about the
danger of racial bodies and racial geographies. Although the statistical
frequency of disease detection differed by nationality, the organizing category of "Orientals" shaped the expectations and practices of the PHS,
allowing them to detain Asian Indian and Japanese steerage passengers
as they had Chinese passengers. Race shaped the inspection treatment
that immigrants received, and the process of inspection carried an expectation regarding which national bodies were most likely to bring disease to U.S. shores.

The right to medicalize arriving immigrants had been rationalized by
U.S. politicians and PHS officers as a national necessity, an issue of health
security. But the anonymous poetry on the barrack walls disavowed the
legitimacy of medical science to regulate entry into the nation. The procedures were viewed instead as the capricious and cruel barriers erected
by an unjust and despotic government. Through their poetry and testimony, Chinese detainees demonstrated a variety of different visions of
mobility, justice, and bodily autonomy.

San Francisco Chinese American activists pragmatically sought middle ground. They opposed discriminatory treatment but summoned
medical expertise in order to challenge the exclusion of those affected by
intestinal parasites. Much as during the 1900–04 bubonic plague epidemic in San Francisco, this strategy was politically effective in adjust-
ing public health policy. Under pressure from Chinese American lobbying efforts and lawsuits, the PHS had to reconsider tropical-medicine
evidence that challenged their definition of *contagious*. In 1917 the PHS
demoted hookworm from a disease that resulted in immediate exclusion
to one that could potentially exclude the sufferer at the discretion of the
medical officer. In 1927 the PHS reclassified liver fluke as well. Though
they were important victories, these adjustments did not interrupt the

racial selection of Asians for bacteriological testing. Rather, they reinforced the legitimacy of the medical management of the nation's borders.

The process of medical screening and, in particular, the treatment for hookworm administered at Angel Island offer a significant hint of the role of public health reform in transforming Chinese American society in San Francisco in the early twentieth century. In the second and third decades of the twentieth century, many of the Chinese women who successfully passed through Angel Island joined husbands, had children, and created domestic lives in urban centers like San Francisco's Chinatown—a contrast with the enduring legacy of Chinese bachelor society. Their children were part of a small and growing class of second-generation Chinese Americans who participated in the process of hygienic self-care through organizations like the YWCA and the YMCA, public schools, and well-baby and child-health clinics. These institutions offered mothers and their children training and consciousness of public health reform. The aim was to cultivate individuals who shared a quest for health and the capacity to achieve it through personal hygiene, vaccination, and professional medical care sought when necessary. Race continued to shape the expectations of the immigrants likely to be "carriers" of disease and disability into the United States. However, the willingness to undertake medical testing and treatment to ensure fitness and health enabled Chinese Americans to be considered potential citizens—like those who had been permitted entry into the nation from Angel Island.

CHAPTER 8

# Healthy Spaces,
# Healthy Conduct

By 1910, after the twin bubonic plague pandemics, the intensity of epidemic crisis had subsided in twentieth-century San Francisco. Occasionally, outbreaks of typhoid, measles, diphtheria, and polio mobilized health officials, but they rarely caused widespread panic or accusations of Chinese villainy. Preschool immunization, water purification, and milk pasteurization programs limited the severity of deadly epidemics. In the overall population, fewer children and adults suffered and fewer still died. The declining mortality rates swelled confidence in the preventive measures instituted by public health reform. So, when outbreaks of typhoid or diphtheria hit, public health officials responded by fine-tuning sanitation procedures, providing public health instruction, and encouraging regular medical screenings.[1]

The incorporation of Chinatown into American society depended on standardizing Chinese conduct and living spaces according to American hygienic norms. The imperatives of health cemented the relationship between conduct and citizenship. In the twentieth century, the emphasis of health regulation shifted from reducing disease to prolonging life and extending the body's capacity. The management of space and the care of the body were perceived to be an index of American cultural citizenship and civic belonging.[2] The American system of cultural citizenship combined class discourses of respectability and middle-class tastes with heteronormative discourses of adult male responsibility, female domestic caretaking, and the biological reproduction legitimated by marriage.[3]

The practices of middle-class domesticity were perceived to cultivate citizen-subjects capable of undertaking the responsibilities of American citizenship.[4] At the turn of the century, American capitalists and social reformers perceived home life as a crucial marker of social behavior and citizenship, and domestic spaces were seen as possessing influential capabilities for shaping "character traits, promoting family stability, and assuring good society." Domestic space and middle-class family life were perceived to be enablers of healthy social conduct and healthy lives.[5]

Middle-class social reformers developed institutions to reform the conduct of the lower classes and new immigrants. The health improvement projects first targeted the white working class and the European immigrants. The government and voluntary organizations fostered institutions such as hospitals and clinics, mother and child welfare agencies, schools, and recreational parks in order to shape the relationship of human bodies to each other and within the environment. In the middle-class American vision of a clean, well-ordered society, these institutional activities were intended to produce healthy citizens in nuclear family arrangements. Motherhood and childhood were two life experiences of intensive interest in the effort to institutionalize the middle-class, heterosexual family as the social norm. Nurses, reformers, and social workers promoted proper maternal conduct and provided resources to ensure healthy babies. Professionals intervened to shape relations between mother and child with regard to nutrition and care of the fetus, infant, or child. Extending the life capacity of children involved transformations of domestic and public space. In the cities the health and survival of children became connected to recreation movements as well as instruction in the management of domestic space. In pursuit of child health and welfare, Progressive-era programs enabled mothering and created foster and orphan care institutions that provided substitutes and models for mothering and reconfigured the spatial arrangements of domestic and public space.[6]

## DEMOGRAPHIC TRANSITIONS
## AND CULTIVATING HEALTHY HABITS

The reconstruction of Chinatown after the 1906 disaster produced dramatic demographic changes in Chinese American society. At first in the decades following the 1906 fire, the San Francisco Chinese population plummeted from 13,954 in 1900 to only 7,744 in 1920. The population loss paralleled steep declines across the country, with the overall Chinese

American population down to 61,639 in 1920, from a peak of 107,488 in 1890. The restrictions of the Chinese Exclusion Act had taken a toll. Fewer new migrants could enter the United States, and many elderly men returned to China to retire. In the late nineteenth century, the immigration of Chinese women had dropped precipitously with the enforcement of the 1875 Page Act and 1882 Chinese Exclusion Act. In the early twentieth century, however, the civil unrest and the economic dislocation in South China and the opportunities for women in family-run small businesses in the United States encouraged Chinese American men to seek the immigration of their wives. From a nadir of 12 in 1900, the number of Chinese women entering the United States picked up steadily, reaching 1,893 in 1924.[7]

Chinese Americans adeptly maneuvered around immigration barriers to enable the entry of women, young men, and children and to reshape twentieth-century Chinese American society. Since the Chinese Exclusion Act did not restrict the immigration of Chinese merchants and individuals who were U.S. citizens by birth, Chinese men made claims to either status and widened the legal loopholes for the immigration of their wives and children. Often Chinese men found clever ways to assume these favored identities that were prescribed by legislators and immigration authorities. Those men who did not directly own small businesses would bribe other Chinese merchants to list their names as business partners. And after San Francisco city records were destroyed in the 1906 fire, Chinese men often claimed U.S. birth and added the names of more sons and daughters than they possessed when they reapplied for birth certificates and Chinese residency certificates. Besieged by claimants, the city government reissued the certificates without investigation. Although the Immigration Service vigorously interrogated all Chinese immigrants in order to curb identity fraud, many wives of illegitimate citizens as well as "paper sons" and "paper daughters" entered the United States. Immigration hurdles were raised once again by the Immigration Act of 1924. The law created quotas that curbed eastern and southern European immigration as well as prohibited the immigration of any "aliens ineligible for citizenship." This clause applied to Chinese, Japanese, Koreans, and Asian Indians. The immigration of Chinese women immediately ceased, but judicial judgments and legislation opened the doors again slightly. The U.S. Supreme Court ruled that Chinese merchants' wives were exempt because of treaty obligations; however, the wives of U.S. citizens were not. In 1930 Congress amended the act to permit the entry of Chinese alien wives married prior to May 26, 1924.[8]

Despite the substantial barriers to legal entry for Chinese women, their increasing presence in San Francisco stimulated increased marriages and childbirths. During the 1920s Chinese women gave birth at a rate 90 to nearly 250 percent higher than women in the city overall. The birthrate for Chinese women did not correspond with the overall rate until 1935. The number of births peaked in 1924, when 451 babies were born to Chinese American mothers, and declined to 397 in 1928 and to 225 in 1935.[9] The baby boom was linked to the arrival of a large number of married Chinese women in the early 1920s. The steady immigration of merchants' wives and paper daughters lifted the Chinese female population in San Francisco by 22 percent between 1910 and 1920 and significantly narrowed the ratio of women to men, from 1 to 27 in 1890 to 1 to 2.8 in 1930. These transformations in immigration, marriage, and birthrates helped the Chinese population in San Francisco rebound to 16,303 in 1930.[10]

These immigration and demographic changes, however, did not readily make Chinese American domestic arrangements conform to the models of nuclear family domesticity. From Sanborn fire insurance maps of city buildings, from structural features, and from manuscript census details, one can reconstruct some of the contours of the kinds of domestic arrangements that flourished in Chinatown. For instance, in 1910 the second-floor apartment at 913–917 Stockton street housed a mix of six males and two females. Chun She Leong was the twenty-seven-year-old Chinese-born wife of She Nam Leong, who was thirty-seven years old and who had been born in California. They had married eleven years before in China, and Chun She had immigrated to San Francisco in 1909. Of their two living children, Soon Lee, an eight-year-old Chinese-born daughter, lived with them. The second child does not appear in census records and probably remained with relatives in China. With the family lived five male lodgers who varied in age from seventeen to thirty. Three had been born in China, one in Hawaii, and a fifth in California. Of the Chinese-born men, two had arrived in the United States in 1906 and 1908, probably as paper sons. All the lodgers and the wife, husband, and daughter shared the name Leong, but it was not known how they may have been related. These domestic arrangements were not unusual among new immigrants in U.S. cities, and they reveal the diversity and entanglement of social and kinship relations in Chinatown that did not strictly demarcate Chinese family society from bachelor society.[11]

In order to nurture a family society and tourist businesses in Chinatown, the Chinese merchant elite established new institutions, including

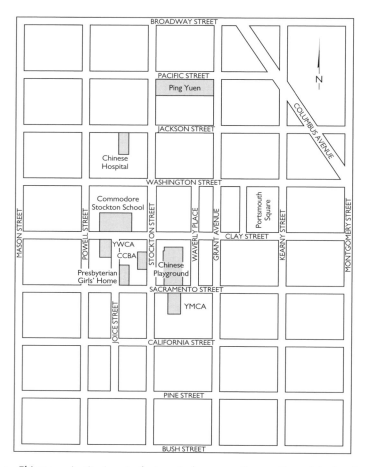

Map 2. Chinatown institutions in the twentieth century. Source: *Map of the San Francisco Chinese Colony* prepared for the *Survey of Social Work Needs of the Chinese Population of San Francisco.* Supervising official: T. Y. Chen; drawn by S. J. Yim, November 1934. (Alleys not shown; map redrawn by Bill Nelson.)

Chinese schools, the Chinese Hospital, the YMCA and YWCA, the Chinese Chamber of Commerce, and the Chinese American Citizens Alliance (CACA). These new institutions, shown in Map 2, reshaped the social and physical geography of Chinatown and sought to cultivate "modern ways of life and health" among the Chinese. Their efforts paralleled the work of Americanizing and self-improvement institutions in European immigrant communities. These same institutions sought to persuade individuals to adopt the habits, behavior, and outlook of the American middle class and to make them recognizable citizens in a nation that denied the Chinese the privileges and possibilities of full participation in society. They shaped the conduct of individuals in nuclear families in order to make citizens.

The establishment of the Chinese YWCA and YMCA in the second decade of the twentieth century was a key step in the movement to reform Chinese habits, hygiene, and morals to resemble modern American Protestant standards. Chinese Christian businessmen supported efforts to rehabilitate the Chinese reputation for dirty appearance and opium smoking. Chinese Christians used YMCA programs to teach the morality of personal hygiene, the cultivation of healthful habits, and the importance of physical fitness to second-generation Chinese boys and young men. The YMCA demonstrated the convergence of modern public health and Protestant Christianity in stipulating civilized behavior. Its programs blended moral training with hygienic care. The YMCA offered regular instruction in sanitation, personal hygiene, exercise, and citizenship in order to cultivate healthy habits and "promote hygienic living." They emphasized self-help and education to transform the conduct of the individual and attain the improvement of the community.[12]

The YMCA also provided immensely practical assistance to its members. Its showers facilitated regular bathing for boys and men in a community in which most apartments did not have bathtubs. Residents often relied on Japanese bathhouses and the YMCA to provide bathing facilities. Although many older Chinese believed that regular tub-baths weakened the body's system and instead preferred sponge baths, Chinese youth were encouraged to and could afford to take daily showers through their YMCA membership.[13] At the YMCA, programs of self-improvement promoted the development of healthy habits, and moral instruction helped create citizen-subjects who were able to regulate themselves.

The Chinese YWCA not only addressed the physical and moral fitness of individual Chinese youth but pitched to women and girls its programs for strengthening the family and domesticity. To immigrant women, the Chinese YWCA offered home visits, English classes, and advice on household sanitation and infant hygiene. Their daughters were taught how to care for baby siblings in preparation for their own eventual motherhood. These training programs emphasized the crucial role of mothers in both race uplift and Americanization projects. The *Chung Sai Yat Po* declared that the YWCA's training of Chinese women, morally and physically, benefited "the family and future citizens of tomorrow and therefore the Chinese community." Jane Kwong Lee, a social worker and coordinator of the Chinese YWCA in the 1930s and 1940s, highlighted individual and national benefits of YWCA programming:

"A girl who is physically and socially fit, a housewife who gives her family the right nutritional food, both help the national morale." [14]

The increasing numbers of married Chinese women and children helped rehabilitate Chinatown's reputation for lascivious immorality and deviant heterosexuality. Nineteenth-century white Americans had been deeply suspicious of the institution of marriage in Chinatown. Although most Chinese men claimed to have wives and children in China, white observers dismissed them as "bachelors" without family responsibilities and as being indifferent to "monogamous morality." [15] The commitment to monogamy had been uncertain at best in nineteenth-century San Francisco society, in which Chinese merchants sought multiple wives and concubines and Chinese men frequented female prostitutes. Twentieth-century Chinese American institutions heralded the increasing presence of Chinese wives and children in San Francisco, calling them crucial to reshaping and channeling Chinese male sexuality into monogamous morality. The perverse reputations of Chinese male and female sexuality were slowly dislodged by the frequency of exclusive Protestant marriage commitments and the birth of children in the apartments that small businessmen had re-created from bachelor bunkrooms. Chinese social workers and Christian institutions emphasized the roles of sanitary housewives and health-conscious mothers in improving the welfare of the Chinese community. [16]

In the 1920s and 1930s, Chinese American social workers took up the discourses of hygiene, domesticity, and gender and reworked them in their advocacy for access to municipal social services and for improved housing. They took statistics indicating the small but increasing number of childbirths as a sign that Chinatown was nurturing a "family society" and held up the educated Chinese American housewives as being most able to apply the norms of American middle-class domestic culture. Their intention was to position Chinese motherhood as a foil against the nineteenth-century image of a male bachelor and female prostitute society. Social workers emphasized the necessity for Chinese housewives to learn "modern" standards of sanitation and urged local institutions to provide courses in hygiene. As mothers and wives, Chinese women were expected to educate children and reform men to exhibit American normative behavior. A married Chinese woman's style of housekeeping would determine the family's successful assimilation to American society. This process of incorporation through discourses of hygiene and nuclear family society enabled Chinese Americans to claim access to American civic polity and social resources. [17]

## CHINATOWN REFORM AND ALLOPATHIC MEDICINE

Hospitals represented another key institutional site for reforming China-town society and shaping the conduct of its residents. While reform institutions such as the YMCA and YWCA sought to inculcate in Chinese subjects conduct that would shape their everyday existence, the Western allopathic hospital removed the ill person and the expectant mother from everyday residence and workspaces and brought them under professional care. Until the opening of the Chinese Hospital in 1925, Chinese residents in San Francisco had limited access to Western, allopathic medical care and regular public health services. During the bubonic plague epidemic, the CCBA had sponsored emergency care by white allopathic physicians. Most Chinese Americans relied upon the services of Chinese herbalists and acupuncture specialists. Their aversion to Western medical practices developed from the correlation of Western physicians with fatal epidemics and from the hospitals' reputation for high mortality rates. Most Chinese had little confidence in the health-preserving skills of Western medical practice and considered hospitalization and care by Western-trained physicians to be "deathbed" care.

The reputation of hospital care was neither ill-deserved nor uncommon for the era. At the turn of the century, the San Francisco public hospital had a reputation for an exceptionally high mortality rate, which often discouraged the white working class and poor from seeking care until they were close to death, perpetuating the cycle of high mortality and fear. Although the poor and working class also generally had access to the charity wards of private hospitals in emergencies, they did not have access to the routine care of Western physicians. This made it more difficult for the poor and working class to "maintain health," a condition that had become increasingly possible for the white middle class.[18] The conception of health in Chinese traditional medicine embraced an idea of bodily equilibrium and sensitivity to changes in the body. Chinese residents in San Francisco regularly accessed traditional Chinese therapeutics and remedies and sought Western allopathic care only in times of grave danger.[19]

In San Francisco, the system of free public health clinics and charitable hospital services ignored the Chinese. At the turn of the century, middle-class social reformers responded to the chronic health problems and high mortality of the city's poor and working class by establishing neighborhood free clinics. Progressive-era organizations, such as the Telegraph Hill Settlement House and the San Francisco Tuberculosis Association, made physicians and visiting nurses accessible to newly arrived European immigrants and white working-class residents. By the end of World War I these private charitable tuberculosis clinics and maternal care programs were taken over by the Public Health Departments to become part of a citywide network of neighborhood municipal health centers and clinics.

Since 1854 Chinese political leaders and merchant elite had repeatedly attempted to build a hospital for their community. The Board of Health had consistently opposed licensing any facility and often condemned the dispensaries for unsanitary conditions. In 1899, the Chinese consul and the CCBA leaders once again raised funds for a hospital. The hospital was promoted to provide medical care to indigent Chinese from Western-trained physicians exclusively.[20] When the Tung Wah Dispensary opened at 828 Sacramento Street in 1900, patients were treated by three white physicians.[21] The bubonic plague epidemic, however, reinforced the perception that the dispensary, like other Western care facilities, was a "deathhouse," a place to go when all other treatments had failed.

After World War I, leading merchants and political leaders campaigned to expand and remodel the dispensary into a "modern hospital." [22] They raised two hundred thousand dollars from Chinese contributors in California, New York, and Hong Kong. When the five-story, fifty-five-bed Chinese Hospital was opened in April 1925, it was hailed for bringing the "benefits of scientific medicine" to the Chinese community.[23] The Chinese Hospital was also intended to provide clinical education for Chinese physicians, nurses, and technicians. At first the hospital drew its staff of physicians from the city's white medical establishment, but within a couple of years several Chinese American physicians, trained at Stanford and the University of California, joined the staff.[24]

Many Chinese American physicians received a cool reception from other Chinese Americans, and the most financially successful served a predominantly white clientele. When Dr. Collin Dong graduated from Stanford Medical School in 1931 and began his practice in San Francisco, he was one of six Western-trained physicians of Chinese origin competing with fifty Chinese acupuncturists and herbalists. Dong recalled that it was "not easy to introduce Western medical concepts to our Chinese patients. They were eclectic, taking our pills sometimes, and other times, they reverted to herbs and acupuncture." [25] Chinese patients selected different therapies as much out of practicality as out of fear. "Everyone was suspicious of strange medications, especially hypodermic injections of any type," remembered Dr. Helen Tong Chinn, who began practicing in Chinatown in 1933.[26]

Traditional Chinese medicine practitioners thrived in the twentieth century. More than half the advertisements in Chinese-language papers promoted herbal cures and practitioners. Chinese residents were far more eager to appeal to traditional Chinese medical practitioners, since a Western medical physician was obligated to report communicable diseases to the Public Health Department, which could order a quarantine and force the patient to "lose time and work." The Chinese traditional practitioners were attentive to the preferences and fears of their patients and operated a small charity clinic next door to the Chinese Hospital. Throughout the 1930s, most Chinese regarded the Chinese Hospital — like the Western care facilities — as a last refuge for the dying, as a place for the "elderly and hopeless cases," leaving it an underutilized facility.[27]

In the 1920s Chinese Americans became successful in developing strategies to protect traditional Chinese medicine from defamation and regulation. In 1925, Chinese medical practitioners and supporters among Chinese American civic organizations like the CACA mobilized to fight a bill in the California legislature that would subject all Chinese medicinal herbs to federal control. They quickly organized the Association to Defend Chinese Medicine (ADCM), raised funds through a twenty-dollar annual membership fee, and developed a public relations campaign to undercut support for the bill. The ADCM compiled articles in English on the benefits of Chinese herbal medicine and distributed copies to hospitals and clinics throughout California, gathered signatures and testimony from white patients, and drew on the lobbying expertise of the CACA. The strategy was to provide evidence of widespread public acceptance and information about the benefits of Chinese herbal medicine. The public relations campaign and political pressure forced the bill to be withdrawn six weeks later. In order to preempt future unilateral regulation by government authorities, the Association to Defend Chinese Medicine developed their own plans for professionalization that paralleled those of allopathic practitioners in the United States. They offered a plan for licensing practitioners, accrediting educational institutions, and requiring practitioners to have facility in both Western and traditional Chinese medicine. In the mid–twentieth century, and particularly after the Kuomintang assumption of power in Taiwan in 1949, programs for autonomous licensing and accreditation of traditional Chinese medicine flourished.[28]

The establishment of the Chinese Hospital, nevertheless, provided an institutional foothold for public and private health agencies in their attempts to reach the Chinese American community. The San Francisco Public Health Department and the Baby Hygiene Committee of the

American Association of University Women adapted their public health programs to take advantage of this institutional presence in Chinatown.

The children's entrance into public schools presented public health officials with the opportunity to secure their broader program for the "conservation of child health and life." Public health officials delivered services to Chinese American children through the Chinese Hospital and the Commodore Stockton School. In the late 1920s the Public Health Department used the Chinese Hospital for preschool immunization drives and health screenings in order to prevent health defects such as "decayed teeth, diseased tonsils and defective eyesight." The hospital's interpreter, a Chinese woman with "social service experience and a modern American viewpoint," provided an invaluable link for reassuring and educating the mothers.[29] Public health nurses conducted monthly health inspections of students in the Commodore Stockton School, in which they used weight and height measurements to determine "physical progress" and "normal development." Through health education in the schools, Chinese American parents and children were made conscious of health norms and hygienic conduct. Teachers instructed children with weekly talks about disease prevention, personal hygiene, and the meaning of their individual growth charts.[30] Through this process of education, screening, and medical intervention, Chinese American school children became subjects of health consciousness and care.

## CHILD WELFARE AND HEALTHY CITIZENSHIP

Chinese Americans were now no longer viewed as the source of harm but rather as a danger to themselves. This transformation in perspective for charities and government in early-twentieth-century San Francisco was most evident in the campaigns to address the high rate of infant mortality among Chinese Americans, a rate that exceeded city averages. Infant mortality emerged as a national and international problem in the early twentieth century, and in the United States women's charities and public health programs developed to address the high rate of infant death. Infant mortality did not arise from a single ailment and did not have a single cause or detection method. In early-twentieth-century United States, the most frequent causes of the deaths of babies under the age of one were premature birth, respiratory infection, pneumonia, and chronic diarrhea. Nationwide, local white women's voluntary associations emerged to reduce the high rates of infant and maternal mortality in the United States, which far outstripped European industrialized nations. Women reformers instructed mothers on how to prevent disease and ensure healthy growth of their babies.[31] In San Francisco, women activists organized health demonstration projects such as home visits by public health nurses to new mothers, free clinics for prenatal and infant care, and the health screening of toddlers and school-aged children.[32] City governments expanded the demonstration projects, and in the 1920s, with the Sheppard-Towner Act, the federal government supported and financed educational services for expectant and new mothers in both cities and rural areas.[33]

Women reformers and their public health allies believed that by transforming the conduct of mothers and by improving the home environment, children would become physically and morally "fit" to undertake the demands of democratic citizenship.[34] Protecting the health of infants functioned within a logic of race improvement and national strength. Questions about the quality of mothering and the health of children figured prominently in turn-of-the-century anxieties about the "suicide" of the white race, and they pushed infant protection programs to improve the health and increase the number of white native-born children.[35] Not surprisingly, San Francisco women activists from the second decade of the twentieth century to the 1930s offered training in infant health care to the mothers and babies of the "moderate circumstanced white-color class of citizens." Voluntary associations recognized the higher rates of infant mortality for Asian Americans and African Americans but were reluctant to expend resources to aid "inferior" mothers.[36]

In the late 1920s, the Public Health Department finally began to offer infant care instruction to Chinese American mothers in San Francisco. The effort to bring maternal instruction to Chinatown was a belated response to the abrupt rise in Chinese births in the early 1920s. Through the Chinese YWCA and the Chinese Hospital's commitment to hygiene and Western medicine, the Public Health Department had sympathetic institutional footholds from which to reach Chinese women. However, it took a decade for preventive measures to take hold, and Chinese infant mortality remained nearly double the overall city rate until the late 1930s.[37] Public health programs offered different strategies to combat the chief causes of infant deaths. Well-baby contests and conferences offered preventive instruction to help mothers avoid fatal pneumonia and diarrhea. In order to reduce deaths from premature birth, public health nurses encouraged delivery by obstetrician and childbirth hospitalization.

In 1928 the Public Health Department sponsored a well-baby contest at the Chinese YWCA. Over sixty mothers entered 176 babies ranging from six months to five years old in the contest, which was largely

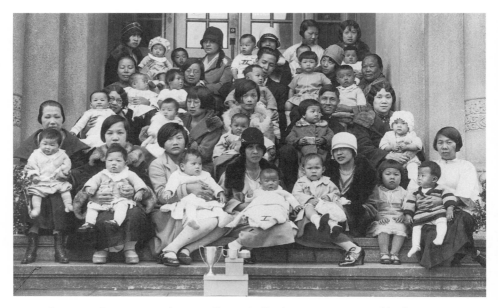

Figure 11. Contestants in the 1928 Chinese Well Baby Contest, sponsored by the YWCA, pose with their parents on the steps of the Chinese YWCA. Courtesy California Historical Society, FN-19823.

a "weighing and measuring project" intended to teach mothers the relationship between height, weight, and the child's health. The Public Health Department combined the contest with individual well-baby conferences that included mothers in order to instruct them in infant hygiene and expected normal growth. Modeled on livestock shows, better-baby and well-baby contests first occurred at state fairs and demonstrated health norms as well as showcased the achievement of eugenic excellence. (See Figure 11.) The very idea of a well-baby clinic as opposed to a clinic for sick infants suggested the idea of health as a state to be measured, judged, and maintained. Mothers were encouraged to seek guidance on the baby's diet, clothing, and care not only to prevent illness but also to facilitate "normal" growth.[38] When the Chinese Health Center opened in 1934, the well-baby conferences became a regular feature of infant care. The Chinese Health Center also offered free vaccinations, physical examinations, and prenatal care. With the hire of the first Chinese visiting nurse, Minnie Lee, the Chinese Health Center became much more effective in reaching Chinese mothers.[39] More than three thousand women and children visited the center in its first year of opera-

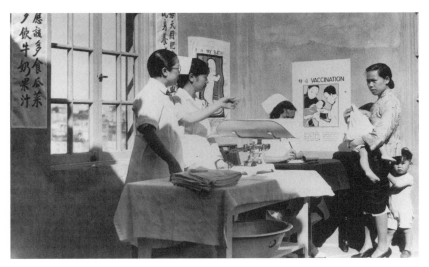

Figure 12. Dr. Rose Goong Wong (far left) coaxes a child in the San Francisco Chinese Health Center, Well Baby Clinic, circa 1934. Courtesy San Francisco History Center, San Francisco Public Library.

tion. Lee's fluency in Cantonese helped her to reassure mothers and educate them in "American" health standards for infants.[40] (See Figure 12.)

In order to combat premature birth, Minnie Lee offered prenatal care and encouraged pregnant women to have obstetricians rather than midwives deliver their babies. Dr. Helen Tong Chinn, a physician at the Chinese Hospital, recalled that it took years of education for mothers to turn to the hospital for obstetric care. Many Chinese mothers and fathers were more comfortable with female midwives and worried about the prurient interest of male obstetricians. The availability of Dr. Rose Goong Wong, an obstetrician and gynecologist who began practicing in San Francisco in 1927, changed the attitude of many expectant parents. She delivered babies both at the Chinese Hospital and in homes. Through the persuasion of Lee's prenatal care and the popularity of Wong's reassuring bedside manner, the rate of hospital deliveries jumped dramatically, from only 20 percent of all Chinese births in 1929 to 56 percent in 1939. Many of the mothers who did seek hospitalization were on state relief and could access charity beds. The high cost of hospitalization discouraged a number of Chinese women, but even the Chinese births at home occurred with a licensed physician attending. Incorporating Chinese mothers into the medical system of obstetrician-assisted deliveries either at home or in the hospital was rounded out by the programs of prenatal and postnatal public health nursing. Public health nurses like Minnie Lee visited mothers at home and instructed them on breast-feeding schedules, food selection and preparation, infant care, and house-keeping in order to remake the tenement into a more American and healthful home.[41]

The Baby Hygiene Committee strove to make the services of public health nursing available to "every mother in San Francisco." In a fund-raising campaign, the committee emphasized the universal value of post-natal home visits even to Chinese shrimp-fishing families at Hunter's Point. The fishing villages were located on the southeastern edge of San Francisco, and the inhabitants were considered to be the San Francisco group most untutored in hygiene.[42] An infant's birth at the Chinese Hospital entitled the baby to the "best services" available though the "power of Medical Science"; however, when "Mother and Babe go home must they be subjected to the conditions of their environment without further scientific aid?" The Baby Hygiene Committee believed that the "right" of proper care was "justly due to this tiny life." The committee promoted its readiness to provide free the service of a public health nurse to "every New Baby and Mother in San Francisco." The nurse would visit the mother's home and impart a "very simple method" to the "Mother, who is naturally anxious to learn, because she wants the best for her child."[43] The Public Health Department's director, J. C. Geiger, linked the precipitous declines in Chinese infant mortality in 1937 and 1938 to incorporating Chinese mothers into the system of hospital births, visiting nurses, and well-baby clinics.[44]

Healthy reproduction indexed national strength and the individual's potential for productive citizenship. The Baby Hygiene Committee articulated the importance of proper diet and clothing and a "sanitary" environment for children in order to ensure that the child could attain the "best possible physical development . . . [and] be an asset to himself, the State, and the community." In order for democracy to survive, the state must have the "wholesome service" that could be provided only by the "healthy individual." The extension of services to every new mother and baby was justified, the committee believed, by the tremendous social consequences of maladjusted individuals: "The undernourished, misunderstood child grows into a warped adult with warped ideas that will undermine our very foundations."[45]

The campaigns to reduce infant mortality demonstrated that public health and social workers expected Chinese Americans to submit to disease screening, develop hygienic habits, and seek Western medical care. Through a persuasive regimen of well-baby clinics, tuberculosis testing sites, and YMCA and YWCA programs in personal hygiene, they trained Chinese Americans to consider the link between the care of individual health and the wider social improvement. The care and cultivation of the healthy body was considered a facet of civic responsibility and participation.[46]

## SUBSTITUTE MOTHERHOOD

The needs of Chinese infants presented a peculiar problem in the otherwise apparently successful operation of the foster care system, which had been organized in 1907 to reduce the high infant mortality of babies in long-term institutional care. The program redirected the resources of charitable social welfare agencies to immediate postnatal institutional care and the placement of babies with individual foster mothers who, under intensive medical supervision, cared for the children. The astonishing drop in the mortality rate, from 52 percent at the program's inception in 1908 to 2.3 percent in 1910, encouraged the reorganization of state services and local charitable agencies. State welfare departments and charity boards dispensed financial assistance for the care of orphans and destitute children and regulated the operations of local agencies. Locally, charitable agencies adapted to the new institutional configuration produced by the policy that made two child welfare organizations— Babies' Aid and the Infant Shelter—the sites for institutional care for orphaned infants, that held the child services organization Associated Charities responsible for placing children with foster mothers until they were adopted, and that enabled the Baby Hygiene Committee to conduct programs to dispense pasteurized milk, medical instruction, and pediatric care to foster children. Since white foster mothers and the Infant Shelter refused to accept Chinese children, two critical links in the prevailing system of tending to destitute and abandoned babies were, in the case of Chinese babies, broken.[47]

The idea that it was important for every child to have a chance at life encouraged the rescue and care of vulnerable babies. In the early twentieth century, local charities had rapidly developed a system of foster care in San Francisco that discriminated against Chinese babies. Many "boarding home mothers" refused to "take Chinese children," and few Chinese families could be licensed to take children because of space and sanitary requirements. The Infant Shelter also turned away Chinese babies by falsely claiming space shortages.[48]

For decades, the Presbyterian Mission Home had accepted the occasional care of Chinese infants who had been orphaned, abandoned, or made state wards. In the 1920s they found room for babies in their Oakland orphanages even though their facilities did not meet California's health and safety standards for infant care.[49] San Francisco and Oakland charities had relied on the Mission Home and its charismatic matron, Donaldina Cameron, to meet all the needs of abandoned or abused Chinese women and children. Agencies depended upon Cameron's contacts and judgment in recommending "high type Chinese homes" to adopt babies.[50] By relying on the Presbyterians, San Francisco Community Chest charities were spared a direct confrontation with the informal practices of race segregation in all of their child-saving institutions. Recognizing the segregated climate of charitable services, Cameron organized a group of Chinese Presbyterian women and men to establish an independent shelter for orphaned Chinese babies. After extensive fund raising, they established Mei Lun Yuen (literally, Garden of Beautiful Family Relationships) in 1933. Dr. Bessie Jeong, a young physician well-known in local Presbyterian missionary circles, served as the first director of the facility and was later replaced by a single Chinese professional woman, Lily Lum, who had graduated from the California Nursing School.[51]

The Community Chest and Babies' Aid administrators assumed responsibility for the Mei Lun Yuen shelter in 1935. The president of Babies' Aid believed that the shelter's operation extended the child-preservation agenda to the Chinese community. The shelter was necessary to protect Chinese children from health dangers and ignorance. According to Mrs. Henry L. Baer, the president of Babies' Aid, "Due to overcrowding and lack of knowledge of child care, mortality in that quarter is too high, and tuberculosis and other diseases threaten not only that population but that of the entire city. It does not seem safe to continue to neglect that crowded district, and this cottage was a beginning which promised to care for a certain number of these dependent and neglected children."[52] The shelter sought to remove Chinese children from neglect, ignorance, and disease and thereby begin to improve the health of the Chinese race as well as to protect the general population. Child welfare agencies who intervened to rescue vulnerable Chinese children also intended their actions to improve the general social conditions in Chinatown. In conjunction with the California State Emergency Relief Administration, the Community Chest enlisted a Chinese social worker who would screen requests for admission to the Mei Lun

Yuen shelter and instruct parents and guardians on child care that would alleviate the necessity for a child's removal from her natural family.[53]

The Presbyterian Mission's choice of the name "Garden of Beautiful Family Relationships" was both utopian and decidedly ironic. The home was supposed to serve as a model family for children whose utopian nuclear family had been disrupted by the death or illness of a parent, abandonment, divorce, or illegitimate birth. Many of these children were vulnerable because of the hospitalization or death of their mothers.[54] By providing scientific child care in spacious and hygienic surroundings within a Chinese cultural setting, the shelter was intended as a substitute for the ideal Chinese mother-child relations. The characteristic "overcrowding" in Chinatown and the presumed "lack of knowledge of child care" contributed to a high infant mortality rate and infant tuberculosis infection.[55] Jeong believed that the Mei Lun Yuen could serve as a "demonstration project" for the Chinese community in teaching the techniques of child hygiene. Jeong expressed her eagerness to impart to "Chinese mothers what wonders may be accomplished through the scientific study and proper care of children."[56]

Social workers justified the separate "Chinese" facilities by stressing the importance of maintaining "distinctive" cultural traditions and language fluency, especially since the Chinese were a "foreign group" that was "perpetuated rather than assimilated." The Mei Lun Yuen provided a rare institutional opportunity for Chinese children to "mingle with their own race," which would help these children, since "Chinese children must return to their families, be able to speak their language, and eat their food." The Mei Lun Yuen cottage was constructed on Babies' Aid property on Thirty-sixth Avenue in the Richmond District, which was a predominantly white residential area.[57] Although Babies' Aid administered the Mei Lun Yuen program, mostly Chinese staff members were hired to run the shelter in order to ensure that the experience would not accelerate cultural loss and alienation of Chinese babies from their relatives and Chinatown cultural world. The staff's challenge was to re-create a Chinese cultural atmosphere within the shelter without provoking the ire of their white middle-class neighbors.[58] White property-owners, however, began circulating a petition that opposed the "use of the new cottage for Oriental children." Miriam Feldelym feared that an "influx" of "Oriental children" violated property restrictions of the segregated, "residential, zoned Richmond district" and would send property values plummeting. The Babies' Aid president, Mrs. Morrison Hawkins, deflected the question of racial integration by addressing worries about maintaining a proper garden and fencing to shield the sight of Chinese babies from white residents. Internally, she advised the staff not to take the children to neighboring parks and to restrict the number of "Oriental" visitors.[59]

The willingness of the Community Chest and the Babies' Aid agencies to proceed with the Mei Lun Yuen home in the face of opposition by white residents demonstrated the increasing importance that the welfare of Chinese children had taken in San Francisco's social welfare organizations. However, despite the institutional support, the shelter suffered from administrative problems and its operation violated health and safety regulations. The new cottage did not meet Public Health Department requirements for proper quarantine facilities and adequate play space for its capacity of sixteen infants.[60] Although Babies' Aid and the Community Chest supported the facility, they were unwilling to invest in making structural improvements, purchase equipment, or hire the professional staff necessary for state certification. The facility closed as an infant shelter in 1939.[61]

When the home reopened in 1940, Helen Wu, a member of the Mei Lun Yuen board for seven years, volunteered to turn the cottage into the first certified Chinese foster care home for school-aged Chinese children awaiting adoption. With her husband living in Alaska, where he was business manager of the family mining company, Wu was eager to move from her house on Fulton Street with her twelve-year-old daughter in order to transform the cottage into a "friendly home" for six Chinese youngsters, ranging in age from three to thirteen. Wu was determined that in her care the children would learn the meaning of "protection and love and security" and would be exposed to a strong maternal presence. She hoped that her work would inspire other Chinese women to become foster mothers and "take homeless youngsters to their hearts."[62] (See Figure 13.)

Jeong and Wu participated in a broader initiative to train Chinese women in the techniques of proper child care and to offer Chinese children access to charitable services. This process of inclusion, however, was incomplete. Although the municipality and private agencies increasingly applied the public health–informed standards of "progress" to the Chinese American community, they considered Chinese social welfare needs to be "special" and, therefore, to require "segregated" solutions. Jeong and Wu attempted to incorporate Chinese women into the cultural citizenship and entitlements of white motherhood. Chinese women's success at accessing resources depended on their interest in adopting mod-

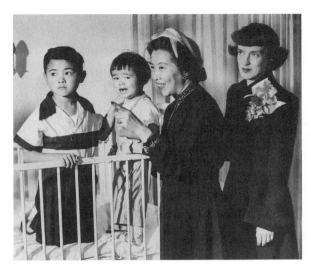

Figure 13. The Babies' Aid and Mei Lun Yuen home assisted orphaned Chinese American children. Helen Wu (standing next to the crib), a member of the Mei Lun Yuen Board, is pictured here with Mrs. Charles Bulolti Jr., a member of the Babies' Aid Board, October 24, 1950. Courtesy California Historical Society, FN-31287.

ern maternal conduct. Both the origins and the failure of the Mei Lun Yuen shelter raised questions about the obstinacy of residential and institutional segregation and the uneven allocation of municipal and charitable resources.

## FOSTERING FAMILIES IN UNSANITARY SPACES

The problems of cultural citizenship, nuclear family formation, and housing conditions became reformulated in 1935 with a survey conducted by a team of eighteen Chinese social workers employed by the California State Emergency Relief Administration (CSERA).[63] During the 1920s, the immigration of "marriageable" Chinese women and the increasing birthrate were considered crucial to the transformation of Chinatown into a family society. The survey distinguished between two kinds of families who lived in the Chinatown tenements. First, and representing the majority, were families in which Chinese-born "housewives" were not "yet familiar with the modern sanitation"; second were those who were forced to live in the tenements "solely for economic reasons." Once "housewives from China can gain the general knowledge of modern sanitation and hygiene" and segregation restrictions were removed, Chinese families would be able to live in improved conditions.[64]

Social workers emphasized the necessity for Chinese housewives to learn "modern" standards of sanitation and urged local institutions to provide courses in hygiene. Their training in modern hygiene would instill an appreciation of the ways in which cramped living conditions and poor hygiene could jeopardize "normal family life" and exacerbate Chinese juvenile delinquency. The practices of public health reform in female housekeeping had molded the so-called norms of American living standards to the extent that the exercise of proper sanitary habits was crucial for the Chinese to "assimilate" to American life.[65]

In their crusade to ensure the "progress" of Chinatown society, the CSERA staff created two categories of Chinese people—the modern, assimilated Chinese and the ignorant, complacent Chinese. "Modern" functioned as a shorthand indication of proper sanitary living conditions and American living standards. The idea of modern technological improvements valorized the use of sophisticated kitchen appliances and indoor plumbing.[66] Not surprisingly, these contrasting categories of "modern" and "ignorant" could be distinguished as much by social class and economic differences as by perceived differences in social behavior and cultural styles. The praise for those Chinese who "chose" to live in "modern" circumstances was reinforced by their financial success, which provided the resources necessary for mobility.

Distinctive from the public neglect that the Chinese American community experienced at the turn of the century, these social welfare perceptions of the needs of Chinese women and children developed out of a different kind of cultural relativism. The impact on Chinese American social and political life was, nevertheless, formidable. In a turnabout from the widespread representation of the Chinese American society as primarily a perverse Chinese bachelor society devoid of family responsibilities, public health reform in the 1920s and 1930s encouraged Chinese residents to pursue normal social reproduction through the raising of children. The development of institutions and services to improve the health of the community turned public attention to the vulnerability of the Chinese American family in San Francisco and the menacing and unsanitary environment of the Chinatown ghetto.

# CHAPTER 9

# Reforming Chinatown

In the twentieth century, Chinatown residents experienced a dramatic sea change in their relationship with the residents of the rest of the city. They went from being reviled and demonized at the turn of the century to being considered deserving and worthy of assistance in the mid–twentieth century. The popular image of Chinatown had shifted from that of an immoral and disease-infested slum to, by the late 1930s, a sanitized tourist destination for middle-class white families. Chinatown's residents were no longer characterized as a bachelor society of working-class men and female prostitutes and instead were seen as a family society of independent nuclear family households. This tremendous shift in popular representation emphasized demographic, commercial, and institutional changes and specifically reflected the impact of public health reform in Chinese American lives.[1]

Since the nineteenth century, city investigators, travelogues, and newspapers had derided the crowded, unventilated, and filthy housing conditions in Chinatown. A century of public health investigations had marked Chinatown housing as representative of a different living style and standards, incompatible with American norms. The cluster of aberrant meanings surrounding Chinatown housing meant that the reform of housing conditions and the formation of families would be fundamental in any move toward acculturation into American society by the Chinese community and toward the reform of Chinatown in the twentieth century. The housing crisis was exacerbated by a system of legal and informal segregation that severely restricted housing options for Chinese American residents.

Despite the increasing numbers of married women and children, the vitality and health of Chinatown's family society was imperiled by their living conditions. Public health officials and social workers feared that crowded apartments disseminated tuberculosis and imperiled infant viability. From the 1920s to 1940s, Chinese mortality rates fluctuated to levels three times the city average for tuberculosis deaths and twice the city rate for infant deaths. These two health crises became the signature threats to Chinese American society in the mid–twentieth century and the grounds on which Chinatown society was rehabilitated in order to participate in American civic culture.[2]

Those most committed to changing Chinatown living and social conditions were university-educated, second-generation Chinese American men and women who came of age in the 1920s and 1930s. Institutions founded in the early twentieth century—particularly the Chinese YMCA and YWCA, Boy Scout Troop 3, and other Protestant youth organizations—socialized this generation in the values of American self-improvement and social reform. Although many succeeded in school and received college degrees, racial discrimination prevented them from finding work outside Chinatown. As nurses, teachers, social workers, and physicians, some university-educated Chinese Americans found work in new Chinese American institutions, including the Chinese Hospital, the Chinese YMCA and YWCA, and Protestant social welfare organizations. During the depression, dozens were employed by New Deal agencies such as the Works Progress Administration (WPA) and the California State Emergency Relief Administration.

Their professional status and experience helped bridge the chasm between the Chinese American community and dominant white society. Through experiences with American voluntary associations and government institutions, second-generation Chinese Americans became familiar with the language, customs, and political strategies necessary to enlist assistance, seek government intervention, and draw on a network of regional and national chapters of voluntary associations. Although national organizations like the YWCA had racially segregated affiliates, they also provided occasions to cross racial divides. Chinese Americans were able to share common socialization, values, and rhetoric with white affiliates and build alliances. They came of age in the post-World-War-I Americanization campaigns that conveyed a vision of hygienic and heteronormative American family life. They recognized that the values of monogamous morality and domesticity were crucial to the formation of the citizen-subject. They were effective in making their community and its needs appear "deserving" to the majority white constituencies. Their socialization fostered an interest in working within the system to highlight needs and seek charitable and government remedies, and the ability to do so.[3]

During the 1930s Chinese American social workers, journalists, and community advocates developed two overlapping strategies to call public attention to Chinatown's social ills. As a political strategy to claim access to government resources, they identified needs and demonstrated the worth of those whose needs were unmet. The identification of needs involved first the statistical comparison to standards and norms of mortality, disease incidence, living arrangements, facilities, and residential space. This strategy identified which groups and neighborhoods had deficient or substandard access to clinics and hospitals, recreation, and housing. However, "need" alone would not necessarily elicit assistance. In order to portray substandard circumstances as tragic and those affected as requiring assistance, community activists and social workers described those adversely affected as "worthy" and "deserving." Not only were these individuals "caught in a web of misfortune," their circumstances inspired action and redress because of their status as dependents—either young children or married women. Sympathy could be invoked and politically marshaled not just because of their status but also because of evidence that these women and children demonstrated—through their morality, conduct, and aspiration—a desire to acculturate to American norms, values, and standards of living.

Using these strategies, Chinese Americans had energetically made claims to municipal, state, and federal resources. They lobbied the Public Health Department to open the Chinese Health Center in 1934 and the Recreation Department to construct the Chinese Playground in 1927. A cadre of eighteen Chinese American social workers were hired to administer welfare assistance to nearly 18 percent of Chinatown's population during the height of the depression. Through WPA-supported studies, Chinese American social workers identified Chinatown's social welfare needs, children's health status, and living conditions.[4]

In the mid-1930s, Chinese American social workers and community activists focused on the devastating contribution of decrepit housing to tuberculosis infection. The rampant spread of tuberculosis in the Chinese community presented a dramatic obstacle to clipping the soaring mortality rates. The understanding and treatment of tuberculosis had changed dramatically since the late nineteenth century. In the 1870s pulmonary tuberculosis, otherwise known as consumption or phthisis, was considered a hereditary predisposition aggravated by a bad environment or improper living. Physicians could not intervene to reverse predisposition but could attempt to strengthen a patient's body with nutrition, tonics, and a change to a drier and less congested environment. By the 1920s and 1930s, tuberculosis was understood as a bacterial disease that was communicable, preventable, and often curable. Robert Koch had identified the tubercle bacillus in 1882 and proved that tuberculosis was communicable when an uninfected individual inhaled bacilli from an infected person's sputum. Factors such as crowding and poor nutrition could predispose a person to it, but the tubercle bacillus was the indisputable cause of the disease. Physicians recommended sanitarium treatment and, increasingly, thoracic surgery for those who did not respond to the more conservative recommendation of rest, nutrition, and fresh air. After Word War II, breakthroughs in antibiotic treatments led to sharp declines in sanitarium stays and to eventual cures.[5]

In the 1930s and 1940s San Francisco public health officials and social workers attributed the high tuberculosis mortality rate among the Chinese to congested housing and disease-spreading practices such as unsanitary community kitchens, consumption of meals from common serving dishes, and the habit of spitting indiscriminately. In October 1934, the Public Health Department opened the Chinese Health Center at 1212 Powell Street to screen for tuberculosis and provide immunization services to Chinatown residents. Public health nurses used tuberculin skin tests and x-ray examinations to identify potential cases. The San Francisco Tuberculosis Association had used these detection techniques in the mobile screening centers it set up in hospitals and health clinics in European immigrant and working-class neighborhoods since the second decade of the twentieth century. For two decades, the San Francisco Tuberculosis Association had conducted annual programs of free fluoroscopic and chest x-ray examinations to identify tuberculosis sufferers as well as to survey the healthy population. Beginning in the 1930s, the Tuberculosis Association offered these free exams to Chinese residents in coordination with the Chinese YMCA and YWCA. For individuals diagnosed with tuberculosis, public health officials arranged physician care, hospitalization in special isolation wards and sanitariums, and training in hygienic habits.[6]

Further improvements in health were stymied by an unsanitary and overcrowded living environment. In order to win sympathy for Chinese

residents, Chinese American activists and their supporters were convinced that they had to transform the representations of Chinese American society. They had to replace nineteenth-century images of the Chinese as inscrutable aliens living in mysterious clan networks of single
men with images of assimilating, Americanized nuclear families. The
agenda of promoting community self-improvement and positive public representations was at the forefront for the group of activists, social workers, and businessmen who launched the *Chinese Digest,* an
English-language newsmagazine for "American Chinese," which published weekly for one year and later monthly, from 1935 to 1941. The
first editor of the *Chinese Digest,* Thomas Chinn, argued that improving living conditions for Chinese Americans required dislodging prevailing Hollywood images of a "sleepy Celestial enveloped in mists of opium
fumes or a halo of Oriental philosophy." He added that "the *Chinese
Digest* is fighting to kill this Celestial bogey and substitute a normal human being who drives automobiles, shops for the latest gadgets and
speaks good English." [7] Chinn's image of the "normal" Chinese American was calculated to resemble the average American middle-class consumer. Chinn recognized that claims to full political access and inclusion
in American society would require that Chinese behavior appear intelligible. For Chinese women and men, long derided for subsisting at an
"Oriental standard of living," there could be no better claim to American citizenship than evidence that their consumption levels had brought
them up to the "American standard of living." Chinn argued, however,
that the pathetic housing conditions in Chinatown were a persistent barrier to living at the American standard. In the *Chinese Digest*'s first editorial, Chinn decried the "menace to health and happiness" and highlighted the public health dangers of tenement housing. The social worker
Lim P. Lee condemned the windowless and cramped rooms in the tenements, where eight to ten people were crammed into a single room. [8]

These observations of overcrowded, unventilated, and dilapidated
housing were not new. As noted in earlier chapters, in the nineteenth
century public health authorities, labor leaders, and women missionaries had derided the living conditions in Chinatown. The difference
was that these nineteenth-century observers had blamed the Chinese
residents for the filth and squalor in which they lived. Lim P. Lee and
Thomas Chinn, however, blamed the housing crisis on American society's corrosive system of racial segregation and social neglect. Lee
faulted a powerful system of legal and extralegal intimidation that
forced Chinese to live in a severely restricted area. The housing crisis

was further exacerbated by slumlords who charged high rents but made no improvements in their property.[9]

Since the nineteenth century, systems of formal and informal segregation had maintained the boundaries of Chinatown, regulating where Chinese American women, men, and children could live. Chinese Americans found it impossible to move outside the boundaries of Chinatown. Attempts to move encountered resistance from white real estate brokers, who refused to show Chinese Americans houses in exclusively white neighborhoods, and from white landlords, who turned down Chinese tenants.[10] Chinese Americans confronted concerns that they practiced "vices peculiar to their own people" and that they would be a "source of danger and contamination" to their white neighbors.[11] Those who were allowed to live in white neighborhoods were informally tested to ensure that "Oriental" homes were "exceptionally neat and clean" and that the Chinese did not live like "peasants or pigs." Chinese Americans had to dislodge the images of animality, filth, deviance, and disease that had proliferated from the representations of Chinatown. Like the nineteenth-century Presbyterian missionaries, twentieth-century white homeowners were comforted by those Chinese who adapted to American living styles and standards in furnishings and decor and by Chinese families who conformed to idealized nuclear-family social dynamics.[12]

Residential segregation produced in Chinatown the environment of high rents, tenement slums, and limited opportunities to move. Landlords and other property owners had developed the racial restrictions that shaped both the twentieth-century segregation system and the Chinatown housing shortages that in turn inflated rentals. The landlords prospered in the prevailing system and were reluctant to invest in improvements. When the Public Health Department successfully condemned substandard buildings, the intervention exacerbated the shortage of affordable housing. Recognizing the disincentives for landlords to renovate tenements, Chinese American social workers sought alternatives to the private housing market.[13]

An opportunity to radically change Chinatown housing emerged in 1937 when Congress passed the Wagner-Steagall Housing Act, which allocated hundreds of millions of dollars for public housing construction nationwide. The enormous commitment to public housing construction was meant to ensure that low-income families would have access to "decent, safe and sanitary dwellings."[14] However, Chinese American activists had to persuade a skeptical public and indifferent politicians to spend a portion of the ten million dollars allocated to San Francisco on a housing project in Chinatown. Despite a century of diatribes against Chinatown's dilapidated and disease-incubating tenements, there was no guarantee that the "alien Chinese" were entitled to federal housing funds. Politicians and civic authorities preferred to concentrate on the housing needs of white working-class and lower middle-class constituencies and neighborhoods.[15]

In 1938 Chinese American social workers, health workers, and teachers formed a committee to lobby for the allocation of public housing funds in Chinatown. In a preliminary report presented to the San Francisco Housing Authority, the WPA social worker Samuel Lee and the *Chinese Digest* editor William Hoy argued that the growing population of low-income Chinese families were confined to cramped tenement rooms with communal kitchens and toilets. They estimated that nearly eleven thousand Chinese lived as families, which eclipsed the population of seven thousand single men. Drawing on survey samples of families on relief, the report unfurled statistics on housing density, the demand on communal toilets, and monthly wage levels to present dry, statistical evidence of the need for fully equipped apartments for low-income families.

The housing crisis, largely ignored by local politicians, captured national attention when Eleanor Roosevelt championed the cause in her nationally syndicated "My Day" column on June 6, 1939. After reading an unpublished report on Chinatown living conditions, she urged San Francisco officials to take action to alleviate the housing crisis.[16] Roosevelt provided a personal gloss on the issue: "I always enjoy my trips to Chinatown when I am in San Francisco, but I have always been conscious that just as in our own picturesque Chinese quarter in New York City, there are undoubtedly dangers to the whole city there because of poor housing and living conditions."[17] In an effort to capture the attention of the white public, Roosevelt resurrected an alarm frequently expressed by nineteenth-century public health advocates that the unhealthy conditions in Chinatown imperiled the entire city.

The following day the Associated Press reported the findings of the study over its international wire service under the headline "San Francisco Chinatown Living Conditions Held Worse Than Any in World."[18] San Francisco's newspapers declared that Chinatown was a "slum largely unfit for human habitation, comparable with the worst in the world and where a majority of the residents live in worse squalor than in any city in China." The report blamed the ignorance of San Franciscans, the neglect of slumlords, and the informal policy of racial residential restrictions for forcing the Chinese to live in crowded, unsanitary slums.[19]

The nationwide publicity startled San Francisco's officials. The San Francisco Housing Authority (SFHA) director, A. J. Cleary, denied the report's "exaggerated" conclusions and expected that the health officer J. C. Geiger would verify the "healthy and cleanly condition" of San Francisco's Chinatown. Cleary argued that the 1906 fire had cleansed Chinatown of its disreputable tenements, and that the buildings since then had met stringent health and housing codes. Geiger, however, refused to provide the SFHA with political cover for ignoring the living conditions in Chinatown. He declared that the conditions in Chinatown were "even worse than described" and boasted of sharing Chinese Health Center reports with the authors of the study. Geiger unequivocally established the link between health and housing. He claimed that the high rate of tuberculosis infection was "so interwoven with the wretched housing" in Chinatown that it was impossible to disentangle the two perils. The mortality rate for tuberculosis infection was more than double the city average, and one-quarter of all tuberculosis cases in the city were diagnosed and treated at the Chinese Health Center. Health officials blamed the high tuberculosis rate on bad ventilation, overcrowded sleeping accommodations, and the impossibility of isolating the sick.[20]

Geiger reported that since the 1930s the Public Health Department had aggressively tried to identify and track tuberculosis cases to their domestic contacts in the Chinese American community. He declared that overcrowding punished infants and was directly related to high rates of infant mortality. Respiratory infections such as pneumonia, chronic bronchitis, and sinus infections far outstripped those in the rest of the city. The public health nurses asked questions such as "What . . . can we expect of our babies who often share rooms used for all living purposes with six or more people?" The high living density was both an index of poverty as well as an enabler of the spread of respiratory infection.[21] The health dangers of Chinatown's overcrowding had been chronicled for a century; however, in the 1930s they were perceived to cruelly converge on the Chinese American community, slaying infants and sabotaging the community's processes of social reproduction.

Some Chinese leaders responded to the publicity with surprising hostility. Kenneth Lee, former secretary of the CCBA, bristled at the suggestion that Chinatown was a slum and residents lived in "squalor." Lee argued that renovations had made these conditions a rarity and that "Chinatown's younger generation . . . live [like] average American families." His confidence that crowding was "almost a thing of the past" and that "only the elders, whose income is limited, remain in cramped quarters" revealed anxieties that images of tuberculosis-breeding slums would keep white tourists from patronizing Chinatown bazaars, restaurants, and nightclubs. The housing exposé coincided with the 1939 Golden Gate International Exposition, when Chinese business leaders were intensively promoting Chinatown as an exotic tourist playground. Even the social worker and public housing advocate Lim P. Lee feared that the publicity about slum conditions might provoke more fear than sympathy from the (white) public. He remained cautious about the action that might result: "Airing our dirty linen to the public view will not help us to solve our social and human problems." [22] Both men preferred images that highlighted Chinese American dignity and striving, over the sensational coverage of tenements and slums.

The editors of the communist labor periodical *People's Daily World* lambasted Kenneth Lee for disingenuously depicting "overcrowding and slum conditions . . . [as] things of the past." The editors suspected Chinese leaders were reluctant to embarrass Chinese landlords, who by 1939 owned three-fifths of all Chinatown property, according to the study. Chinatown property ownership had shifted dramatically since 1906, when Chinese owned less than 10 percent of all property. During the property boom of 1927 to 1930, Chinese businesspeople bought up buildings at inflated prices and then justified steep rents to pay their heavy mortgage burdens. White communist organizers argued that Chinese landlords preferred the captive market created by housing segregation and were wary of competition from public housing.[23]

Surprisingly, the Chinese Americans most eager to parlay the sensationalist news coverage into policy changes were the young businessmen and professionals in the Chinese Junior Chamber of Commerce. The organization was established in 1938 as an affiliate of the white Junior Chamber of Commerce. Myron Chan, George Chow, and Chingwah Lee gathered thirty young Chinese American businessmen and professionals to form a Chinatown branch and elected Dr. Theodore Lee as their first president. In November 1939 they joined forces with the Chinatown housing project committee, chaired by Chee S. Lowe, which included members of the Chinese American Citizens Alliance, the Chinese Chamber of Commerce, and the CCBA.[24]

Chinese American activists repackaged the data from a decade of housing and health surveys and challenged the city to rescue the Chinese community from threats of social disintegration and disease. They emphasized that overcrowded and unventilated housing generated the breeding ground for respiratory diseases and tuberculosis. In spotlighting the precarious condition of Chinese American families, they reported that young couples delayed marriage plans and deferred childbearing because of space limitations. And those children who were born experienced retarded physical development because of the unhealthy conditions. Cramped quarters were perceived to breed disease as well as criminality. They predicted that those children who did live to maturity would become juvenile delinquents in such an environment.[25]

Social workers described the unsuitable and unsanitary Chinatown housing as a shocking legacy of Chinese bachelor society. Chinese bachelors lived in tiny cubicles and barracks and were said to have "little desire to improve their living quarters." The bachelors lived "in back of, above or below their places of employment or they huddle into bachelor tenements," often with a dozen men sharing a small room and sleeping on the bunks in rotation after putting in fourteen-hour workdays.[26] Chinese American families had to adjust to the architecture of sleeping barracks and communal toilets. Social reformers argued that families could not tolerate the "abject squalor and filth and lack of sanitary facilities" endured by Chinese bachelors. The accusation of bachelor indifference harbored suspicions that, bereft of the presence of wives and children, Chinese men had no interest in improving basic sanitary conditions. The very necessity for space, light, separate toilets, and kitchens characterized the specific gender and sexual coding of monogamous heterosexual family life.[27]

In the prevailing political calculus, Chinatown public housing advocates denigrated the circumstances and indifference of Chinese bachelors while upholding the needs of "deserving" nuclear families. Since only low-income working nuclear families were eligible for New Deal public housing, the emphasis on "Chinatown's families" was a pragmatic move to overturn the stereotypes of bachelor society and to ensure Chinese American eligibility for public housing placement. The strategy was aimed at recrafting the sensationalist portraits of decadent, bachelor Chinatown with a somber portrayal of the needs of deserving families. The plight of children held the center of a sympathetic needs assessment. The conditions of tiny, "dark, poorly ventilated rooms" were considered grim for adults but an incontestable "health hazard" for the growing number of Chinese babies.[28] Although Chinese bachelors were not eligible for placement in public housing, they shaped the boundaries of those considered "worthy" and "deserving" of public housing assistance. The aberration of Chinese bachelor society acted as a foil for the astonishing

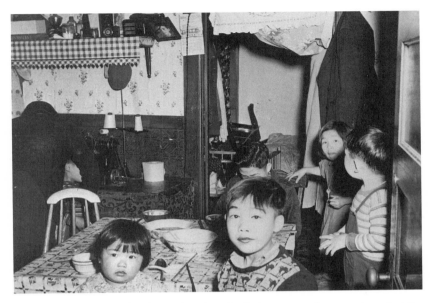

Figure 14. This photo of a Chinese American family in a cramped tenement apartment was included in the San Francisco Real Property Survey conducted circa 1939. Courtesy San Francisco History Center, San Francisco Public Library.

progress of the Chinese American nuclear family. Housing was seen as the only remaining obstacle to public health reform and normal social reproduction. The Junior Chamber's fears of "the imminent breakdown of the family" depicted the Chinese as victims of social disintegration, victims who merited assistance.[29] (See Figure 14.)

Despite the national publicity and the support of businesspeople, the SFHA remained reluctant to approve a housing project for Chinatown and divert funds away from housing projects that would serve white working-class constituents. Rather than wait for the SFHA's approval, the white Junior Chamber commissioned the architect Mark Daniels Sr., who had designed the Chinese Pavilion at the 1939 San Francisco Exposition, to draw up plans for a Chinatown public housing project. With his experience he was well suited to design buildings with Chinese architectural features, including pagoda-style roofs and ornate front gates, which would "further augment the district's world-famed tourist attraction value." Slum clearance and the construction of sanitary new apartments with an "Oriental atmosphere" would only heighten the new businesslike image of Chinatown's sanitized exoticism.[30]

In October 1939, the white Junior Chamber launched a speakers' campaign to drum up political support for a public housing solution to Chinatown's housing crisis. Representatives of the Junior Chamber and a coalition of Chinese American social workers, journalists, and civic leaders who created the Chinatown Housing Committee fanned out to meetings of local civic, business, and social welfare organizations. In tandem, they galvanized San Francisco civic and improvement clubs to write letters and lobby federal and local housing authorities.[31] The public education campaign focused on the Junior Chamber poster "Chinatown Housing: Which Shall It Be?" which graphically displayed side-by-side the options available to San Francisco residents. On one half, under the headline "Poor Housing breeds filth, disease, crime, and fire hazard" were startling photographs of the dirty toilet stalls, dilapidated sinks, and peeling walls that were "typical" of Chinatown conditions. On the other half, under the headline "Good Housing breeds health, safety, and good citizenship," were drawings of multistoried apartment buildings with pagoda-style roofs and balconies and a rendering of an interior that was spacious and orderly. The poster warned that 85 percent of Chinatown housing was "substandard" and that 25 percent of San Francisco's tuberculosis cases were in Chinatown. The poster suggested that "if we give the Chinese proper housing we reduce the danger of plague, aid health as well as business and, at the same time, retain the lure of San Francisco's famed Chinatown."[32]

Unlike other public housing projects, which faced resistance from neighboring property owners who feared plummeting property values and increased crime, the Chinatown public housing project even drew the support of the Nob Hill Protective Association. The protective association sought to stem the "intrusion" of the Chinese into their neighborhood. Historically, Nob Hill had been an exclusively white, upper-middle-class neighborhood. Before the depression, Chinese residents had been contained in the district bounded by Powell Street on the west, by Broadway on the north, by Kearny on the east, and by Bush Street on the south. During the depression, the eastern edge of Nob Hill had slowly become part of Chinatown as wealthier Chinese paid premium rents to lease apartment houses.[33] Joseph Bauers, a spokesman for the Nob Hill Protective Association, explained that his members were waging a "losing battle against encroachment on their territory" by the Chinese and hoped that a new housing project would relieve the pressure on the district's racial boundaries. Bauers endorsed the implicit segregation argument of the Junior Chamber's president, Arthur J. Dolan Jr., that "better housing would keep the Chinese in Chinatown." [34]

The intensive lobbying persuaded the SFHA to propose a Chinatown project where 250 dwelling units were planned at a cost of $1.25 million.[35] However, the exorbitant property prices in Chinatown presented another obstacle for Chinatown housing advocates. The property costs exceeded the $1.50-per-square-foot maximum set by the U.S. Housing Authority (USHA). The USHA administrators were sympathetic to the problem of high land values in Chinatown and offered to cover excess costs if the city paid for one-third of the land costs above the federal land acquisition budget. For the first time the city was required to appropriate its own funds for public housing construction. The board of supervisors had to approve the unusual supplemental appropriation of $75,000 in order to build public housing for the Chinese in Chinatown.[36] Lim P. Lee, alarmed at the possibility that high land costs would drive the board to locate a Chinese housing project on the outskirts of the city, warned that "housing in some isolated spots would be disastrous to the social life of the Chinese." Thriving Chinatown businesses would be cut off from Chinese consumers and even the tourist trade would be irreparably harmed. Lee played up the tourist card by claiming that construction of "modern, sanitary dwellings in Chinese design" within Chinatown would "pay for itself in a short time by increased tourist trade." [37]

In order to save the Chinatown housing project, the Junior Chamber and its civic allies orchestrated hearings before the board of supervisors to persuade the supervisors to pass the special appropriation. Chinatown housing advocates touted the cost-effectiveness of public housing construction over the expenses of tuberculosis care. In a presentation before the board, Lee declared that San Francisco taxpayers were spending $104,000 annually to care for Chinese tuberculosis patients at city hospitals and sanitariums, in addition to that spent on indigent aid to their dependent children. He warned that the number of Chinese tuberculosis patients admitted to San Francisco General Hospital had nearly doubled in six years and would continue to increase annually. Since decaying housing spread tuberculosis, Lee and the Junior Chamber representatives argued that Chinatown public housing would save taxpayers money. The annual expenses for tuberculosis care exceeded the onetime investment in public housing construction.[38]

The political tie between tuberculosis care expenses and public housing investments won over the editors at the *San Francisco Chronicle* and the *News*. They applauded the "humanitarian" and fiscally prudent benefits of destroying Chinatown's "breeding grounds for white plague germs" by providing "modern housing." They optimistically believed that public housing would miraculously bring tuberculosis infection rates to normal levels, saving the city from the "excessive cost of health services and removing a dangerous source of infection for all the rest of the population." In their zeal for immediate solutions, they conflated a limited public housing project with extensive slum clearance and apartment reconstruction for all residents. Correlation of tuberculosis infection directly with the living environment made the investment in public housing a panacea for all of Chinatown's ills and won political support from the board of supervisors, who agreed to cover the higher land costs for the Chinatown housing project.[39]

In the weeks and months that followed, local and national publications transformed the representations of San Francisco's Chinese population. They were now depicted as the patient victims of pernicious circumstances, worthy of public assistance, and their housing crisis was portrayed as the "big responsibility" of the city. The *Woman's Home Companion* celebrated plans for the new housing project and for the relief it would provide Chinatown families who were "jammed into living quarters that are both un-American and un-Chinese." The writer insisted that slum housing was "no way to treat our good friends the Chinese and we knew it and they knew it."[40] The discourse of Chinese American worthiness even persuaded conservative opponents of public housing, such as the San Francisco Federation of Taxpayers. Mr. Kleiber, the president of the Federation of Taxpayers, favored low-rent housing for Chinese residents because of the "sterling character of the Chinese people." He explained that "there is no better type of foreign-born resident than the Chinese. They build our railroads, harvest our crops and live according to a legal code which puts our own to shame." Kleiber's portrayal of Chinese Americans as industrious and law-abiding enhanced their standing as cultural citizens who deserved better than "the squalid conditions of Chinatown."

However, Kleiber's embrace of deserving Chinese Americans foundered on the question of segregation. The common presumption that the Chinatown housing project would serve exclusively Chinese tenants was shattered by the SFHA's admission that it could not officially endorse segregation. Without assurances of segregated occupancy, Kleiber withdrew his support for extra city funds to pay for the Chinatown project. He reasoned that cheaper land was available if the SFHA could not ensure an explicitly segregated solution to the Chinatown housing crisis.[41]

The SFHA's hypocrisy, however, became obvious when World War II postponed the construction of the Chinatown housing project, and contradictions between the SFHA's policy of segregation and rhetoric of antidiscrimination came to the surface. Since the opening of Holly Courts, the first SFHA housing project, in 1940, the SFHA pretended to offer apartments to any needy applicants. Although twenty Chinese families applied for admission to Holly Courts, the Chinese applicants, along with black, Japanese, and Filipino applicants, were refused apartments. The SFHA justified tacit segregation on a "neighborhood pattern" policy applied to federal housing projects nationwide in order to placate white segregation advocates. The policy was designed to "preserve the same racial composition which existed in the neighborhood," prevent the "commingling of races," and thereby maintain the "public peace and good order."[42] This policy promoted racially exclusive claims on housing projects, since there was a patent unwillingness to acknowledge racial diversity in any residential district. During the 1940s most housing projects were reserved for white tenants. When wartime housing shortages emerged, the SFHA made a concession to black war workers by directing them exclusively to the Westside Courts Project, which opened in 1943.[43] Similar struggles over racial integration and segregation in public housing exploded in Detroit, Philadelphia, and Chicago.[44]

In July 1949, Congress authorized extension of the public housing program and recommitted funds for war-deferred and new public housing projects. The SFHA devoted its first federal funds to construction of the Chinatown housing project as a "token of esteem for San Francisco's citizens of Chinese descent." The 1941 construction estimate of $1.5 million doubled to over $3.25 million.[45] In the fall of 1949, the SFHA demolished dozens of stores and tenements on Pacific Avenue to make way for construction. Forty-one families and 158 single men were evicted from the three-block site. The SFHA had hired Mary Mai Chong to conduct a census of affected families and tenants and to offer only low-income families temporary placement in the other SFHA apartments. Only two families had requested replacement housing from the SFHA; the others had chosen to stay in the Chinatown area and search for housing on their own. Although low-income families that were evicted had priority for placement in the about-to-be-constructed Ping Yuen apartments, the single men were left to fend for themselves. Many of these men could seek assistance and charity only from their district associations.[46]

Three long, six-story, reinforced concrete buildings with open-air corridors rose on Pacific Avenue between Grant and Stockton Avenues. The one-, two-, and three-bedroom apartments were outfitted with bathtubs and the latest modern kitchen appliances, and they housed 232 families. The project's Chinese name, *Ping Yuen,* which means "Tranquil Garden," and the buildings' "Oriental" architectural features—the dragon decorations and Chinese characters on the facade—gave aesthetic confirmation to the project's special status as the first public housing project in the United States planned exclusively for Chinese families. A replica of the Paliou Gate at the Yellow Monastery in Beijing provided the entrance to the housing complex. More than six hundred families applied for apartments, but the SFHA and a Chinese American selection committee gave priority to veterans and U.S. citizens.[47]

When the Ping Yuen project opened in October 1951, the apartment complex was hailed as a triumph of the modernization of Chinatown. The Public Health Department's director, J. C. Geiger, proclaimed that the "modern" apartment buildings would "automatically improve health conditions in the district," reducing the tuberculosis and infant mortality rates. The Ping Yuen project was widely understood in terms of its impact on the larger Chinatown District and its Chinese American residents. It fulfilled the promise of "progress" in housing, sanitation, and greater access to "modern" services.[48]

Five thousand people attended dedication ceremonies, which celebrated the project's opening with parades, speeches, and fireworks. For Chinese American activists who had struggled for fifteen years for its completion, Ping Yuen symbolized a recognition of full citizenship, equality, and a pledge of civic inclusion. The *Chinese Press* proclaimed that "Ping Yuen is America's pledge that a century-old wrong is being righted." Chinese Americans summoned the American history of discrimination and contemporary global politics to glorify the local triumph of public housing construction. In the wake of the communist takeover of government in mainland China and the outbreak of the Korean War, stridently anticommunist Chinese American leaders declared Ping Yuen a symbol of American equality. Lim P. Lee argued that the apartments represented a "dynamic challenge to Communist charges that American democracy" has no place for the poor and for racial minorities. In a rhetoric steeped in patriotism and wartime sacrifice, Dr. Theodore Lee, chairman of the Chinatown Housing Committee,

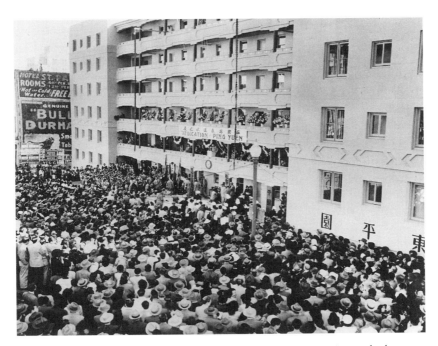

Figure 15. The dedication ceremony for Ping Yuen East Housing Project took place on October 21, 1951. Courtesy San Francisco History Center, San Francisco Public Library.

saw the structures as a reward for the loyalty and fidelity demonstrated by American citizens of Chinese ancestry during World War II. As a monument to the American way of life, the apartments would also "make better citizens" of a new generation of Chinese Americans.[49] (See Figure 15.)

Godfrey Lehman of the Council for Civic Unity saw a different symbolism in the buildings. Lehman appreciated the project's sanitary advantages and applauded the move of more than two hundred Chinese families from "disease incubating, decaying tenements into clean, modern apartments." However, he gave a stinging rebuke to the project's purpose. For Lehman, the Chinese characters embellishing the buildings facades might as well have declared that this "project is for Chinese only. Negroes, whites, even other peoples of Oriental descent—go live in your own projects."[50] Although in 1950 the Council for Civic Unity and the American Civil Liberties Union had forced the SFHA to renounce racial segregation in future public housing projects, the policy change had not applied immediately to war-deferred projects like Ping Yuen.[51] Lehman was disturbed that Chinese American community leaders refused to open Ping Yuen to applicants of all races as a symbolic gesture of desegregation.

Lehman, like many of his white liberal colleagues, refused to recognize that Chinese Americans' access to public housing had been won not through a campaign for racial integration but a crusade to demonstrate a racial minority's needs and worth. Although the Council for Civic Unity had predicted that desegregated public housing would accommodate twice as many Chinese American families as the Ping Yuen project, Chinese American activists had been skeptical.[52] From decades of experience, Chinese American leaders had realized that the prospect of acquiring a public housing project that recognized the entitlement of Chinese Americans to the social provisions of American society was a far more realistic goal than any attempt at dismantling the system of residential segregation in either private or public housing. The political reality of segregation shaped the Chinese public housing movement's strategy for a Chinatown project.

Ping Yuen functioned as a demonstration project for enabling nuclear family domesticity. The proper environment of multiple rooms with explicit purposes would enhance the conviviality and viability of the Chinese family and make their relationships and social dynamics familiar and intelligible to the white public. The *San Francisco News* declared the arrival of "real homes" for the first time in the "history of Chinatown": "Families which have endured the shocking housing of Chinatown never planned for family living will have a real living room where they can gather and visit and where the children can invite their friends. Each home will have its own kitchen and bath, and enough bedroom space for all the family. Each has been designed to receive plenty of fresh air and its windows will invite the sunshine."[53] The dedication ceremonies at the opening of the first Ping Yuen apartment building showcased the Chinese American model of respectable domesticity and the idea that it could flourish with proper domestic space. Mayor Elmer Robinson presented a gold key to Ping Yuen's "first family," Henry G. and Alice Wong and their two children, four-year-old Beverly and four-month-old Calvin. From over six hundred applications for 232 apartments, the family was selected because of Henry Wong's service as a navy sailor in World War II and the family's need for more space. Henry worked as a waiter in a Chinatown restaurant and Alice was a resourceful, university-educated housewife. The Wongs and their two young children had lived in a cramped two-room tenement. There was no space for separate bedrooms for parents and children, no room to entertain, no specific cook-

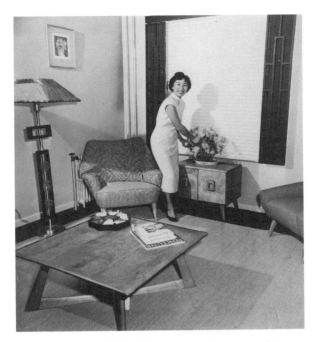

Figure 16. The model Pearl Lau arranges flowers in a living room in Ping Yuen East, 1951. Photo by Bob Campbell, *San Francisco Chronicle* Library. Courtesy California Historical Society, FN-31288.

ing and dining facilities, and they shared a bath and toilet with other families. As the featured tenants of Ping Yuen East, the Wongs had their pick of two-bedroom apartments.[54] The Wongs represented the idea of the young couple and their children who were rewarded for the husband's war veteran status and the couple's work ethic and attempts at nuclear-family domesticity in order to be among the ranks of the "deserving Chinese" who could escape from the "warrens of Chinatown" to proper public housing.[55] Following the dedication ceremonies, the public was invited to inspect two model apartments furnished and decorated by Chinatown merchants. The apartment, shown to the press by the model Pearl Lau, stressed modern "functionalism" in design but had "strong Chinese accents in lamps, draperies and ornaments."[56] (See Figures 16 and 17.)

The idea that young nuclear families were "deserving" had dire consequences for the men who lived in the residential hotels and tenements that were leveled to make way for the three Ping Yuen buildings. What happened to the 158 men who were evicted and made homeless in 1949?

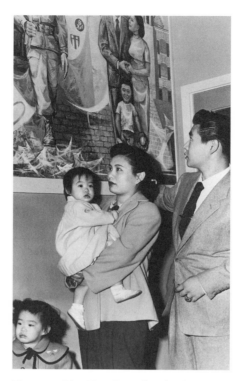

Figure 17. Ping Yuen East's first family, Alice
and Henry Wong and their children, Beverly
(standing) and Calvin (in Alice's arms), poses
in front of the Ping Yuen mural, 1951. Courtesy San Francisco History Center, San Francisco Public Library.

Although the 41 evicted families were accommodated in a variety of
public and private housing, the bachelors got lost in the frame of the
Ping Yuen dedication ceremonies, when 232 patriotic Chinese American
families were accommodated in the new sanitary apartments with the
latest modern appliances. In the mid–twentieth century this new articulation of citizenship adapted the trope of the American middle-class family to Chinese American entitlement claims.[57]

Chinese American activists were delighted that their claims to social
provision were politically and publicly recognized. Although the effort
to prove the existence of middle-class Chinese Americans enjoyed uneven success in private housing, Chinese American activists did succeed
in reshaping the image of Chinese American society in their quest for ac-

cess to federal entitlements like public housing. The markers of citizenship and the nuclear family that Chinese leaders and social workers had so carefully cultivated became the very eligibility requirements that the SFHA imposed on Chinese applicants for the Ping Yuen project. Veterans were given priority, and only nuclear families were eligible for public housing placement. Although such eligibility practices were not unique among public housing placements in postwar United States, they did divide Chinatown residents according to the familiar normal/aberrant dichotomies. Americanized nuclear families joined other favored Americans on the "normal" side of the dichotomy, while single Chinese laboring men remained aberrant.

Chinese American activists discovered that redeveloping housing in Chinatown drew wide political acceptance. Within the context of a segregated society where the individual claims of racial minorities were frequently ignored, Chinese American activists proceeded along an avenue for social justice by means of lobbying for group needs. In the following decades, activists continued to use this path of making racial claims to social provisions such as public housing. In the late 1950s, they mobilized for the construction of an addition to Ping Yuen farther down Pacific Avenue. Throughout the 1950s, Chinese Americans in San Francisco parlayed their political voice and votes into crusades for additional public assistance to improve housing and community facilities for families and, in the 1970s, enlarged their agenda to include the single and widowed elderly who lived in Chinatown.[58]

This strategy, based upon group claims and intent on preserving the Chinatown ghetto as the center of the community, contested liberal political assumptions of individualism and unfettered mobility. However, the movement this strategy spawned carried much of the cultural baggage of mainstream U.S. politics. Foremost, Chinese American activists fundamentally favored the process of "Americanization." Furthermore, by placing the viability of the nuclear family at the center of entitlement claims, they and their supporters reaffirmed the assumption that only the nuclear family could ensure proper assimilation to American society. All other social relations and networks were rendered deviant and decidedly un-American.

## SEGREGATION AND CULTURAL REPRESENTATIONS

In October 1950, the *San Francisco News* reported the demise of the cultural buttress of segregation, the accumulated traditions and ignorance that contradicted rationality and liberal modernity: "San Francisco's 'Great Wall'—the boundaries which in the past have confined Chinatown through custom, superstition and fear—is crumbling as the latest addition to the American family, the Chinese-American, is melting into the areas outside." [59] Despite optimistic predictions, residential segregation as a way of life for Chinese men and women did not disappear for another two decades. The attempts of Chinese social workers and political activists to combat the class fears that they believed undergirded segregation were of little avail. In many of the welfare and housing reports produced after the 1930s, both Chinese and white writers carefully depicted Chinese society as increasingly dominated by modern nuclear families with middle-class habits and sensibilities. Assimilation to these middle-class norms was expected to help Chinese Americans "integrate" into American society.

Jane Lee, interviewed in 1974 for the Combined Asian American Resources Oral History Project, recalled her family's experiences moving into a house in Oakland. Her father, Man Quong Fong, a reputable retail pharmacist, recognized that his white neighbors could prohibit his family from moving into the house they had bought. Lee recalled being tested by her white neighbors to determine whether her family acted like "peasants or pigs." To their astonishment, the neighbors discovered that the Fong family were "human," tidy, and polite and that they spoke English fluently. At first only a handful of neighbors allowed their children to play with Jane and her siblings: "Most stayed away and thought we had the plague or something." In time, though, the neighbors decided that the Fong children and parents were "normal" and gradually accepted them, if somewhat reluctantly, into the neighborhood. [60]

These new representations, however, did little to alleviate the hysteria, lawsuits, and violence that greeted the arrival of many Chinese middle-class families into white neighborhoods during the 1940s and 1950s, as racial covenants lost their power to maintain segregation. The large migration of African Americans into San Francisco during World War II, chronic housing shortages in traditionally minority districts, and the increasing fragility of Chinatown boundaries during the depression and afterward contributed to the growing use of and conflict over residential covenants during and immediately following the war. Neighborhood improvement associations sprang up in older residential neighborhoods such as Pacific Heights, the Marina, and Cow Hollow to maintain racially exclusive, upper-middle-class neighborhoods of single-family residences. For example, the Pacific Heights Improvement Association was formed in 1942 to maintain zoning restrictions and to "prevent, if possible, the encroachment of Non-Caucasion [sic]" tenants or property owners.[61] Immediately after the war, a series of cases of Chinese, Filipino, and black families attempting to move into restricted neighborhoods received widespread publicity, galvanizing the improvement associations and rival white-led antidiscrimination groups.

The confrontation between minority home owners and neighborhood residents was often tumultuous, but legal decisions usually failed to clarify the use of racial covenants. In 1944, the attempt by Mabel Tseng to occupy a building she owned at 1150 Clay Street, in the Nob Hill neighborhood, was met with resistance from white neighbors and resulted in a lawsuit filed by twenty-eight white property-owners. Restrictive covenants, devised in 1931, reserved the block on Clay Street between Taylor and Mason Streets exclusively for white residents. Having no representation in court, Tseng lost the suit by default. Superior Judge Foley immediately signed a permanent injunction banning Tseng from her home. The American Civil Liberties Union (ACLU) intervened and the attorney John Brill, a member of the Northern California ACLU Executive Committee, represented Tseng and appealed the injunction.[62] In June 1946 the superior court judge James Conlan upheld the restrictive residential covenant, in his opinion stating that the admission of non-Caucasians to the area would constitute a "lowering of social and living standards." Furthermore, Conlan signed a permanent injunction forbidding nonwhites from occupying property bounded by Washington, Sacramento, Mason and Jones Streets while allowing nonwhites to continue to own these properties, since freedom of property ownership was considered an inalienable right.[63]

A few months prior to Conlan's decision upholding racial restrictions on Nob Hill, the enforcement of racial covenants in Portola Heights, a relatively new residential district, was successful opposed. In February 1946, the Portola Heights Boosters Club announced that three families had violated the restrictive covenant of the development, a master deed similar to those initiated earlier in the century in districts like St. Francis Wood and which stated that, with the exception of servants, only whites could reside in Portola Heights. At a meeting of sixty home owners, the boosters club revealed that two families of Filipino men married to white women and a third composed of a Chinese couple had bought homes in Portola Heights. Charles Coates and Walter Knickerbocker, both members of the club, tried to persuade the gathering to file suit to enforce the restrictive covenant. One resident, Albert Thomas, opposed the covenant and, along with several other families, formed the Portola Heights Neighborhood Committee to provide an organized opposition to the covenant. Affiliated with and assisted by the Council for Civic Unity, the Portola Heights Neighborhood Committee publicized attempts to bring suit against the Chinese and Filipino-white couples. The grassroots mobilization in Portola Heights resulted in the withdrawal of the lawsuit.[64] Battles over the occupancy of private property continued to rage until well after a 1948 U.S. Supreme Court ruling invalidating racial covenants. Not until the enforcement of the Fair Housing Act in the late 1960s did many of the twentieth-century strategies of legal and extralegal segregation crumble.

Grassroots and legal strategies of segregation generally succeeded in limiting the housing options of Chinese Americans. This political reality shaped the Chinese public housing movement's strategy for a Chinatown public housing project. Chinese American activists recognized that dismantling the segregation system in private housing was a far less achievable goal than winning an exclusively Chinese American public housing project.

In fact, the struggle for entitlement to public housing and the campaign to promote images of the assimilated Chinese middle-class were ironically combined in an infamous segregation battle in San Francisco's southern suburbs. A local Realtor and opponent of desegregation, Harry Carskadon, claimed that "any attempt to move Negroes or Chinese into areas occupied by the white race will result in a serious depreciation of property values . . . [and] social equalization."[65] Carskadon advocated segregated low-income public housing as the only conceivable means to solve the housing shortage for minorities. At a moment when racial minorities saw the public housing program as an entitlement worth fighting for, white segregationists like Carskadon viewed it as an instrument to appease racial minorities and maintain segregation.

In a letter published in the *San Francisco Chronicle,* Ngai Ho Hong, secretary of the San Francisco chapter of the Chinese American Citizens Alliance, contested Carskadon's use of "racial minority classification." Hong argued that Chinese American men like himself, who had proved their manhood and citizenship by serving as soldiers in World War II, should not be judged by race. Instead, Hong emphasized that citizenship entitled them to "complete freedom" of mobility, a right that several Chinese families had exercised by moving "from San Francisco's Chinatown to adjoining areas because they desire to lead a comfortable home life in healthful and pleasant surroundings instead of having to live in substandard housing conditions."[66] In a variation of wartime propaganda, Hong applied the fight for freedom and democracy abroad to a fight for equality on the home front.

Such attempts to develop a new image of Chinese society—as a community of nuclear families eager to assimilate to American consumer and patriotic culture—did not persuade white segregationists. Claims to citizenship and veteran status did little to dislodge the tenacious adherence to "exclusive white occupancy." Carskadon opposed the movement of wealthy members of nonwhite racial groups onto the Peninsula because he firmly believed that "you cannot mix white people with any different color." He feared that physical proximity would challenge notions of white racial superiority, dislodging perceptions of racial differences in hygiene, morality, and habits. Such developments would allow "social equalization" across race lines and allow a shared middle-class culture to develop.[67]

The Chinatown public housing movement illuminated the ambivalent process by which ghettos created through racial segregation became valorized as ethnic cultural enclaves. During the middle of the twentieth century, descriptions of Chinatown as a site of danger, deviance, and epidemic disease were eclipsed by visions of sanitized exoticism. Entrepreneurs and political leaders, both white and Chinese, promoted Chinatown as a site for the profitable tourist consumption of middle-class white families. Throughout the century, Chinatown transformed from the site of opium dens and prostitutes' cribs to the location for Cantonese restaurants and curio shops. This transformation paralleled the shift in representations of Chinese social structures from those of a bachelor society populated by female prostitutes and single men to a family society of independent nuclear households.

As Chinese American activists were increasingly successful in projecting an image of Chinese society as "normal," they elicited greater interest from government agencies, white politicians, and journalists in the health and social problems of Chinese residents. The mission to redevelop Chinatown through slum clearance and public housing construction reaffirmed the commitment of Chinese American residents to the territory in which they were forced to live. In a climate of continued racial hostility, the redevelopment of Chinatown was perhaps the only possibility for improving the health and living conditions of a large number of Chinese American residents. In the process, Chinese American activists and residents began to associate the Chinatown ghetto with the economic viability, cultural integrity, and social cohesion of the Chinese American community. After decades of white harassment and violence, Chinatown remained the only site of tangible safety and community. It became increasingly impossible to abandon Chinatown. For some Chinese American activists, the maintenance of the Chinatown ghetto became necessary to ensure the cohesion of Chinese American society.

# Norms as a Way of Life

All of this activity in the name of public health begs the questions: Whose public? and Whose health? This examination of public health discourses and practices opens a window to the complicated processes that produce racial meanings and practices in the wider society. Exploring such analytical categories as race through the prism of "public health" helps us understand how Chinese men and women, among others, are absent in the definition of both "public" and "health."[1] In late-nineteenth-century San Francisco, race implicitly structured the concept of public health. The health of Chinese women and men mattered only instrumentally. Medical professionals represented the Chinese as a pestilence, a danger for the white public. Physicians sent them to the "pesthouse" not the hospital. Until the early twentieth century, San Francisco health authorities prescribed the containment of epidemic disease over care of the individuals afflicted, when the patient was Chinese.

Chinese American activists in the mid–twentieth century proceeded upon a strategy of assimilation to American "norms" in domestic arrangements, consumption patterns, and social conduct in the arduous struggle to be perceived as "normal" in their social habits and living styles. This strategy produced both the recognition of citizenship for the Chinese American family community and the disbursal of government resources for the infrastructure and services to sustain the normalized Chinese Americans in their health. With the construction of the Ping Yuen housing project, a new public health clinic, and recreation facilities, and with the new range of health and welfare services, Chinese Americans had achieved a degree of civic inclusion and social progress unimaginable five decades before. By the end of World War II, San Francisco Chinese Americans as self-governing individuals had established a claim on local and national resources.[2]

However, public health's dichotomy of normal and aberrant persisted, simply shifting to a dividing line within the Chinatown community, dividing respectable Chinese American families from Chinese bachelors. Over time, this dividing line shifted again and again. As the segregation system for prospective homeowners crumbled in the 1950s and 1960s, Chinatown again became synonymous with aberration. Those who lived in Chinatown—new immigrants and the elderly—were considered not ready for assimilation, or unwilling to assimilate, and were contrasted with the assimilating Chinese Americans who had left Chinatown.[3]

In the twentieth century, the definition of "progress" was tied to this process of contrasting normal and aberrant. At times, "progress" was contingent on the contrast of past and present conditions, but just as often it relied on a contemporaneous normal/aberrant dichotomy. White workers, missionaries, and public health officials, as well as Chinese American activists and social workers, shared the unsettling belief that progress and the standards of living that it ensured were incomplete and vulnerable to undermining threats and terrifying reversals. Such observations evoked both self-indulgent tributes of social superiority for those who progressed and scathing critiques of those who "chose," through their recalcitrant conduct or living conditions, to refuse the promise of modernity.

Underlying the debates over conduct and progress was the insistence that modern, civilized citizen-subjects must be protected from the aberrant population. This need for protection and the fear of contamination already culturally informed the prevailing system of segregation. When the system was adapted to include Chinese American families in the fold of normative and reformed society, Chinese Americans fit easily into the accommodating political and administrative strategy of "separate but equal."

The complex racial system that developed with public health reform made the Chinese American struggle for assimilation and "normality" severely difficult. Over the course of the century, the process of assimilation was frequently interrupted and often rendered impossible by the perceived intractable and incommensurate racial differences of culture and social organization. Scientific medicine and public health discourse had effectively located the differences of race in the body, in social morality, and in living conditions. It was exceedingly difficult for Chinese Americans to be seen as individuals, independent of the weight of collective meanings and group expectations. However, some Chinese Americans were increasingly able to provide an alternative representation of difference—a version of respectable domesticity that, by the mid–twentieth century, appeared to provide less of a critical threat to American norms.

This shifting configuration of race, health, domesticity, and citizenship has profound implications for contemporary scholarship and analysis. The community claims for Chinese American citizenship and cultural belonging depended upon the performance of normative hygiene and heterosexual family forms, which ignored the needs and even existence of Chinese bachelors. On the level of political critique, this paradox demonstrates that the terms of assimilation that privilege nuclear family domesticity allow only limited inclusion and enable the resilience of exclusionary strategies in U.S. liberal democracy. On the epistemological level, for the fields of ethnic studies, American studies, and history, it reveals how the formation of the human subject in society depends on the performance of norms of conduct and nuclear family domesticity. The process of normalization shapes our historical projects and analysis by rendering the politics, cultures, and experiences of citizen-subjects as the privileged social actors.[4]

In U.S. political history, both the transformations of national integration and local governance participated in the simultaneous processes of normalization and citizenship in the 1870s to 1930s. New concepts of the citizen and the human subject became the frame by which the process of normalization was organized on the individual, local, and national levels. The broad process of normalization through liberal government and local disciplinary practices shaped the ways in which equality and inequality became understood. At the turn of the century, new categories of racial and sexual identity became increasingly significant in defining differences and dangers to the norm. Recent work in the history of labor, social welfare, urbanization, and family life have demonstrated how standardization moved from governing the technological developments in the workplace and marketplace to shaping social life and the political order. Politically and culturally, diverse groups in U.S. society articulated universal standards of the conduct and consciousness by which life is organized and managed. The concept of the standard of living traveled from economic spheres to cultural and social spheres to become both the aspiration and judgment of lives and social environment.[5]

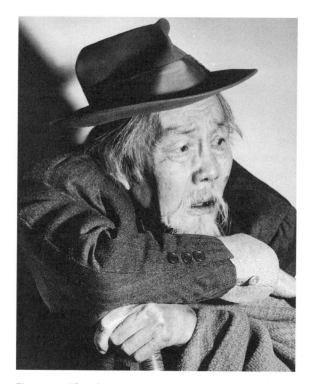

Figure 18. The Chinese bachelor "Dr." Lee Ten Lai, pictured here after his arrest by federal narcotics agents in
1955, claimed to have been an opium addict for fifty years.
He was released because of his ill health. Art Fresno, November 3, 1955. Courtesy California Historical Society,
FN-31289.

The liberal-pluralist formula of status inclusion emphasizes rational
and civilized conduct and abridges the opportunities and resources of
those who are considered unreformed and unreformable, or denies them
opportunity and resources altogether. (See Figure 18.) The question remains, reform to what standard or model of living? The living standards
forged through norms and aberrations generate a dialectic of respectable domesticity and queer domesticity with opposing standards of living. The terms and possibility of exclusion or inclusion depend upon the
performance of norms of gender, sexuality, and domestic space. In order
to be a candidate for inclusion, the previously unreformed have to prove
that their conduct makes them worthy of participation in society and
governance. The specificity of San Francisco's Chinatown and the dy-

namic tension between Chinese bachelor society and Chinese American family society has been crucial to the telling of this story. But even while Chinatown as the site of acute medical menace and immorality in San Francisco has gradually disappeared, the dialectics of public health reform persist, with the focus shifting to other bodies and other geographies. Nevertheless, the analysis of how public health operates in relationship to race, domesticity, and citizenship has ramifications for other historical situations where disease, danger, and deviance become attributed to marginalized social groups.

In public health discourse, people, practices, and place were often conflated. A more recent example is the association of gay men, sodomy, and bathhouses, which informed the San Francisco Health Department's decision to close gay bathhouses in 1984.[6] In that case the AIDS epidemic triggered anxieties about the sexual practices of gay men. Since bathhouses had been perceived as the site where anal intercourse was practiced, they became the target of the Health Department's attentions. The medical authorities employed the knowledge that unprotected anal intercourse was highly likely to transmit the HIV virus to eradicate the perceived site of this sexual practice. In so doing all the rhetoric about safer sex was abandoned. The issue was not the use of condoms but rather the elimination of certain sexual practices and the public site where they were perceived to take place.

Public health measures of security, however, need not be the only way in which one can practice self-care and cultivate social well-being. The repertoires of safe sex conduct generated within community-based gay health associations did far more than shield individual bodies from HIV infection. In the 1980s and early 1990s, gay community safer-sex initiatives emphasized the erotics of safer sex as well as the ethics of affinity with those that were suffering with AIDS. Unlike the dominant society's defensive strategy of health preservation, sex phobia, and targeting diseased pariahs, these grassroots approaches grappled with the devastating human suffering of AIDS, on the one hand, and celebrating the erotic and social relations of gay community, on the other hand. Public health modifications and adaptations of these safer sex repertoires focused on high-risk groups and high-risk activities. Inevitably, many of the dominant society's approaches replaced the ethics of affinity and erotic practices with a schema of defenses. Mercilessly equating certain conduct and behavior with irresponsibility, immorality, and terrible death, safer sex in these terms became another type of public health protection. Public health officials are bewildered by the large number of young urban gay men who, in the age of prophylactics that suppress HIV, have not responded "rationally" because they refuse to disengage fully from the contact that promotes the sharing of bodily fluids. These officials fail to recognize that there is a variety of ways by which people may assess, manage, embrace, or ignore risks.[7]

Deeply embedded in strategies of public health protection is a fear of and moral judgment against the ill person. In such a conceptualization, health is a possession and a status that must be protected at all costs. The ill person can be a pariah by misbehaving, by not protecting the healthy from his or her infection. Illness, however, need not divide people, create pariah status, or even explain the likely routes of infection. Tellingly, those caring for persons with AIDS-related conditions learned very early in the process of AIDS treatment that the presumably healthy person might pose an even greater risk of infection to those with compromised immunity defenses. An ethics of care rather than one of protective fear could embrace the ambivalent interdependence of human contact and illness.[8]

In the late twentieth century, the exclusive authority of physicians and health professionals came under closer scrutiny and greater challenge. In the 1980s, in struggles over HIV-AIDS and breast cancer, those directly impacted by the illness challenged physicians, policy makers, and research scientists to rethink and redirect their resources for disease eradication and prevention. Contemporary affinity groups for those suffering from specific diseases have predecessors in the early-twentieth-century associations for the eradication and cure of tuberculosis and polio and the advocacy groups for cancers and blood and genetic diseases that proliferated at the end of that century.

Within Chinese communities in San Francisco, subcultures of acupuncture and herbal medicine have flourished. There was, in the nineteenth century, immense variability in how persons accessed care and therapies and how they made their decisions based on availability, familiarity, and knowledge. In the twentieth century, the regulation of traditional Chinese medicine and the standardization and licensing of practitioners produced different kinds of therapies, experiences, and expectations in governing. For those accessing care, changes occurred in how well-being was conceived, how disease was conceptualized, and how care and affinity and living were expressed and understood.

The transformations in the twentieth century that led to inclusion beg the questions: What is the harm in these processes of governance by normalization? and Can public health operate without intensive focus on norms? Over the course of the twentieth century in San Francisco, there appeared to be a widening of possibilities for tolerance, diverse therapies, and conceptualizations of care. The norm expanded and incorporated those previously excluded. Social progress is measured by this progressive expansion and improvement over time and space. The problem, then, lies in understanding how governing society by norms becomes the hegemonic style of governance. Standardization and normalization, however, devalue and diminish that which does not fit, which deviates. In a normalized society it is increasingly impossible to think outside the normalizing process and imagine the governing of society and the form of politics differently.[9]

There is an immense and incommensurate variety of struggles and strategies that people have explored in order to confront and cope with the disease, distress, and death that we live with. People have struggled within heterogeneous domestic, work, and social arrangements and spaces and explored the contrasts, inequalities, vulnerabilities, and terrors within each. In this book, I have attempted to interrupt the impulse of normalizing governance in order to view those outside the confines of standardized production or respectable domesticity in ways different from the normalizing frame. The normalizing framework interprets those outside the norm as harboring pathogens, immorality, and disorder, which must be squelched in order for the rest to survive and thrive. Normalizing strategies often fail to recognize human variety, and put some lives at risk in order to satisfy the fears of the always vulnerable norm. Is it possible for knowledge, ethics, and governance to be expressed differently than in a relentless preoccupation with and pursuit of norms?

I do not want to employ epidemic logic to justify the value of these questions, so I will not revert to claims that particular kinds of normalizing practices will result in unforeseen epidemic calamities or that health, individually or collectively, will be threatened. Disease and the sorrows and terrors of illness are, we know, a part of the human condition. Although we recognize and are astonished by the substantial transformations of the human condition in the past 150 years as a result of the innovations of scientific medicine, sanitation infrastructure, and public health practices, we are also aware that infectious diseases will continue to emerge, affect, disable, and kill. Not only the diseases we are familiar with but also those we have yet to learn about will impact human histories. In this new century, drug-resistant tuberculosis, malaria, HIV, *E. coli* bacteria, and hepatitis will disable and destroy thousands of lives. Pharmaceutical science and public health have courageously and diligently intensified the quest to identify, alleviate, and suppress these and many other illnesses. However, in this new century the goal of a sickness-free society will remain an elusive one. Its allure satisfies a noble vision of human progress, but its utopian impulse underwrites public health as a panacea for human inequity, hardship, and distress. Scientific medicine may change the world as we know it again and again, but it will never accomplish perfection in human conditions and societies.

Public health reform is far more than the instruments to suppress epidemic disease and enhance human vitality. It promotes a strategy of governance and citizenship with its own ethical and knowledge formations. As such, it is worth investigating whose lives are enabled, which possibilities are enhanced, and what kinds of cultures and communities thrive in this form of governance. Would it be possible to think of citizenship, with its obligations and access to resources, as not dependent upon modifying behaviors by elevating certain social relations and demonizing others? Rather than distinguishing the alien from the citizen, could full access to civic participation be understood through physical presence in a locality in which participation is not abridged or denied because of race, class, nationality, gender, or sexuality?[10]

It is possible for our politics to embrace a sense of interdependence and the widening circles of complicit action and regard for each other. Government by normalization and standardization will undoubtedly continue apace. But it need not be the only available strategy of governance. The question for the new century is whether it is possible to embrace multiple modernities rather than judge all lived experiences from the vantage point of a single and universal standard that inevitably includes some and excludes others.

# Notes

## INTRODUCTION: PUBLIC HEALTH, RACE, AND CITIZENSHIP

1. San Francisco Board of Health (SFBH hereafter), *Annual Report of the Board of Health of the City and County of San Francisco* (San Francisco, 1876–77), pp. 13–14. John L. Meares, M.D., served as city health officer from 1876 to his death in 1888. "Dr. John Meares: Obituary," *Pacific Medical and Surgical Journal* 31, no. 2 (February 1888): 89–90.

2. SFBH, *Annual Report,* 1876–77, pp. 13, 15. Similar assessments of Chinatown as a "moral and social plague spot," "sanitary curse," and region "contaminating the atmosphere" can be found in SFBH, *Annual Report,* 1878–79, p. 5; SFBH, *Annual Report,* 1879–80, p. 2; SFBH, *Annual Report,* 1880–81, p. 5. For a thorough analysis of this imagery in the formation of knowledge of Chinatown and its inhabitants, see chapter 1.

3. J. C. Geiger, M.D., et al., *The Health of the Chinese in an American City—San Francisco* (San Francisco: San Francisco Department of Public Health, 1939), pp. 4, 6, 18; J. C. Geiger, M.D., et al., *The Health of the Chinese in an American City—San Francisco* (San Francisco: San Francisco Department of Public Health, 1945), pp. 1–6.

4. George Rosen, *A History of Public Health* (New York: MD Publications, 1958); John Duffy, *The Sanitarians: A History of American Public Health* (Urbana: University of Illinois Press, 1990); Judith Waltzer Leavitt, *The Healthiest City: Milwaukee and the Politics of Health Reform* (Princeton: Princeton University Press, 1982); Charles E. Rosenberg, *The Cholera Years: The United States in 1832, 1849, and 1866* (Chicago: University of Chicago Press, 1962); Barbara Rosencrantz, *Public Health and the State: Changing Views in Massachusetts, 1842–1936* (Cambridge: Harvard University Press, 1972).

5. I draw a distinction between modernity as a historical phenomenon and ideological project and modernism as a literary and aesthetic practice. For the former see, Anthony Gidden, *The Consequences of Modernity* (Stanford: Stanford University Press, 1990); Stuart Hall et al., eds., *Modernity and Its Futures* (Hempstead: Open University, 1993); Barbara Marshall, *Engendering Modernity: Feminism, Social Theory, and Social Change* (Cambridge: Polity Press, 1994); Geoff Eley, "German History and the Contradictions of Modernity: The Bourgeoisie, the State, and the Mastery of Reform," in *Society, Culture, and the State in Germany,* ed. Geoff Eley (Ann Arbor: University of Michigan Press, 1996), pp. 67–104; J. Baudrillard, "Modernity," *Canadian Journal of Political and Social Theory* 11, no. 3 (1987): 63–72; Jurgen Habermas, "Modernity, an Incomplete Project," in *The Anti-Aesthetic: Essays on Postmodern Culture,* ed. Hal Foster (Seattle: Bay Press, 1983), pp. 3–15.

6. William J. Novak, *The People's Welfare: Law and Regulation in Nineteenth Century America* (Chapel Hill: University of North Carolina Press, 1996), pp. 1–18, 191–234; Rosencrantz, *Public Health and the State;* Leavitt, *The Healthiest City.*

7. I draw upon Michel Foucault's concept of "governmentality" to understand the state and social project of public health. Governmentality refers to the relations that regulate the conduct of human subjects as a population and as individuals in the interests of ensuring the security and prosperity of the nation-state. Foucault, "Governmentality," in *The Foucault Effect: Studies in Governmentality,* ed. Graham Burchell, Colin Gordon, and Peter Miller (Chicago: University of Chicago Press, 1991), pp. 99–102; Foucault, *History of Sexuality,* vol. 1: *An Introduction* (New York: Vintage Books, 1990), pp. 39–145. A number of scholars have elaborated on the fact that the creation of the idea of the general population as an object of study and intervention was crucial to nineteenth- and twentieth-century liberal rationalities of government in western European and North American liberal democracies. See Thomas Osborne, "Security and Vitality: Drains, Liberalism, and Power in the Nineteenth Century," in *Foucault and Political Reason: Liberalism, Neo-Liberalism, and Rationalities of Government,* ed. Andrew Barry, Thomas Osborne, and Nikolas Rose (Chicago: University of Chicago Press, 1996); Mary Poovey, *Making a Social Body: British Cultural Formation, 1830–1864* (Chicago: University of Chicago Press, 1995), pp. 1–8.

8. Robert Crawford, "The Boundaries of the Self and the Unhealthy Other: Reflections on Health, Culture, and AIDS," *Social Science Medicine* 38, no. 10 (1994): 1347–65; Catherine Gallagher, "The Body versus the Social Body in the Works of Thomas Malthus and Henry Mayhew," *Representations* 14 (spring 1986): 83–106; Poovey, *Making a Social Body.*

9. I draw on Alexander Saxton, Ronald Takaki, and Tomas Almaguer's insights on nineteenth-century class politics, political economy, and the formation of white race culture in California. Alexander Saxton, *The Rise and Fall of the White Republic: Class Politics and Mass Culture in Nineteenth Century America* (New York: Verso, 1990); Saxton, *The Indispensable Enemy: Labor and the Anti-Chinese Movement in California* (Berkeley and Los Angeles: University of California Press, 1970); Ronald Takaki, *Iron Cages: Race and Culture in 19th*

*Century America* (Seattle: University of Washington Press, 1979); Tomas Almaguer, *Racial Fault Lines: The Historical Origins of White Supremacy in California* (Berkeley and Los Angeles: University of California Press, 1994).

10. My understanding of racial formations has been drawn from the conceptualizations of the political and social formation of race developed by Michael Omi and Howard Winant, *Racial Formation in the United States from the 1960s to the 1980s* (New York: Routledge, 1986); David Theo Goldberg, "The Social Formation of Racist Discourse," in *Anatomy of Racism,* ed. David Theo Goldberg (Minneapolis: University of Minnesota Press, 1990), pp. 295–318; Goldberg, *Racist Culture: Philosophy and the Politics of Meaning* (Cambridge: Blackwell, 1993). I have also been influenced by comparable theoretical work on the social formation of gender. In particular, see Denise Riley, *"Am I That Name?": Feminism and the Category of "Women" in History* (Minneapolis: University of Minnesota Press, 1988); Joan Wallach Scott, *Gender and the Politics of History* (New York: Columbia University Press, 1988).

11. Colette Guillaumin, "The Idea of Race and Its Elevation to Autonomous, Scientific, and Legal Status," in *Sociological Theories: Race and Colonialism* (Paris: UNESCO, 1980), pp. 37–68; Guillaumin, *Racism, Sexism, Power and Ideology* (London: Routledge, 1995), pp. 61–107, 133–52; Guillaumin, "Race and Nature: The System of Marks," *Feminist Issues* 8 (fall 1988): 25–44; M. De Lepervanche, "The Naturalness of Inequality," in *Ethnicity, Class, and Gender in Australia,* ed. G. Bottomley and M. De Lepervanche (Sydney: Allen and Unwin), pp. 49–71; Thomas C. Holt, "Marking: Race, Race-Making, and the Writing of History," *American Historical Review* 100, no. 1 (February 1995): 1–20; Barbara Fields, "Slavery, Race, and Ideology in the United States of America," *New Left Review* (May-June 1990): 95–118; Nancy Leys Stepan, "Race and Gender: The Role of Analogy in Science," in *Anatomy of Racism,* ed. David Theo Goldberg (Minneapolis: University of Minnesota Press, 1990), pp. 38–57; Aiwha Ong, "Cultural Citizenship as Subject Making: New Immigrants Negotiate Racial and Cultural Boundaries," *Current Anthropology* 37, no. 5 (December 1996): 737–62.

12. For science and race, see the essays in Sandra Harding, ed., *The 'Racial Economy of Science': Toward a Democratic Future* (Bloomington: Indiana University Press, 1993); William Stanton, *The Leopard's Spots: Scientific Attitudes toward Race in America, 1815–59* (Chicago: University of Chicago Press, 1960); Nancy Leys Stepan, *Idea of Race in Science: Great Britain, 1880–1960* (Hampden, Conn.: Archon Books, 1982); Martin Barker, "Biology and the New Racism," in *Anatomy of Racism,* ed. David Theo Goldberg (Minneapolis: University of Minnesota Press, 1990). For philosophy and morality see Goldberg, *Racist Culture;* Sander L. Gilman, *Difference and Pathology: Stereotypes of Sexuality, Race, and Madness* (Ithaca: Cornell University Press, 1985).

13. For select examples of other local formations of race and class difference and public health in the United States, Africa, Asia, and Europe, see Tera W. Hunter, *To 'Joy My Freedom: Southern Black Women's Lives and Labors after the Civil War* (Cambridge: Harvard University Press, 1997); Stuart Galishoff, "Germs Know No Color Line: Black Health and Public Policy in Atlanta, 1900–1918," *Journal of History of Medicine* 40 (1985): 22–41; Vanessa Gamble,

*Germs Have No Color Line: Blacks and American Medicine, 1900–1940* (New York: Garland Press, 1989); David McBride, *From Tuberculosis to AIDS: Epidemics among Urban Blacks since 1900* (Albany: State University of New York Press, 1991); Georgina D. Feldberg, *Disease and Class: Tuberculosis and the Shaping of Modern North American Society* (New Brunswick, N.J.: Rutgers University Press, 1995); Randall Packard, *White Plague, Black Labor: Tuberculosis and the Political Economy of Health and Disease in South Africa* (Pietermaritzburg: University of Natal Press, 1989); William Deverell, "Plague in Los Angeles: Ethnicity and Typicality," in *Over the Edge: Remapping the American West,* ed. Valerie Matsumoto and Blake Allmendinger (Berkeley and Los Angeles: University of California Press, 1999), pp. 172–200; Lara Marks and Michael Worboys, eds., *Migrants, Minorities, and Health: Historical and Contemporary Studies* (London: Routledge, 1997); Alan I. Marcus, *Plague of Strangers: Social Groups and the Origins of City Services in Cincinnati, 1819–1870* (Columbus: Ohio State University Press, 1991); Cathy Kudlick, *Cholera in Postrevolutionary Paris* (Berkeley and Los Angeles: University of California Press, 1996).

14. Harriet Deacon, "Racial Segregation and Medical Discourse in Nineteenth Century Cape Town," *Journal of Southern African Studies* 22, no. 2 (June 1996): 287–308; Vijay Prashad, "Native Dirt/Imperial Ordure: The Cholera of 1832 and the Morbid Resolutions of Modernity," *Journal of Historical Sociology* 7, no. 3 (September 1994): 243–60; Maynard W. Swanson, "The Sanitation Syndrome: Bubonic Plague and the Urban Native Policy in the Cape Colony, 1900–1909," *Journal of African History* 18, no. 3 (1977): 387–410; Veena Oldenburg, *The Making of Colonial Lucknow, 1856–1877* (Princeton: Princeton University Press, 1984), pp. 96–144; Reynaldo Illeto, "Cholera and Origins of American Sanitary Order in the Philippines," in *Discrepant Histories: Translocal Essays on Filipino Cultures,* ed. Vincente Rafael (Philadelphia: Temple University Press, 1995), pp. 51–82; Warwick Anderson, "Excremental Colonialism, Public Health, and the Poetics of Pollution," *Critical Inquiry* 21, no. 3 (spring 1995): 640–69; Kelvin Santiago-Valles, "On the Historical Links between Coloniality and the Violent Production of the Native Body and the Manufacture of Pathology," *Centro* 7, no. 1 (1995): 108–18.

15. Gwendolyn Mink, *The Wages of Motherhood: Inequality in the Welfare State, 1917–1942* (Ithaca: Cornell University Press, 1995).

16. Nikolas Rose, "Governing Advanced Liberal Democracies," in *Foucault and Political Reason: Liberalism, Neo-Liberalism, and the Rationalities of Government,* ed. Andrew Barry, Thomas Osborne, and Nikolas Rose (Chicago: University of Chicago Press, 1996), pp. 37–64; A. Ong, "Cultural Citizenship as Subject Making," pp. 737–62; Lisa Lowe, *Immigrant Acts: On Asian American Cultural Politics* (Durham, N.C.: Duke University Press, 1996).

17. James Holston and Arjun Appadurai, "Cities and Citizenship," *Public Culture* 8 (1996): 187–204; Linda Kerber, "The Meanings of Citizenship," *Dissent* 44 (1997): 33–37; Bryan S. Turner, "Contemporary Problems in the Theory of Citizenship," in *Citizenship and Social Theory,* ed. Bryan S. Turner (London: Sage, 1993).

18. Rogers M. Smith, *Civic Ideals: Conflicting Visions of Citizenship in U.S.*

*History* (New Haven: Yale University Press, 1998); Nancy Cott, "Marriage and Women's Citizenship in the United States, 1830–1934," *American Historical Review* 103, no. 5 (December 1998): 1440–74; Sucheng Chan, ed., *Entry Denied: Exclusion and the Chinese Community in America, 1882–1943* (Philadelphia: Temple University Press, 1991); Kitty Calavita, *Inside the State: The Bracero Program, Immigration, and the INS* (New York: Routledge, 1992); Ellen Carol DuBois, "Outgrowing the Compact of the Fathers: Equal Rights, Woman Suffrage, and the United States Constitution, 1820–1878," *Journal of American History* 74 (December 1987): 836–62; Amy Dru Stanley, "Conjugal Bonds and Wage Labor: Rights of Contract in the Age of Emancipation," *Journal of American History* 75 (September 1998): 471–500; Rowland Berthoff, "Conventional Mentality: Free Blacks, Women, and Business Corporations as Unequal Persons, 1820–1870," *Journal of American History* 76 (December 1989): 753–84.

19. Uday S. Mehta, "Liberal Strategies of Exclusion," in *Tensions of Empire: Colonial Cultures in a Bourgeois World,* ed. Frederick Cooper and Ann Laura Stoler (Berkeley and Los Angeles: University of California Press, 1997), pp. 59–86.

20. Rose, "Governing Advanced Liberal Democracies," p. 40.

21. The problem of thinking of multiple overlapping public spheres and counterpublics has been addressed by Nancy Fraser, "Rethinking the Public Sphere: A Contribution to the Critique of Actually Existing Democracy," in *The Phantom Public Sphere,* ed. Bruce Robbins (Minneapolis: University of Minnesota Press, 1993), pp. 1–32; Ooskar Negt and Alexander Kluge, *Public Sphere and Experience: Toward an Analysis of the Bourgeois and Proletarian Public Sphere* (Minneapolis: University of Minnesota Press, 1993); Thomas C. Holt, "Afterword: Mapping the Black Public Sphere," *The Black Public Sphere: A Public Culture Book* (Chicago: University of Chicago Press, 1995), pp. 325–26. Philip Ethington develops an argument for the formation of the public sphere in nineteenth-century San Francisco. Ethington, *The Public City: The Political Construction of Urban Life in San Francisco, 1850–1900* (New York: Cambridge University Press, 1994).

22. Chinese American activists were able to reverse the relations of governing by rearticulating the norms cultivated by citizens into a demand that citizens can make of authorities. Rose, "Governing Advanced Liberal Democracies," p. 59; A. Ong, "Cultural Citizenship as Subject Making"; Barbara Cruikshank, *The Will to Empower: Democratic Citizens and Other Subjects* (Ithaca: Cornell University Press, 1999).

23. Judith Farquhar, *Knowing Practice: The Clinical Encounter of Chinese Medicine* (Boulder, Colo.: Westview Press, 1994); Paul U. Unschuld, *Medicine in China: A History of Ideas* (Berkeley and Los Angeles: University of California Press, 1985); Marta Hanson, "Inventing a Tradition in Chinese Medicine: From Universal Canon to Local Medical Knowledge in South China, 17th Century to 19th Century" (Ph.D. diss., University of Pennsylvania, 1997); Paul D. Buell, "Theory and Practice of Traditional Chinese Medicine," in *Chinese Medicine on the Golden Mountain: An Interpretive Guide,* ed. Henry G. Schwartz (Seattle: Wing Luke Memorial Museum, 1984), pp. 25–50; Nathan Sivin, "The History of Chinese Medicine: Now and Anon," *Positions: East Asian Critique*

6, no. 3 (1998): 731–62; Mary P. Sutphen, "Not What, but Where: Bubonic Plague and the Reception of Germ Theories in Hong Kong and Calcutta, 1894–1897," *Journal of the History of Medicine and Allied Sciences* 52, no. 1 (January 1997): 81–113; Birdie J. Andrews, "Tuberculosis and the Assimilation of Germ Theory in China, 1895–1937," *Journal of the History of Medicine and Allied Sciences* 52, no. 1 (January 1997): 114–57; Carol Benedict, *Bubonic Plague in Nineteenth Century China* (Stanford: Stanford University Press, 1997); Frederick Dunn, "Traditional Asian Medicine and Cosmopolitan Medicine as Adaptive Systems," in *Asian Medical Systems: A Comparative Study*, ed. Charles Leslie (Berkeley and Los Angeles: University of California Press, 1976), pp. 133–58; Ruth Rogaski, "From Protecting Life to Defending the Nation: The Emergence of Public Health in Tianjin, 1859–1953" (Ph.D. diss., Yale University, 1996); Kerrie L. Macpherson, *A Wilderness of Marshes: The Origins of Public Health in Shanghai, 1843–1893* (Hong Kong: Oxford University Press, 1987).

24. Much of the historical research on traditional Chinese medicine in the United States has followed the herbal medical practice of the Ah-Fong physicians of Idaho and a handful of other Chinese physicians in California and the Pacific Northwest who left substantial pharmacological records. Paul D. Buell, "Chinese Medicine on Gold Mountain: Tradition, Adaptation, and Change," in *Disease and Medical Care in the Mountain West: Essays on Region, History, and Practice*, ed. Martha L. Hildreth and Bruce T. Moran (Reno: University of Nevada Press, 1998), pp. 95–109; Christopher Muench, "One Hundred Years of Medicine: The Ah-Fong Physicians of Idaho," in *Chinese Medicine on the Golden Mountain: An Interpretive Guide*, ed. Henry G. Schwartz (Seattle: Wing Luke Memorial Museum, 1984), pp. 51–80; Christopher Muench, "Chinese Medicine in America: A Study in Adaptation," *Caduceus: A Museum Quarterly for Health Sciences* (spring 1988): 4–35; Paul D. Buell and Christopher Muench, "A Chinese Apothecary in Frontier Idaho," *Annals of the Chinese Historical Society of the Pacific Northwest* 1 (1983): 39–48; Liu Haiming, "The Resilience of Ethnic Culture: Chinese Herbalists in the American Medical Profession," *Journal of Asian American Studies* 1, no. 2 (June 1998); Jeffrey Barlow, *China Doctor of John Day* (Portland, Ore.: Binford and Mort, 1979); Chun-wai Chan and Jade K. Chang, "The Role of Chinese Medicine in New York City's Chinatown," *American Journal of Chinese Medicine* 4 (1976): no. 1, pp. 31–45, and no. 2, pp. 129–46.

25. Kay J. Anderson, "Engendering Race Research: Unsettling the Self-Other Dichotomy," in *Bodyspace: Destabilizing Geographies of Gender and Sexuality*, ed. Nancy Duncan (London: Routledge, 1996), pp. 197–211; Cindy Patton, "Refiguring Social Space," in *Social Postmodernism: Beyond Identity Politics*, ed. Linda Nicholson and Steven Seidman (New York: Oxford University Press, 1995), pp. 216–49; Ghassan Hage, "The Spatial Imaginary of National Practices: Dwelling—Domesticating—Being—Exterminating," *Environment and Planning D: Society and Space* 14 (1996): 463–85.

26. Robert G. Lee, *Orientals: Asian Americans in Popular Culture* (Philadelphia: Temple University Press, 1999); Matthew Frye Jacobson, *Whiteness of a Different Color: European Immigrants and the Alchemy of Race* (Cambridge: Harvard University Press, 1998); David Roediger, *The Wages of Whiteness:*

*Race and the Making of the American Working Class* (London: Verso, 1991); Richard Dyer, "White," *Screen,* no. 29 (autumn 1988): 44–64; Vron Ware, *Beyond the Pale: White Women, Racism, and History* (London: Verso, 1992); Toni Morrison, *Playing in the Dark: Whiteness and the Literary Imagination* (Cambridge: Harvard University Press, 1992); George Lipsitz, "The Possessive Investment in Whiteness: Racialized Social Democracy and the 'White Problem' in American Studies," *American Quarterly* 47, no. 3 (September 1995): 369–87; Richard Dyer, *White* (London: Routledge, 1998); W. Anderson, "Excremental Colonialism, Public Health, and the Poetics of Pollution," pp. 640–69; Vincente Rafael, "White Love: Surveillance and Nationalist Resistance in U.S. Colonization of the Philippines," in *Cultures of U.S. Imperialism,* ed. Don Pease and Amy Kaplan (Durham, N.C.: Duke University Press, 1994).

27. Kay J. Anderson, *Vancouver's Chinatown: Racial Discourse in Canada, 1875–1980* (Montreal: McGill-Queen's University Press, 1991), p. 30. See also Susan Craddock, "Sewers and Scapegoats: Spatial Metaphors of Smallpox in Nineteenth Century San Francisco," *Social Science Medicine* 41, no. 7 (1995): 957–68.

28. For examples in the historiography of the public health reform of San Francisco and Chinese immigrants, see Joan B. Trauner, "The Chinese as Medical Scapegoats in San Francisco, 1870–1905," *California History* 57 (1978): 70–87; Craddock, "Sewers and Scapegoats"; Elmer Clarence Sandmeyer, *The Anti-Chinese Movement in California* (Urbana: University of Illinois Press, 1939); Chasla M. Loo, *Chinatown: Most Time, Hard Time* (New York: Praeger, 1991); Fitzhugh Mullan, *Plagues and Politics: The Story of the United States Public Health Service* (New York: Basic Books, 1989); Alan M. Kraut, *Silent Travelers: Germs, Genes, and the "Immigrant Menace"* (New York: Basic Books, 1994), pp. 78–96; Charles McClain, "Of Medicine, Race, and American Law: The Bubonic Plague Outbreak of 1900," *Law and Social Inquiry* 13, no. 3 (1988): 447–513; Guenter B. Risse, "'A Long Pull, a Strong Pull, and All Together': San Francisco and the Bubonic Plague, 1907–1908," *Bulletin of the History of Medicine* 66 (summer 1992): 263–64; Susan Craddock, "Diseases on the Margin: Morphologies of Tuberculosis and Smallpox in San Francisco, 1860–1940" (Ph.D. diss., University of California at Berkeley, 1994); Linnea Klee, "The 'Regulars' and the Chinese: Ethnicity and Public Health in 1870s San Francisco," *Urban Anthropology* 12, no. 2 (summer 1983): 181–207; J. Gerard Power, "Media Dependency, Bubonic Plague, and the Social Construction of the Chinese Other," *Journal of Communication Inquiry* 19, no. 1 (spring 1995): 89–110.

29. Elizabeth Blackmar, "Accountability for Public Health: Regulating the Housing Market in Nineteenth Century New York City," in *Hives of Sickness,* ed. David Rosner (New Brunswick: Rutgers University Press, 1995), pp. 42–64; Eileen Boris, *Home to Work: Motherhood and the Politics of Industrial Homework in the United States* (New York: Cambridge University Press, 1994); Lawrence Glickman, "Inventing the 'American Standard of Living': Gender, Race, and Working-Class Identity, 1880–1925," *Labor History* 34, no. 2–3 (1993): 221–35.

30. Richard Fung, "Burdens of Representation, Burdens of Responsibility,"

in *Constructing Masculinity,* ed. Maurice Berger et al. (London: Routledge, 1995), pp. 291–99; Jennifer Ting, "Bachelor Society: Deviant Heterosexuality and Asian American Historiography," in *Privileging Positions: The Sites of Asian American Studies,* ed. Gary Okihiro et al. (Pullman: Washington State University Press, 1995), pp. 271–79.

31. Ting, "Bachelor Society"; Susan L. Johnson, "Sharing Bed and Board: Cohabitation and Cultural Difference in Central Arizona Mining Towns, 1863–1873," in *Women's West,* ed. Susan Armitage and Elizabeth Jameson (Norman: University of Oklahoma Press, 1987).

32. Sucheng Chan, "The Exclusion of Chinese Women, 1870–1943," in *Entry Denied: Exclusion and the Chinese Community in America, 1882–1943,* ed. Sucheng Chan (Philadelphia: Temple University Press, 1991); Benson Tong, *Unsubmissive Women: Chinese Prostitution in Nineteenth Century San Francisco* (Norman: University of Oklahoma Press, 1994).

33. I am deeply indebted to Nancy Cott's formulation of "monogamous morality" and its framing of "civilized behavior" and respectable domesticity in her comment. Nancy Cott, comment to Nayan Shah, "Paradoxes of Inclusion and Exclusion in American Modernity: Formations of the Modern Self, Domicile, and Domesticity" (paper presented to the conference "Project to Internationalize the Study of American History," Joint Project of New York University and the Organization of American Historians, Villa La Pietra, Florence, Italy, July 4–7, 1999). For further explorations of ideas of civilization and practices of hygiene in the formation of respectable domesticity, see Lori Ginzberg "Social Movements" (paper presented to the conference "Project to Internationalize the Study of American History," Joint Project of New York University and the Organization of American Historians, Villa La Pietra, Florence, Italy, July 4–7, 1999), manuscript in author's possession; Mariana Valverde, *The Age of Light, Soap, and Water: Moral Reform in English Canada, 1885–1925* (Toronto: McClelland and Stewart, 1991); Gail Bederman, *Manliness and Civilization: A Cultural History of Gender and Race in the United States, 1880–1917* (Chicago: University of Chicago Press, 1995); Nancy Tomes, *Gospel of Germs: Men, Women, and the Microbe in American Life* (Cambridge: Harvard University Press, 1998); Timothy Burke, *Lifebuoy Men, Lux Women: Commodification, Consumption, and Cleanliness in Modern Zimbabwe* (Durham, N.C.: Duke University Press, 1996).

34. Amy Kaplan, "Manifest Domesticity," *American Literature* 70, no. 3 (September 1998); Vincente L. Rafael, "Colonial Domesticity: White Women and United States Rule in the Philippines," *American Literature* 67 (December 1995): 639–66; Norbert Elias, *The Civilizing Process,* vol. 1: *The History of Manners,* trans. by E. Jephcott (New York: Pantheon Press, 1978).

35. Roddey Reid, *Families in Jeopardy: Regulating the Social Body in France, 1750–1910* (Stanford: Stanford University Press, 1993); Pierre Bourdieu, "On the Family as a Realized Category," *Theory, Culture, Society* 13, no. 3 (1996): 19–26; Ann Laura Stoler, *Race and the Education of Desire: Foucault's History of Sexuality and the Colonial Order of Things* (Durham, N.C.: Duke University Press, 1996).

36. For two exemplary articulations of this critique, see Gayatri Spivak,

"Subaltern Studies: DeConstructing Historiography," in *Other Worlds* (New York: Methuen, 1987); Evelyn Brooks Higginbotham, "African American Women's History and the Metalangue of Race," *Signs* (winter 1992): 251–74.

37. R. G. Lee, *Orientals;* Sucheng Chan, *Asian Americans: An Interpretive History* (Boston: Twayne, 1988); Ronald Takaki, *Strangers from a Different Shore* (New York: Little, Brown, and Company, 1989); Gary Y. Okihiro, *Margins and Mainstreams: Asians in American History and Culture* (Seattle: University of Washington Press, 1994); Ling Chi Wang, "The Structure of Dual Domination: Toward a Paradigm for the Study of Chinese Diaspora in the U.S.," *Amerasia Journal* 21, nos. 1–2 (1995): 149–70. Cultural critics and sociologists have also developed extensive critiques of race analysis in the context of Asians in the United States. Lowe, *Immigrant Acts;* David Palumbo-Liu, *Asia/American: Historical Crossings of a Racial Frontier* (Stanford: Stanford University Press, 1999); Shirley Hune, "Rethinking Race: Paradigms and Policy Formation," *Amerasia Journal* 21, nos. 1–2 (1995): 29–40; Michael Omi and Howard Winant, *Racial Formation in the United States from the 1960s to the 1990s* (New York: Routledge, 1994).

38. William Wei, *The Asian American Movement* (Philadelphia: Temple University Press, 1993); Glenn Omatsu, "The 'Four Prisons' and the Movements of Liberation: Asian American Activism from the 1960s to the 1990s," in *The State of Asian America: Activism and Resistance in the 1990s,* ed. Karin Aguilar-San Juan (Boston: South End Press, 1994); Curtis Choy, *Fall of the I-Hotel,* 58 minutes (San Francisco: NAATA/Crosscurrents, original version 1983; revised 1993), documentary film.

## CHAPTER 1. PUBLIC HEALTH AND THE MAPPING OF CHINATOWN

1. "The Chinese Quarter: Chinatown Overhauled by Health Inspectors—a Terrible State of Affairs Found to Exist—Crowded into Garrets and Cellars—Radical Sanitary Regulations Needed," *Daily Alta California,* May 16, 1870; "Moving on Their Works: Health Officer Dr. J. L. Meares Notifies the Chinese to Set Their Houses in Order," *San Francisco Examiner,* February 24, 1880.

2. SFBH, *Annual Report,* 1880–81, p. 5; SFBH, *Annual Report,* 1881–82, p. 9; SFBH, *Annual Report,* 1879–80, p. 2.

3. K. J. Anderson, *Vancouver's Chinatown,* p. 31.

4. Thomas W. Laqueur, "Bodies, Details, and the Humanitarian Narrative," in *The New Cultural History,* ed. Lynn Hunt (Berkeley and Los Angeles: University of California Press, 1989); Poovey, *Making a Social Body;* Osborne, "Security and Vitality," pp. 99–122; Margaret Cohen, ed., *Spectacles of Realism: Body, Gender, and Genre* (Minneapolis: University of Minnesota Press, 1995).

5. Stuart Hall, "Gramsci's Relevance for the Study of Race and Ethnicity," *Journal of Communicative Inquiry* 10, no. 2 (1986): 5–27; Lorraine Daston, "Historical Epistemology," in *Questions of Evidence: Proof, Practice, and Persuasion across the Disciplines,* ed. James Chandler, Arnold I. Davidson, and Harry Harootunian (Chicago: University of Chicago Press, 1994), pp. 282–89; Thomas C. Holt, "Reflections on Race-Making and Racist Practice: Toward a

Working Hypothesis" (paper prepared for the Newberry Seminar in American Social History, Chicago, May 30, 1991), pp. 17–18; Stuart Hall, "Race, Articulation, and Societies Structured under Dominance," in *Sociological Theories: Race and Colonialism* (Paris: UNESCO, 1980); T. J. Jackson Lears, "The Concept of Cultural Hegemony: Problems and Possibilities," *American Historical Review* 56 (June 1985). For another example of the conflation of race, culture, behavior, and a ghetto location, see Robin D. G. Kelley, *Yo Mama's Disfunktional: Fighting the Culture Wars in Urban America* (Boston: Beacon Press, 1998), particularly chapter 1.

6. *Gamsaan* was the Yale Cantonese transliteration, and *Jinshan* the Mandarin pinyin transliteration. Similarly, *Tongyan gaai* is *Tangren jie* in pinyin. Dupont Street was renamed Grant Avenue in 1908 during the reconstruction of San Francisco. *Daily Alta California,* November 21, 1853; Thomas W. Chinn, Him Mark Lai, and Philip P. Choy, *A History of the Chinese in California: A Syllabus* (San Francisco: Chinese Historical Society of America, 1969), pp. 10–11; Paul M. Ong, "Chinese Labor in Early San Francisco: Racial Segmentation and Industrial Expansion," *Amerasia* 8, no. 1 (1981): 70–75.

7. "Common Council," *Daily Alta California,* August 19, 1854.

8. *Daily Alta California,* August 15, 19, and 22, 1854.

9. Ibid., August 17 and 22, 1854.

10. Ibid., August 15, 1854; and "Spread of the Cholera," *Daily Alta California,* August 19, 1854. Cholera epidemics in the early nineteenth century became the occasion for intense debates about the administration of public health and national borders, and, more generally, about the role of government in ensuring social and political order in France and the United States. See Rosenberg, *The Cholera Years;* François Delaporte, *Disease and Civilization: The Cholera in Paris,* trans. Arthur Goldhammer (Boston: MIT Press, 1986).

11. *Daily Alta California,* August 15 and 22, 1854; Rosenberg, *The Cholera Years;* Delaporte, *Disease and Civilization;* Kudlick, *Cholera in Postrevolutionary Paris.*

12. "Common Council, Board of Aldermen, August 21," *Daily Alta California,* August 22, 1854.

13. Ibid.

14. Him Mark Lai, "Historical Development of the Chinese Consolidated Benevolent Association/Huiguan System," *Chinese America: History and Perspectives* (San Francisco) (1987): 13–51; Shih-shan Henry Tsai, *China and Overseas Chinese in the U.S., 1868–1911* (Fayetteville: University of Arkansas Press, 1983), pp. 31–38; William Hoy, *Chinese Six Companies* (San Francisco: Chinese Consolidated Benevolent Association, 1942); Yong Chen, *Chinese San Francisco, 1850–1943: A Trans-Pacific Community* (Stanford: Stanford University Press, 2000), pp. 71–73.

15. The meeting was chaired by the Chinese merchant A Hing; a white journalist, William Howard, editor of the *Golden Gate News,* served as secretary and submitted the petition as part of the Common Council's official record. Letter to William Rabe from William Howard, August 21, 1854, with petition, printed in *Daily Alta California,* August 22, 1854.

16. Editorial, *Daily Alta California*, August 17, 1854.

17. "More Chinese Emigrants," *Daily Alta California*, August 15, 1854; "The Exchange Chinamen," *Daily Alta California*, August 22, 1854; "Health of the City," *Daily Alta California*, August 26, 1854.

18. Sucheng Chan, *This Bittersweet Soil: The Chinese in California Agriculture, 1860–1910* (Berkeley and Los Angeles: University of California Press, 1986), pp. 37–78; Takaki, *Strangers from a Different Shore*, esp. pp. 86–94; Roger Daniels, *Asian American: Chinese and Japanese in the United States since 1850* (Seattle: University of Washington Press, 1988), pp. 9–69.

19. Census records did not account for the range of Spanish-speaking migrants (from Chile, Peru, Mexico, Spain, and the Caribbean), but they were not a significant portion of the population in the period 1860 to 1920. William Issel and Robert Cherny, *San Francisco, 1865–1932: Politics, Power, and Urban Development* (Berkeley and Los Angeles: University of California Press, 1986), p. 56; Douglas Henry Daniels, *Pioneer Urbanites: A Social and Cultural History of Black San Francisco* (Berkeley and Los Angeles: University of California Press, 1990), p. 13.

20. C. M. Bates, "Health Officer's Report," included in San Francisco Board of Supervisors (SFBS hereafter), *San Francisco Municipal Report* (San Francisco, 1869–70), p. 233.

21. David Sibley, *Geographies of Exclusion: Society and Difference in the West* (London: Routledge, 1995), p. 28; Peter Stallybrass and Allon White, *The Politics and Poetics of Transgression* (London: Methuen, 1986), pp. 132–33.

22. Bates, "Health Officer's Report," 1869–70, p. 233.

23. Saxton, *The Indispensable Enemy*, pp. 72–77; Neil Larry Shumsky, "Tar Flat and Nob Hill: A Social History of Industrial San Francisco during the 1870s" (Ph.D. diss., University of California at Berkeley, 1972).

24. "The Chinese on the Pacific Coast. The Statement of the Anti-Coolie Association," *Daily Alta California*, June 24, 1869.

25. California State Board of Health (CSBH hereafter), *Biennial Report of the State Board of Health of California* (Sacramento, 1870–71), pp. 44–47 and the appendix, p. 55.

26. Among the most famous popular accounts are B. E. Lloyd, *Lights and Shades in San Francisco* (San Francisco: A. L. Bancroft and Co., 1876), pp. 236–66; Walter Raymond, *Horrors of the Mongolian Settlement, San Francisco, California: Enslaved and Degraded Race of Paupers, Opium Eaters, and Lepers* (Boston: Cashman, Keating, and Co., 1886); Rudyard Kipling's series of articles for the *Allahbad "Pioneer"* (1889), reprinted in Rudyard Kipling, *Rudyard Kipling's Letters from San Francisco* (San Francisco: Colt Press, 1949), pp. 31–32; William Walter Bode, *Lights and Shadows of Chinatown* (San Francisco: Crocker, 1896); G. B. Densmore, *The Chinese in California: Description of Chinese Life in San Francisco. Their Habits, Morals, Manners* (San Francisco: Petit and Russ, 1880), pp. 20, 23, 117; J. W. Buel, *Metropolitan Life Unveiled; or, the Mysteries and Miseries of America's Great Cities* (St. Louis: Historical Publishing Company, 1882).

27. Bates, "Health Officer's Report," 1869–70, p. 233.

28. SFBS, *Report of the Special Committee of the Board of Supervisors of San Francisco on the Condition of the Chinese Quarter and the Chinese in San Francisco, July 1885* (San Francisco, 1885), p. 19.

29. CSBH, *Biennial Report,* pp. 44–47. Logan's medical explanations of the dangers of underground spaces reappeared in popular travelogues through the late nineteenth century. See Lloyd, *Lights and Shades in San Francisco,* p. 257; Bode, *Lights and Shadows of Chinatown,* pp. 7, 13; Kipling, *Letters from San Francisco,* pp. 31–32; Buel, *Metropolitan Life Unveiled,* p. 276.

30. CSBH, *Biennial Report,* p. 46.

31. Ibid., p. 47.

32. Ibid., p. 46.

33. Judith Walkowitz, *City of Dreadful Delight: Narratives of Sexual Danger in Late Victorian London* (Chicago: University of Chicago Press, 1992); Margaret Cohen and Christopher Prendergast, eds., *Spectacles of Realism: Body, Gender, and Genre* (Minneapolis: University of Minnesota Press, 1995); Laqueur, "Bodies, Details, and the Humanitarian Narrative," pp. 176–204.

34. Bode, *Lights and Shadows of Chinatown,* p. 14; Densmore, *The Chinese in California,* p. 25.

35. CSBH, *Biennial Report,* pp. 44–47; SFBS, *San Francisco Municipal Report, 1869–70,* p. 233.

36. Raymond, *Horrors of the Mongolian Settlement,* pp. 52–53.

37. CSBH, *Biennial Report,* p. 47; M. P. Sawtelle, "The Plague Spot," *Medico-Literary Journal* 1, no. 4 (December 1878): 10–12; SFBH, *Annual Report, 1871–72,* p. 4; SFBH, *Annual Report, 1872–73,* p. 21; SFBH, *Annual Report, 1879–80,* p. 2.

38. This narrative of Kalloch's 1879 election relies on the historical research and analysis of Saxton, *The Indispensable Enemy;* Issel and Cherny, *San Francisco, 1865–1932,* pp. 127–30; Sandmeyer, *The Anti-Chinese Movement in California,* pp. 73–75.

39. Frank Roney, *Frank Roney, Irish Rebel and California Labor Leader,* ed. Ira Cross (Berkeley and Los Angeles: University of California Press, 1931), cited in Saxton, *Indispensable Enemy,* pp. 141–42.

40. Doctor Hugh Huger Toland was a prominent figure in the development of an understanding of the Chinese medical threat. In the mid-1870s his testimony to the California State Senate and U.S. congressional committees on the transmission of syphilis from Chinese female prostitutes to white adolescent males became the authoritative medical opinion on the subject and was cited in almost every subsequent report on Chinese female prostitution. See chapter 3. He died on February 27, 1880, in the midst of the controversial declaration that Chinatown was a sanitary nuisance. Letter to the Board of Supervisors from I. S. Kalloch, February 27, 1880, printed in the *San Francisco Examiner,* February 28, 1880.

41. "Moving on Their Works: Health Officer Dr. J. L. Meares Notifies the Chinese to Set Their Houses in Order."

42. The report of the committee has been reprinted in Workingmen's Party of California, Anti-Chinese Council, comp. (WPC hereafter), "Board of Health: Resolutions of Condemnation," in *Chinatown Declared a Nuisance!* (San Fran-

cisco: Workingmen's Party of California, 1880), pp. 3–4. Curiously I have not found a reference to this report in the SFBH, *Annual Report,* 1879–80; or SFBS, *San Francisco Municipal Report,* 1879–80.

43. WPC, *Chinatown Declared a Nuisance!* p. 4.

44. Ibid., p. 6.

45. Ibid., pp. 5–6.

46. "The Workingmen in Session," *San Francisco Examiner,* February 26, 1880.

47. "Again Solicited to Cooperate," *San Francisco Examiner,* February 28, 1880.

48. Andrew Gyory, *Closing the Gate: Race, Politics, and the Chinese Exclusion Act* (Chapel Hill: University of North Carolina Press, 1998); Charles J. McClain, *In Search of Equality: The Chinese Struggle against Discrimination in Nineteenth-Century America* (Berkeley and Los Angeles: University of California Press, 1994), pp. 145–220; S. Chan, *Asian Americans;* Sandmeyer, *The Anti-Chinese Movement in California.*

49. SFBS, *Report of the Special Committee,* p. 3.

50. J. B. Harley, "Deconstructing the Map," *Cartographica* 26 (1989): 1–20; Harley, "Maps, Knowledge, and Power" in *The Iconography of Landscape: Essays on the Symbolic Representation, Design, and Use of Past Environments,* ed. Denis Cosgrove and Stephen Daniels (New York: Cambridge University Press, 1988), pp. 277–312.

51. SFBS, *Report of the Special Committee,* pp. 3, 4, 32.

52. SFBS, *Official Map of "Chinatown" in San Francisco* (San Francisco: Bosqui Engraving and Printing, 1885), in Maps Collection, Bancroft Library. Copy 1 has manuscript annotation.

53. Ibid., p. 8.

54. Jean Comaroff and John Comaroff, *Ethnography and the Historical Imagination* (Boulder, Colo.: Westview Press, 1992), pp. 265–94; Gareth Stedman Jones, *Outcast London: A Study of the Relationship between the Classes in Victorian Society* (Oxford: Clarendon Press, 1971).

55. SFBS, *Report of the Special Committee,* p. 9.

56. Ibid., pp. 18–25.

57. Ibid., pp. 4–5, 67.

58. Densmore, *The Chinese in California,* pp. 117–21.

59. Curt Abel-Musgrave, *The Cholera in San Francisco: A Contribution to the History of Corruption in California* (San Francisco: San Francisco News Company, 1885), p. 5.

60. Raymond, *Horrors of the Mongolian Settlement,* p. 2.

61. Fernando Coronil, "Beyond Occidentalism: Towards Nonimperial Geohistorical Categories," *Cultural Anthropology* 11, no. 1 (February 1996): 51–87; Frederick Cooper and Ann Stoler, *Tensions of Empire: Colonial Cultures in a Bourgeois World* (Berkeley and Los Angeles: University of California Press, 1997).

62. Mary Louise Pratt, *Imperial Eyes: Travel Writing and Transculturation* (New York: Routledge, 1992), p. 64.

63. Robert Miles, *Racism* (London: Routledge, 1989); Goldberg, *Racist*

*Culture;* Winthrop D. Jordan, *White over Black: American Attitudes towards the Negro, 1550–1812* (New York: W. W. Norton, 1968).

64. For a theoretical elaboration of the processes of representation and repetition in relation to the performative and incomplete production of identity, see Homi K. Bhabha, "Signs Taken for Wonders: Questions of Ambivalence and Authority under a Tree outside Delhi, May 1817," in *"Race," Writing and Difference,* ed. Henry Louis Gates Jr. (Chicago: University of Chicago Press, 1986), pp. 163–84; Homi K. Bhabha, *The Location of Culture* (New York: Routledge, 1994); Judith Butler, "Imitation and Gender Insubordination," in *Inside/Out: Lesbian Theories/Gay Theories,* ed. Diana Fuss (New York: Routledge, 1991), pp. 13–31.

65. Stuart Creighton Miller, *The Unwelcome Immigrant: The American Image of the Chinese, 1785–1882* (Berkeley and Los Angeles: University of California Press, 1969), pp. 145–204; Sandmeyer, *The Anti-Chinese Movement in California,* pp. 25–39.

66. K. J. Anderson, *Vancouver's Chinatown,* pp. 81–82.

## CHAPTER 2. REGULATING BODIES AND SPACE

1. SFBH, *Annual Report, 1871–72,* p. 3.

2. For further discussion of both the stimulus to and constraints on the growth of urban government in San Francisco and in other nineteenth-century American cities, see Issel and Cherny, *San Francisco, 1865–1932;* Terence J. McDonald, *The Parameters of Urban Fiscal Policy: Socioeconomic Change and Political Culture, 1860–1906* (Berkeley and Los Angeles: University of California Press, 1986); Ethington, *The Public City;* Christine Meisner Rosen, *The Limits of Power: Great Fires and the Process of City Growth in America* (Cambridge: Cambridge University Press, 1986); Robin Einhorn, *Property Rules: Political Economy in Chicago, 1833–1872* (Chicago: University of Chicago Press, 1991), pp. 137–43; Eric J. Monkkonen, *America Becomes Urban: The Development of U.S. Cities and Towns, 1780–1980* (Berkeley and Los Angeles: University of California Press, 1988).

3. John Harley Warner, "From Specificity to Universalism in Medical Therapeutics: Transformation in 19th Century United States," in *Sickness and Health in America: Readings in the History of Medicine and Public Health,* ed. Judith Waltzer Leavitt and Ronald L. Numbers (Madison: University of Wisconsin Press, 1978, 1987), pp. 87–102; Elias, *The Civilizing Process.*

4. Osborne, "Security and Vitality," pp. 99–122; Rose, "Governing Advanced Liberal Democracies," pp. 37–64; Peter Miller and Nikolas Rose, "Political Rationalities and Technologies of Government," in *Texts, Contexts, and Concepts,* ed. S. Hanninen (Helsinki: Finnish Political Science Association, 1989); Colin Gordon, "Governmental Rationality: An Introduction," in *The Foucault Effect: Studies in Governmentality,* ed. Graham Burchell, Colin Gordon, and Peter Miller (Chicago: University of Chicago Press, 1991), pp. 19–20.

5. Poovey, *Making a Social Body;* Bernard S. Cohn and Nicholas B. Dirks, "Beyond the Fringe: The Nation State, Colonialism, and the Technologies of

Power," *Journal of Historical Sociology* 1, no. 2 (June 1988): 224–29; Nikolas Rose, "Governing by Numbers," *Accounting Organization and Society* 16, no. 7 (1991): 673–92; Osborne, "Security and Vitality," p. 102.

6. Joel Tarr and Gabriel DuPuy, introduction to *Technology and the Rise of the Networked City in Europe and America,* ed. Joel A. Tarr and Gabriel DuPuy (Philadelphia: Temple University Press, 1988), p. xiii.

7. Issel and Cherny, *San Francisco, 1865–1932,* pp. 124–25, 175–76, 184. In the courts the Spring Valley Water Works Company and San Francisco government struggled to define water distribution as private property or as a public service. Throughout the late nineteenth century, the courts and the city attempted to define the public use of water, its rates, and who was obligated to pay taxes for the construction and maintenance of water pipes. Katha G. Hartley, "*Spring Valley Water Works v. San Francisco:* Defining Economic Rights in San Francisco," *Western Legal History* 3, no. 2 (summer-fall 1990): 287–308.

8. In 1865 a population of approximately 110,000 consumed 2.3 million gallons; in 1870, with the population at nearly 150,000, the consumption increased to 6 million. In 1880 nearly 234,000 people consumed between 16 and 17 million gallons. John P. Young, *San Francisco: A History of the Pacific Coast Metropolis* (San Francisco: S. J. Clarke Publishing), 2:586; George E. Waring Jr., comp., *Report on the Social Statistics of Cities* (Washington, D.C.: Government Printing Office, 1887), p. 806.

9. C. M. Bates, "Health Officer's Report,"in SFBS, *San Francisco Municipal Report,* 1868–69, p. 217; Marsden Manson, *System of Sewerage for the City and County of San Francisco* (San Francisco: Bosqui Engraving and Printing, 1893), p. 64.

10. Joel A. Tarr, "Sewerage and the Development of the Networked City in the United States, 1850–1930," in *Technology and the Rise of the Networked City in Europe and America,* ed. Joel A. Tarr and Gabriel DuPuy (Philadelphia: Temple University Press, 1988), p. 160; Jon Peterson, "The Impact of Sanitary Reform on American Urban Planning," *Journal of Social History* 13 (fall 1979): 85; SFBS, *San Francisco Municipal Report,* 1868–69, p. 217; Leavitt, *The Healthiest City;* Stuart Galishoff, *Newark: The Nation's Unhealthiest City, 1832–1895* (New Brunswick: Rutgers University Press, 1988); Alan I. Marcus, *Plague of Strangers: Social Groups and the Origins of City Services in Cincinnati, 1819–1870* (Columbus: Ohio State University Press, 1991).

11. SFBH, *Annual Report,* 1872–73, p. 20; John J. Hoff, *Report of the City Surveyor* (San Francisco: O'Meara and Painter, 1856), pp. 9–11; SFBH, *Annual Report,* 1871–72, pp. 9–10.

12. Hastings S. Hall, *Health and Disease—How to Obtain One and Avoid the Other* (San Francisco: Towne and Bacon, 1867), pp. 78–79; Klee, "The 'Regulars' and the Chinese," pp. 181–207.

13. Stanley K. Schultz and Clay McSchane, "To Engineer the Metropolis: Sewers, Sanitation, and City Planning in Late Nineteenth-Century America," *Journal of American History* 65, no. 2 (1978): 389–411; Stuart Galishoff, "Drainage, Disease, Comfort, and Class: A History of Newark's Sewers," *Societas* 6, no. 2 (1976): 121–38; Martin V. Melosi, "Out of Sight, Out of Mind:

The Environment and the Disposal of Municipal Refuse, 1860–1920," *Historian* 35, no. 4 (1973): 621–40; Melosi, "Sanitary Services and Decision Making in Houston, 1876–1945," *Journal of Urban History* 20 (May 1994): 365–406.

14. Young, *San Francisco,* 1:158–59, 311.

15. William P. Humphreys, *Report on the System of Sewerage for the City of San Francisco* (San Francisco: n.p., 1876), pp. 1, 27–28; Young, *San Francisco,* 2:569; Hoff, *Report of the City Surveyor,* pp. 10–11; Manson, *System of Sewerage,* pp. 27, 36–38, 43–63; Geoffrey Giglierano, "The City and the System: Developing a Municipal Service, 1800–1915," *Cincinnati Historical Society Bulletin* 35 (1977): 223–47.

16. SFBS, *San Francisco Municipal Report,* 1868–69, p. 217; SFBH, *Annual Report,* 1871–72, pp. 9–10.

17. Hoff, *Report of the City Surveyor,* p. 12; Humphreys, *Report,* p. 18; SFBH, *Annual Report,* 1876–77, pp. 4–5; SFBH, *Annual Report,* 1878–79, p. 5; SFBH, *Annual Report,* 1879–80, p. 3; SFBS, *San Francisco Municipal Report,* 1868–69, p. 217.

18. Mayor Washington Bartlett, "Inaugural Address, 1883," SFBS, *San Francisco Municipal Report,* 1882–83, p. 83; Manson, *System of Sewerage,* p. 72.

19. Stewart E. Perry, *San Francisco Scavengers: Dirty Work and the Pride of Ownership* (Berkeley and Los Angeles: University of California Press, 1978), pp. 2–5, 16–20. Garbage collection in San Francisco developed into a system unique for a U.S. city of its size. Throughout the country, 80 percent of cities that are the size of San Francisco have a municipal sanitation department, and in the remaining 20 percent the city contracts with a firm to pick up household refuse. San Francisco residents, however, must deal directly with garbage collection companies and pay directly for the service. Two firms regulated like public utilities have provided San Francisco with garbage collection services since 1921. Both—the Sunset Scavenger Company and the Golden Gate Disposal Company—have their origins in protective associations of independent scavengers, and the workers continue to be recognized as partners in the collectives. The Public Health Department administers the licenses and sets rates and regulations. Although during the 1920s and 1930s there were as many as sixty-four firms competing for the garbage collection business, by 1939 the firms had consolidated into two companies.

20. The scavengers were accused of dumping refuse in "vacant lots," on "sidewalks," in "cesspools," and "in front of churches and school houses," instead of proceeding to the city dump south of San Francisco. The proximity of these illegal and improper dumping sites to "churches and schoolhouses," where proper social conduct and "civilized" behavior were cultivated, presented a particularly galling affront. The night scavengers were characterized as "men who have no regard for the public or themselves." C. M Bates, "Health Officer's Report," in SFBH, *Annual Report,* 1871–72, pp. 8, 10; Shumsky, "Tar Flat and Nob Hill," p. 133.

21. U.S. Congress, Senate, *Report of the Joint Special Committee to Investigate Chinese Immigration,* 44th Cong., 2nd sess., 1877, S. Rept. 689, p. 649; reprinted in Chinese Consolidated Benevolent Association, *Memorial of the Six Chinese Companies Testimony of California's Leading Citizens before the Joint*

*Special Congressional Committee* (San Francisco: Alta Print, December 8, 1877), pp. 37–38.

22. McDonald, *The Parameters of Urban Fiscal Policy*, pp. 66–78.

23. SFBH, *Annual Report*, 1878–79, p. 4; SFBH, *Annual Report*, 1872–73, p. 20; Shumsky, "Tar Flat and Nob Hill," p. 277.

24. Osborne, "Drains and Vitality," pp. 114–16; David Armstrong, "Public Health Spaces and the Fabrication of Identity," *Sociology* 27, no. 3 (August 1993): 393–410.

25. Novak, *The People's Welfare*, pp. 1–18, 191–234; Ernst Freund, *The Police Power: Public Policy and Constitutional Rights* (Chicago: Callaghan and Company, 1904), pp. 132–41; Frank G. Goodnow, "Summary Abatement of Nuisances by Boards of Health," *Columbia Law Review* (1902): 203–22.

26. *Daily Alta California*, August 22, 1854.

27. "Moving on Their Works: Health Officer Dr. J. L. Meares Notifies the Chinese to Set Their Houses in Order."

28. SFBH, *Annual Report*, 1876–77, pp. 13, 15. Similar comments about so-called Chinatown as a "moral and social plague spot," "sanitary curse," and region "contaminating the atmosphere," can be found in SFBH, *Annual Report*, 1878–79, p. 5; SFBH, *Annual Report*, 1879–80, p. 2; SFBH, *Annual Report*, 1880–81, p. 5. John L. Meares, M.D., was born in Wilmington, North Carolina, in 1822. He studied medicine at Jefferson College in Philadelphia, served as a surgeon in the Confederate Army, and came to California in 1871. He died in San Francisco in 1888. Meares's obituary was printed in the *Pacific Medical and Surgical Journal* (*PMSJ* hereafter) 31, no. 2 (February 1888): 89–90.

29. SFBH, *Annual Report*, 1876–77, pp. 8–9.

30. Ibid., pp. 8, 14.

31. Craddock, "Sewers and Scapegoats"; Trauner, "The Chinese as Medical Scapegoats in San Francisco."

32. SFBH, *Annual Report*, 1877–78, p. 4; SFBH, *Annual Report*, 1878–79, p. 67; SFBH, *Annual Report*, 1881–82, p. 9. Enforcement statistics justified the special scrutiny. For instance, from July 1884 to June 1885, 2,597 health code violations in the city were recorded; of these, 1,061 citations were given for buildings in the Chinese quarter. SFBH, *Annual Report*, 1884–85, p. 5.

33. In the late 1890s, Chinatown's special status was shared by the Latin Quarter, where Italian, Portuguese, and Latin American immigrants lived. SFBH, *Annual Report*, 1895–96, p. 7; SFBH, *Annual Report*, 1896–97, p. 182; SFBH *Annual Report*, 1897–98, p. 196.

34. SFBH, *Annual Report*, 1873–74, p. 19; SFBH, *Annual Report*, 1871–72, p. 5.

35. SFBH, *Annual Report*, 1874–75, p. 5. See also SFBH, *Annual Report*, 1872–73, p. 11.

36. Dr. H. H. Toland's testimony in California Legislature, Special Committee on Chinese Immigration, *Chinese Immigration: Its Social, Moral, and Political Effect* (Sacramento, 1876), p. 105; Arthur Stout's testimony, in U.S. Congress, Senate, *Report of the Joint Special Committee*, p. 647; John Meares's testimony, in U.S. Congress, Senate, *Report of the Joint Special Committee*, p. 139.

37. Augustus Ward Loomis, "The Medical Art in the Chinese Quarter," *Overland Monthly* 2, no. 6 (1869): 496–506.

38. "Chinese Practice in San Francisco," *PMSJ*, n.s. 3 (November 1869): 278–79; "Chinese Therapeutics," *PMSJ*, n.s. 4 (June 1870): 45; "Chinese Medicine," *PMSJ* 19, no. 4 (September 1876): 161–65; Charlotte Blake Brown, M.D., "Obstetric Practice among the Chinese in San Francisco," *PMSJ* 23, no. 1 (July 1883): 15–21; "Chinese Treatment of Diphtheria," *Occidental Medical Times (OMT* hereafter) 4, no. 12 (December 1890): 640. Observations of Chinese medical practices in San Francisco were interchangeable with the observations of American medical missionaries in China, reinforcing the notion of an unchanging society, culture, and technology. See J. G. Kerr, "Medical Missions in China and Japan," *PMSJ* 21, no. 1 (November 1878): 249; William Tisdale, "Chinese Physicians in California," *Lippincott's Magazine,* no. 63 (March 1899): 411–16; Stewart Culin, *Chinese Drug Stores in America* (Philadelphia: n.p., 1887).

39. Paul Starr, *The Social Transformation of American Medicine: The Rise of the Sovereign Profession and the Making of a Vast Industry* (New York: Basic Books, 1982).

40. SFBH, *Annual Report,* 1874–75, p. 16.

41. By removing Chinese death figures, Gibbons calculated mortality figures of 19.1 per 1,000 in 1873–74 and 17.5 per 1,000 in 1874–75. If the Chinese had been included, the rates would have crept up to 20.0 per 1,000 in 1873–74 and 18.1 per 1,000 in 1874–75. The difference would have been marginal in relation to Gibbons's own comparison to other cities. His own tables showed that Philadelphia, Chicago, Providence, and Cincinnati had mortality rates that hovered between 19.6 and 20.3 per 1,000 during this period; these were substantially better than New York's and Boston's rates, which were as high as 28.4 per 1,000. Ibid., pp. 5–8.

42. Leavitt, *The Healthiest City;* Rosencrantz, *Public Health and the State;* James H. Cassedy, *Demography in Early America: The Beginnings of the Statistical Mind, 1600–1899* (Cambridge: Harvard University Press, 1982); Thomas McKeown, *The Modern Rise of Population* (New York: Academic Press, 1976).

43. Craddock, "Sewers and Scapegoats," pp. 957–68: Duffy, *The Sanitarians;* D. R. Hopkins, *Princes and Peasants: Smallpox in History* (Chicago: University of Chicago Press, 1983).

44. In 1880, there were 507 cases recorded and 92 deaths, and in 1887–88 there were 568 cases recorded and 69 deaths. SFBS, *San Francisco Municipal Report,* 1868–69; SFBH, *Annual Report,* 1876–77, 1879–80, and 1887–88.

45. SFBS, *San Francisco Municipal Report,* 1868–69; *California Medical Gazette* (August 1868): 39; E. M. Morse, "Something about the Smallpox Epidemic," *California Medical Gazette* (1869): 131; "The Chinese on the Pacific Coast. The Statement of the Anti-Coolie Association," *Daily Alta California,* June 24, 1869.

46. Gibbons attributed smallpox cases to "contact" with the "passengers or baggage of vessels from China," SFBH, *Annual Report,* 1872–73, pp. 12–13. The following year Gibbons blamed all cases of smallpox in the city on the Chinese. In 1875, when he claimed that there were no cases of smallpox among the

Chinese that year, Gibbons remarked that "fortunately no cases have arrived from China to propagate [smallpox] among the [Chinese]. Nearly all the cases that have been reported during the year have either just arrived overland, or have been in contact with the disease in persons who have." SFBH, *Annual Report, 1873–74,* pp. 18–19; SFBH, *Annual Report, 1874–75,* p. 18.

47. SFBH, *Annual Report, 1872–73,* pp. 12–13; SFBS, *San Francisco Municipal Report, 1869–70,* p. 230.

48. "The Quarantine Station at San Francisco," *OMT* 3, no. 1 (January 1889): 34.

49. Craddock, "Sewers and Scapegoats," pp. 961–62; *San Francisco Chronicle,* May 20, 1876; *Western Lancet* 9 (1880).

50. "The National Board of Health and the San Francisco Quarantine," *PMSJ* 25, no. 1 (January 1883): 38–39; Letter to Dr. T. J. Turner, Secretary, National Board of Health, Washington, D.C., from F. A. Bee, Chinese Consul, San Francisco, June 6, 1882, reprinted in National Board of Health, "Appendix N: Quarantine at San Francisco, California," *Annual Report* (Washington, D.C.: Government Printing Office, 1882), pp. 571–72.

51. *Berkeley Beacon,* undated, reprinted in "Appendix N: Quarantine at San Francisco, California," p. 572.

52. Letter to J. L. Cabell, President, National Board of Health, Washington, D.C., from Drs. Simpson, Gibbons, and Douglass, Committee of the San Francisco Board of Health, San Francisco, July 25, 1882, reprinted in "Appendix N: Quarantine at San Francisco, California," pp. 577–78.

53. Letter to Charles Folger, Secretary of the Treasury, Washington, D.C., from Drs. Sutherland, Van Sant, and Wood, San Francisco, July 15, 1882, reprinted in "Appendix N: Quarantine at San Francisco, California," pp. 573–74.

54. Letter to the editor from C. J. Wharry, May 3, 1888, *PMSJ* 31, no. 6 (June 1888): 350.

55. "Quarantine at San Francisco," *PMSJ* 31, no. 6 (June 1888): 347–49.

56. Meares's testimony, in U.S. Congress, Senate, *Report of the Joint Special Committee,* p. 128. Also see SFBH, *Annual Report, 1876–77,* pp. 14–15.

57. SFBS, *San Francisco Municipal Report,* 1871–72, pp. 563–66, 606–11. See also Sandmeyer, *The Anti-Chinese Movement in California,* p. 54.

58. SFBH, *Annual Report, 1876–77,* p. 14.

59. SFBH, *Annual Report, 1880–81,* pp. 5–6; SFBH, *Annual Report, 1873–74,* p. 19; Dr. M. M. Chapman, "Public Hygiene and State Medicine: Suggestions for Chinatown," *Medico-Literary Journal* 2, no. 8 (May 1880): 4; Dr. William S. Whitewell, "The Chinatown Ulcer," *PMSJ* 31, no. 9 (September 1888): 534–35.

60. SFBH, *Annual Report, 1876–77,* pp. 13–14. For a discussion of imagery of the unscrupulous, untrustworthy, and inscrutable Chinese, see Miller, *The Unwelcome Immigrant;* Sandmeyer, *The Anti-Chinese Movement in California;* Takaki, *Iron Cages,* pp. 215–50; William Wu, *The Yellow Peril: Chinese Americans in American Fiction, 1850–1940* (Hamden, Conn.: Archon Books, 1982).

61. SFBH, *Annual Report, 1876–77,* pp. 10–11.

62. Ibid., pp. 14–15; SFBH, *Annual Report, 1871–72,* p. 14.

63. Linda Singer, *Erotic Welfare: Sexual Theory and Politics in the Age of Epidemic* (New York: Routledge, 1993), p. 29.

64. SFBH, *Annual Report*, 1876–77, pp. 4–10; SFBH, *Annual Report*, 1878–79, p. 4.

65. SFBH, *Annual Report*, 1887–88, p. 5.

66. "Doings of the Board of Health," *California Medical Gazette* (July 1868): 16–17; "Report of the Smallpox Hospital of San Francisco," *California Medical Gazette* (August 1868): 37–40; Morse, "Something about the Smallpox Epidemic," p. 131; "The Smallpox," *California Medical Gazette* (March 1869): 158.

67. Sandmeyer, *The Anti-Chinese Movement in California*, p. 54; Henry Gibbons Sr., "On the Danger from Pestilence in California," *PMSJ* 22, no. 6 (November 1879): 253.

68. SFBH, *Annual Report*, 1876–77, pp. 11–15; SFBH, *Annual Report*, 1880–81, p. 8.

69. SFBH, *Annual Report*, 1880–81, p. 8.

70. SFBH, *Annual Report*, 1882–83, pp. 6–7; SFBH, *Annual Report*, 1881–82, p. 10.

71. SFBH, *Annual Report*, 1887–88, pp. 5–7.

72. For further reading on smallpox vaccination and processes of medicalization, see Dorothy Porter and Roy Porter, "The Politics of Prevention: Anti-Vaccination and Public Health in Nineteenth-Century England," *Medical History* 32 (1988): 231–32; C. Heuerkamp, "The History of Smallpox Vaccination in Germany: A First Step in the Medicalization of the General Public," *Journal of Contemporary History* 20 (1985): 617–35.

73. SFBS, *Report of the Special Committee*, p. 26.

74. WPC, *Chinatown Declared a Nuisance!* p. 13.

75. SFBH, *Annual Report*, 1880–81, p. 6.

76. In 1886 the city government estimated that 240 out of 320 laundries were operated by Chinese. *Yick Wo v. Hopkins*, 118 U.S. 356 (1886); John Stephens, "A Quantitative Study of San Francisco's Chinatown, 1870 and 1880," in *The Life and Influence and the Role of the Chinese in the U.S., 1776–1960* (San Francisco: Chinese Historical Society, 1976); Paul Man Ong, "An Ethnic Trade: The Chinese Laundries in Early California," *Journal of Ethnic Studies* 8, no. 4 (1980): 95, fn. 5, 108; Ong, "The Chinese, Laundry Laws, and the Use and Control of Urban Space" (M.A. thesis, University of Washington, 1975).

77. San Francisco City Ordinance no. 1679, June 10, 1882. Invalidated by the circuit court in July 1882, *In Re Quong Woo*, 7 Sawyer, 526, and upheld in *In Re Quong Woo*, 13 U.S. 229 (1882).

78. San Francisco City Ordinance no. 1767, April 8, 1884; Sandmeyer, *The Anti-Chinese Movement in California*, p. 76.

79. Alfred Clarke, *Report of Alfred Clarke, Special Counsel for the City and County of San Francisco, in the Laundry Order Litigation* (San Francisco: W. M. Hinton and Co., 1885).

80. *Yick Wo v. Hopkins*, p. 356; *In Re Wo Lee*, 26 U.S. 434 (1886).

81. McClain, *In Search of Equality*, pp. 45–48, 101–132; *Yick Wo v. Hop-*

kins, p. 356; *In Re Wo Lee*, p. 424; *Soon Hing v. Crowley,* 113 U.S. 703 (1885); *In Re Sam Kee,* 31 U.S. 681 (1887).

82. *Barbier v. Connolly,* 113 U.S. 27 (1885); *Neal v. Delaware,* 103 U.S. 370, 407–8 (1881); *Slaughterhouse Cases,* 83 U.S. 36 (1872); William Nelson, *The Fourteenth Amendment: From Political Principle to Judicial Doctrine* (Cambridge: Harvard University Press, 1988); Earl Maltz, *Civil Rights, the Constitution, and Congress, 1863–1869* (Lawrence: University of Kansas Press, 1990); James Kettner, *The Development of American Citizenship, 1608–1870* (Chapel Hill: University of North Carolina Press, 1978), pp. 346–49.

83. *San Francisco Bulletin,* May 12, 1886, p. 2.

84. The campaign was orchestrated by the Chamber of Commerce and supported by commercial bankers, building and loan associations, real estate agents, and retail businessmen. "Letter to the Honorable Mayor from the Board of Health," included in SFBH, *Annual Report,* 1896–97, p. 159; Issel and Cherny, *San Francisco, 1865–1932,* pp. 152–53.

85. SFBH, *Annual Report,* 1896–97, pp. 5–9; Dr. John Williamson, "The Development of the Local Public Health," speech delivered to the Commonwealth Club, Minutes of the Section on Public Health, January 28, 1928, p. 2, in Ray Lyman Wilbur Collection, Ms. 3, Box 61, Folder 4, Lane Medical Library, Stanford University.

86. SFBH, *Annual Report,* 1895–96, p. 159.

87. "Chinatown," *Pacific Medical Journal* 39, no. 11 (November 1896): 652. The *Pacific Medical Journal* was formerly the *Pacific Medical and Surgical Journal.*

88. SFBH, *Annual Report,* 1896–97, pp. 192–93.

89. "Filthy Chinese Laundries," *Pacific Medical Journal* 40, no. 4 (April 1897): 232.

90. John Meares, in U.S. Congress, Senate, *Report of the Joint Special Committee,* pp. 127–32.

91. "The County Hospital. Chinese Patients to be Excluded—Meeting of the Board of Health," *Daily Alta California,* November 20, 1881.

92. "The San Francisco City Hospital and Chinese Consumptives," *OMT* 5, no. 8 (August 1891): 469–70.

93. Ibid.; Mary Coolidge, *Chinese Immigration* (New York: Henry Holt and Company, 1909), pp. 267–68.

94. For details about early Chinese hospitals, see *Oriental,* March 9, 1888, cited in Him Mark Lai, "Chinese Language Sources Bibliography Project: Preliminary Findings," *Amerasia Journal* 5, no. 2 (1978): p. 97; *The Chinese Hospital of San Francisco* (Oakland: Carruth and Carruth, 1899), pp. 1–2; "The San Francisco City Hospital and Chinese Consumptives," pp. 469–70; Coolidge, *Chinese Immigration,* p. 268.

95. For instance, in the most comprehensive population survey of Chinatown, the authors admitted that they could not count all the Chinese city residents outside the boundaries they had selected, but that they could enumerate the instances of white women cohabiting with Chinese men within the boundaries of Chinatown. Willard B. Farwell and John Kunkler, "Report of the Spe-

cial Committee," in Willard B. Farwell, *The Chinese at Home and Abroad, Together with the Report of the Special Committee of the Board of Supervisors of San Francisco on the Condition of the Chinese Quarter and the Chinese in San Francisco, July 1885* (San Francisco: Bancroft, 1885), pp. 6, 15, 16.

96. *San Francisco Examiner*, February 9 and 12, 1890; *San Francisco Evening Bulletin*, February 9 and 12, 1890. For the ordinance designating the area for offensive trades, see Order 1587, sec 2, in San Francisco Board of Supervisors, *General Orders of the Board of Supervisors* (San Francisco, 1890), p. 17. The section of town was bounded by Kentucky, First, I, Seventh, and Railroad Avenues.

97. *San Francisco Morning Call*, May 21, 1890; *San Francisco Examiner*, May 21, 1890.

98. *In Re Lee Sing et al.*, 43 U.S. 360–61 (1890); Charles J. McClain, "*In Re Lee Sing:* The First Residential-Segregation Case," *Western Legal History* 3, no. 2 (summer-fall 1990): 179–96.

99. For comparisons with the U.S. South, Kenya, and South Africa during the late nineteenth and early twentieth centuries, see C. Vann Woodward, *Strange Career of Jim Crow* (New York: Oxford University Press, 1955); John W. Cell, *The Highest Stage of White Supremacy: The Origins of Segregation in South Africa and the American South* (Cambridge: Cambridge University Press, 1982); Luise White, *The Comforts of Home: Prostitution in Colonial Nairobi* (Chicago: University of Chicago Press, 1990); Swanson, "The Sanitation Syndrome," pp. 387–410.

100. McClain, "*In Re Lee Sing*," pp. 179–98; Marc Weiss, "The Real Estate Industry and the Politics of Zoning in San Francisco, 1914–1928," *Planning Perspectives* 3 (1988): 311–24.

101. Barbara J. Flint makes this argument eloquently in her dissertation, "Zoning and Residential Segregation: A Social and Political History, 1910–1940" (Ph.D. diss., University of Chicago, Department of History, 1977).

102. Clement E. Vose, *Caucasians Only: The Supreme Court, the NAACP, and the Restrictive Covenant Cases* (Berkeley and Los Angeles: University of California Press, 1959), p. 3.

103. Ibid., pp. 17–19.

104. Woodward, *The Strange Career of Jim Crow*, pp. 100–101. The use of covenants throughout California was documented through the research of Eliot G. Mears's team in the mid-1920s, which led to the publication of Mears, *Resident Orientals on the American Pacific Coast* (1927; reprint, New York: Arno Press, 1978). Manuscript research notes and correspondence concerning the segregation practices of real estate boards are located in Survey of Race Relations Collection, Box 2, Herbert Hoover Library, Stanford University.

105. "Declaration of the Conditions, Covenants, and Charges affecting St. Francis Wood, Extension Number 1, San Francisco California," *Articles of Incorporation and By-Laws of St. Francis Wood Homes Association*, Mason-McDuffie Company, San Francisco, October 11, 1912, supplement amended June 29, 1922, Mason-McDuffie Collection, BANC MSS 89/12C, Bancroft Library, University of California at Berkeley (BL hereafter). Other residential

neighborhoods include Ashbury Terrace, Lincoln Manor, Windsor Terrace, and Ingleside Terrace.

106. Mason-McDuffie Company, *St. Francis Wood Homes* (San Francisco: Mason-McDuffie Company, ca. 1912), p. 5, Mason-McDuffie Collection, BANC MSS 89/12C, BL.

107. David Montejano, *Anglos and Mexicans in the Making of Texas, 1836–1986* (Austin: University of Texas Press, 1987), pp. 220–34; K. J. Anderson, *Vancouver's Chinatown*, pp. 8–33, 73–105.

108. "Speech of Aaron A. Sargent, of California, in the Senate of the United States May 2, 1876," in Chinese Pamphlets Collection, Chinese Pamphlets Box 1, p. 3, California State Library, Sacramento.

109. Ibid.


## CHAPTER 3. PERVERSITY, CONTAMINATION, AND THE DANGERS OF QUEER DOMESTICITY

1. Estelle Freedman and John D'Emilio, *Intimate Matters: A History of Sexuality in America* (New York: Harper and Row, 1988); Stoler, *Race and the Education of Desire;* Foucault, *History of Sexuality;* Jeffrey Weeks, *Sex, Politics, and Society* (London: Longman, 1981); George L. Mosse, *Nationalism and Sexuality: Middle Class Morality and Sexual Norms in Modern Europe* (Madison: University of Wisconsin Press, 1985); Reid, *Families in Jeopardy;* Bourdieu, "On the Family as a Realized Category," pp. 19–26.

2. Ting, "Bachelor Society," pp. 271–79; Fung, "Burdens of Representation, Burdens of Responsibility," pp. 291–99; Johnson, "Sharing Bed and Board."

3. I use "queer" as an analytical category to examine social formations, gender expressions, and spatial arrangements that counter and transgress the normal and conventional. See Michael Warner, *Fear of a Queer Planet: Queer Politics and Social Theory* (Minneapolis: University of Minnesota Press, 1993); Gayatri Gopinath, "Homo-Economics: Queer Sexualities in a Transnational Frame," in *Burning Down the House: Recycling Domesticity,* ed. Rosemary George (Boulder, Colo.: Westview Press, 1998), pp. 102–24; Chandan R. Reddy, "Homes, Houses, Non-Identity: Paris Is Burning," in *Burning Down the House: Recycling Domesticity,* ed. Rosemary George (Boulder, Colo.: Westview Press, 1998), pp. 355–79; Janet R. Jakobsen, "Queer Is? Queer Does?" *GLQ: A Journal of Lesbian and Gay Studies* 4, no. 4 (fall 1998): 511–536.

4. Freedman and D'Emilio, *Intimate Matters;* Jonathan Ned Katz, *The Invention of Heterosexuality* (New York: Penguin Books, 1995); George Chauncey, *Gay New York* (New York: Basic Books, 1994); Kevin J. Mumford, *Interzones: Black/White Sex Districts in Chicago and New York in the Early Twentieth Century* (New York: Columbia University Press, 1997); Joanne Meyerowitz, *Women Adrift: Independent Wage Earners in Chicago, 1880–1930* (Chicago: University of Chicago Press, 1988); Chad Heap, "Slumming: The Politics of American Culture and Identity, 1910–1940" (Ph.D. diss., University of Chicago, 2000); Gayle Rubin, "Thinking Sex: Notes for a Radical Theory on the Politics of Sexuality," in *Pleasure and Danger: Exploring Female*

*Sexuality,* ed. Carol Vance (Boston: Routledge and Kegan Paul, 1984), pp. 267–319; Audre Lorde, "The Uses of the Erotic: The Erotic as Power," in *Sister/Outsider: Essays and Speeches* (Trumansburg, N.Y.: Crossing Press, 1984), pp. 53–59; Lauren Berlant and Michael Warner, "Sex in Public," *Critical Inquiry* 24, no. 2 (winter 1998): 547–66.

5. California Legislature, Special Committee on Chinese Immigration, *Chinese Immigration: Its Social, Moral, and Political Effect* (Sacramento, 1876); U.S. Congress, Senate, *Report of the Joint Special Committee.*

6. The notion of the syphilitic prostitute emerged as a persistent figure in debates over morality, health, and the social order in capitalist western Europe and North America. Sander Gilman, "AIDS and Syphilis: The Iconography of Disease," in *AIDS: Cultural Analysis, Cultural Activism,* ed. Douglas Crimp (Cambridge: MIT Press, 1988), pp. 87–107; Mary Spongberg, *Feminizing Venereal Disease: The Body of the Prostitute in Nineteenth-Century Medical Discourse* (New York: New York University Press, 1997).

7. Farwell, *The Chinese at Home and Abroad,* p. 14. For a similar combination of sexual slavery and syphilis, see J. Marion Sims, "Address to the American Medical Association Annual Meeting," *Transactions of the American Medical Association* 27 (1876): 106.

8. Jacqueline Baker Barnhart, *The Fair but Frail: Prostitution in San Francisco, 1849–1900* (Reno: University of Nevada Press, 1986).

9. Judith Walkowitz, *Prostitution in Victorian Society: Women, Class, and the State* (New York: Cambridge University Press, 1980); Luise White, "Prostitution, Differentiation, and the World Economy: Nairobi, 1899–1939," in *Connecting Spheres: Women in the Western World, 1500 to the Present,* ed. Marilyn Boxer and Jean Quataert (New York: Oxford University Press, 1987); White, "Prostitution, Identity, and Class Consciousness during World War II," *Signs: Journal of Women in Culture and Society* 11, no. 2 (winter 1986): 255–73.

10. Timothy J. Gilfoyle, "The Urban Geography of Commercial Sex: Prostitution in New York City, 1790–1860," *Journal of Urban History* 13 (August 1987): 384–87; Neil Larry Shumsky and Larry M. Springer, "San Francisco's Zone of Prostitution, 1880–1934," *Journal of Historical Geography* 7, no. 1 (1981): 71–89; Neil Larry Shumsky, "Tacit Acceptance: Respectable Americans and Segregated Prostitution, 1870–1910," *Journal of Social History* 19 (summer 1986): 665–79.

11. San Francisco Common Council, *Ordinances and Joint Resolutions of the City of San Francisco* (San Francisco: Mason and Valentine, 1854); Frank H. Soule et al., *Annals of San Francisco and History of California* (1855; reprint, Palo Alto: Lewis Osborne, 1966), p. 550; SFBS, *San Francisco Municipal Report,* 1862–63, pp. 139–40; Brenda E. Pillors, "The Criminalization of Prostitution in the United States: The Case of San Francisco, 1854–1919" (Ph.D. diss., University of California at Berkeley, 1982), p. 96; Sucheng Chan, "The Exclusion of Chinese Women, 1870–1943," in *Entry Denied: Exclusion and the Chinese Community in America, 1882–1943,* ed. Sucheng Chan (Philadelphia: Temple University Press, 1991), p. 97.

12. SFBS, *San Francisco Municipal Report,* 1864–65, p. 139.

13. SFBS, *San Francisco Municipal Report,* 1865–66, pp. 124–26; Ryan,

*Women in Public,* pp. 110–11; S. Chan, "The Exclusion of Chinese Women," pp. 97–98; Barnhart, *The Fair but Frail,* pp. 49–50.

14. Densmore, *The Chinese in California,* p. 81; Farwell, *The Chinese at Home and Abroad.*

15. Densmore, *The Chinese in California,* p. 81; Tong, *Unsubmissive Women.*

16. For more on the *mui tsai* system of female bondservants and the confusion with sexual slavery, see Judy Yung, *Unbound Feet: A Social History of Chinese Women in San Francisco* (Berkeley and Los Angeles: University of California Press, 1995); Maria Jaschok, *Concubines and Bondservants: A Social History* (London: Zed Books, 1988).

17. George Anthony Peffer, *If They Don't Bring Their Women: Chinese Female Immigration before Exclusion* (Urbana: University of Illinois Press, 1999), pp. 87–100. Peffer offers a detailed study of the substantial bureaucratic changes in census enumeration between the 1870 and 1880 censuses, as well as biographical background on the 1870 census enumerators, which deepens historical understanding of the political biases and bureaucratic constraints in developing a tabulation and identification of families and female prostitution in San Francisco. See also Carroll Wright and William C. Hunt, *History and Growth of the United States Census* (Washington, D.C.: Government Printing Office, 1900), pp. 156–57, 169–71; Margo J. Anderson, *The American Census: A Social History* (New Haven: Yale University Press, 1988).

18. Farwell, *The Chinese at Home and Abroad,* pp. 8–9.

19. Ibid., p. 16.

20. Historians Sucheng Chan and George Peffer have determined that the Page Law substantially limited the number of Chinese women who immigrated into the United States. S. Chan, "The Exclusion of Chinese Women," pp. 98–109; Peffer, "Forbidden Families: Emigration Experiences of Chinese Women under the Page Law, 1875–1882," *Journal of American Ethnic History* 6 (1986): 28–46.

21. Lucie Cheng Hirata, "Free, Indentured, Enslaved: Chinese Prostitutes in Nineteenth Century America," *Signs* 5 (autumn 1979): 3–29; S. Chan, "The Exclusion of Chinese Women," p. 107; Tong, *Unsubmissive Women.*

22. SFBS, *San Francisco Municipal Report,* 1859–60, p. 42.

23. Mrs. C. M. Churchill, "The Social Evil: Which Do You Prefer?" broadside, BL; CSBH, *Biennial Report,* 1870–71, pp. 45, 48; Mary Ryan, *Women in Public: Between Banners and Ballots, 1825–1880* (Baltimore: Johns Hopkins University Press, 1990), pp. 124–25; James Boyd Jones, "A Tale of Two Cities: The Hidden Battle against Venereal Disease in Civil War Nashville and Memphis," *Civil War History* 31, no. 3 (September 1985): 270–76; John C. Burnham, "Medical Inspection of Prostitutes in America in the Nineteenth Century: The St. Louis Experiment and Its Sequel," *Bulletin of the History of Medicine* 45, no. 3 (May-June 1971): 203–18.

24. At least eight individuals—doctors, clergymen, and police officers— were questioned by the California state senators on the relationship between Chinese prostitutes and the spread of syphilis, particularly to the population of white boys and young men. The testimony was printed in California Legislature,

Special Committee on Chinese Immigration, *Chinese Immigration;* see the testimony of Rev. Otis Gibson, p. 35; F. A. Gibbs, chairman of the Hospital Committee, p. 88; Dr. H. H. Toland, pp. 102–5; Dr. J. C. Shorb, pp. 106–8; David C. Woods, superintendent of the Industrial School, p. 113; James Duffy, Sacramento police officer, p. 125; James Coffey, Sacramento police officer, p. 126; and Matthew Kracher, former Sacramento chief of police, p. 131.

25. California Legislature, Special Committee on Chinese Immigration, *Chinese Immigration,* p. 103.

26. U.S. Congress, Senate, *Report of the Joint Special Committee,* p. 14; Farwell, *The Chinese at Home and Abroad,* pp. 12–13; WPC, *Chinatown Declared a Nuisance!* pp. 4–5; American Federation of Labor, *Some Reasons for Chinese Exclusion: Meat vs. Rice, American Manhood against Asiatic Cooliesism. Which Shall Survive?* (Washington: American Federation of Labor, 1901), p. 28; Dr. M. P. Sawtelle, "The Foul Contagious Disease: A Phase of the Chinese Question," *Medico-Literary Journal* 1, no. 3 (November 1878): 8; Densmore, *The Chinese in California,* p. 81; Raymond, *Horrors of the Mongolian Settlement,* pp. 55, 57; Charles Frederick Holder, "Chinese Slavery in America," *North American Review* 165 (September 1897): 288–94.

27. Sims, "Address to the American Medical Association Annual Meeting," p. 107.

28. California Legislature, Special Committee on Chinese Immigration, *Chinese Immigration,* p. 107.

29. Laqueur, "Bodies, Details, and the Humanitarian Narrative," pp. 176–204; Gilman, "AIDS and Syphilis," pp. 87–107.

30. Dr. M. P. Sawtelle, "State Sanitation," *Medico-Literary Journal* (February 1880): 2–3. More background on Dr. Sawtelle and her analysis of sexuality and domesticity appears in chapter 4.

31. Stallybrass and White, *The Politics and Poetics of Transgression,* p. 22.

32. Sawtelle, "The Foul Contagious Disease," p. 5.

33. Sawtelle, "State Sanitation," p. 3.

34. Sawtelle, "The Foul Contagious Disease," pp. 4–5; Sawtelle, "State Sanitation," pp. 2–3.

35. Stoler, *Race and the Education of Desire,* pp. 147–64; Napur Chaudhrui, "Memsahibs and Motherhood in Nineteenth Century Colonial India," *Victorian Studies* 31, no. 4 (1988): 517–36; Robert Schell, "Tender Ties: Women and the Slave Household, 1652–1834," in *The Societies of Southern Africa in the 19th and 20th Centuries,* University of London Institute of Commonwealth Studies no. 17 (London: University of London, 1992); Jim Swan, "Mater and Nannie: Two Mothers and the Discovery of the Oedipus Complex," *American Imago* 31, no. 1 (spring 1974): 1–64.

36. Sarah E. Henshaw, "Chinese Housekeepers and Chinese Servants," *Scribner's Monthly* 12 (1876): 736.

37. Thomas Logan, cited in CSBH, *Biennial Report,* 1870–71, p. 46.

38. Thomas King, cited in Canada, Royal Commission on Chinese Immigration, *Report of the Royal Commission on Chinese Immigration: Report and Evidence* (Ottawa: Royal Commission on Chinese Immigration, 1885), p. 194.

39. C. C. Cox and J. T. Tobin, cited in Canada, Royal Commission on Chinese Immigration, *Report of the Royal Commission on Chinese Immigration: Report and Evidence,* pp. 14, 228.

40. Elaine Kim, "Such Opposite Creatures: Men and Women in Asian American Literature," *Michigan Quarterly Review* 29, no. 1 (winter 1990): 68; Ting, "Bachelor Society."

41. H. H. Kane, *Opium Smoking in America and China: A Study of Its Prevalence and Effects, Immediate and Remote, on the Individual and the Nation* (New York: G. P. Putnam's Sons, 1882).

42. Opium dens were concentrated in the areas with a large number of houses with Chinese prostitutes, such as Bartlett Alley (2), Dunscombe Alley (6), Jackson Street (6), and Dupont Street (3), as well as in zones of white prostitution on Spofford Alley, Washington Street, Waverly Place, and Sacramento Street. City officials identified in 1885 nearly thirty resorts, most of which accommodated fewer than fourteen bunks. Of these, five were on the first floor of buildings and the rest were in basements and subbasements. The investigators reported that all of the resorts were "filthy." Farwell, *The Chinese at Home and Abroad,* pp. 26–27.

43. WPC, *Chinatown Declared a Nuisance!* pp. 12–13.

44. W. S. Whitwell, "The Opium Habit," *PMSJ* 30, no. 6 (June 1887): 321–38; David T. Courtright, *Dark Paradise: Opiate Addiction in America before 1940* (Cambridge: Harvard University Press, 1982); Kane, *Opium Smoking in America and China.*

45. Kane, *Opium Smoking in America and China;* Peter Ward Fay, *Opium War, 1840–1842* (New York: W. W. Norton, 1976).

46. Elizabeth Anne McCauley, "Taber and Company's Chinatown Photographs: A Study in Prejudice and Its Manifestations," *Bulletin of the University of New Mexico Art Museum,* no. 13 (1980–81): 12–13.

47. Whitwell, "The Opium Habit," p. 329; "The Opium Curse," *PMSJ* 35, no. 12 (December 1892): 745–46.

48. George H. Fitch, "A Night in Chinatown," *Cosmopolitan* 2, no. 6 (February 1887): 356.

49. Pierre Bourdieu, *Distinction: A Social Critique of the Judgement of Taste,* trans. Richard Nice (Cambridge: Harvard University Press, 1984).

50. Kane, *Opium Smoking in America and China,* p. 8; Charles E. Terry and Mildred Pellens, *The Opium Problem* (New York: n.p., 1928), p. 73; Winslow Anderson, "The Opium Habit in San Francisco," *Medical and Surgical Reporter* 57 (1887): 784.

51. Kane, *Opium Smoking in America and China,* p. 14; Farwell, *The Chinese at Home and Abroad,* p. 15.

52. Lloyd, *Lights and Shades in San Francisco,* pp. 261–62.

53. Fitch, "A Night in Chinatown," p. 356.

54. Allen S. Williams, *The Demon of the Orient and His Satellite Fiends of the Joint: Our Opium Smokers as They Are in Tartar Hells and American Paradises* (New York: Allen S. Williams, 1883), pp. 18–19; Williams relates a parallel tale later in the book about a *New York Times* reporter who had a similar

experience of revulsion after recognizing that the same pipe was shared by Chinese and white smokers. See pp. 66–67.

55. Kane, *Opium Smoking in America and China*, p. 78.

56. Terry and Pellens, *The Opium Problem*, pp. 50, 74; William J. Courtney, *San Francisco Anti-Chinese Ordinances, 1850–1900* (San Francisco: Rand E. Research Associates, 1974), pp. 2–3.

57. *San Francisco Chronicle*, July 25, 1881, cited in Kane, *Opium Smoking in China and America*, pp. 10–14.

58. Curtis Marez, "The Other Addict: Reflections on Colonialism and Oscar Wilde's Opium Smoke Screen," *English Literary History* 64 (spring 1997): 257–87; Marez, "The Coquero in Freud: Psychoanalysis, Race, and International Economies of Distinction," *Cultural Critique* 26 (1994): 65–93.

59. "The Opium Curse," p. 745; Whitwell, "Opium Habit," pp. 334–36.

60. Farwell, *The Chinese at Home and Abroad*, p. 103.

61. In the United States, of the forty-one colonies and states that prohibited interracial marriage, twenty-two also prohibited some form of interracial sex. All miscegenation laws explicitly specified an interdiction of marriage between whites and blacks; in addition, twelve states banned marriages between whites and American Indians; fourteen states barred marriages of whites with Chinese, Japanese, and Koreans; nine states banned marriages of whites with Malays (Filipinos); and seven outlawed the marriages of whites with either "Hindus" or "Asiatic Indians." Peggy Pascoe, "Miscegenation Law, Court Cases, and Ideologies of Race in Twentieth Century America," *Journal of American History* 83, no. 1 (June 1996): 44–69; Byron Curti Martyn, "Racism in the United States: A History of Miscegenation Legislation and Litigation" (Ph.D. diss., University of Southern California, 1979); Megumi Dick Osumi, "Asians and California's Anti-Miscegenation Laws," in *Asian and Pacific American Experiences: Women's Perspectives*, ed. Nobuya Tsuchida (Minneapolis: Asian Pacific American Learning Resource Center and General College, University of Minnesota, 1982), pp. 2–8; Peggy Pascoe, "Race, Gender, and Intercultural Relations: The Case of Interracial Marriage," *Frontiers* 12, no. 1 (1991): 5–18.

62. *Compiled Laws of California* (Garfielde and Snyder 1853), p. 175; *Civil Code of the State of California*, 1874, p. 30, and 1876, p. 594.

63. Constitutional Convention of California, *Debates and Proceedings of the Constitutional Convention of California*, 1878–79 (Sacramento, 1880), 1:632.

64. Stout defined the "American people" either as the "Anglo-Saxon" race or the "Caucasian type." His typology of races included Caucasians, aboriginal Americans (sometimes referred to as American Indians, considered a variant of the Mongolian race), Mongolians (or sometimes Asiatics), and Negroes. Stout drew from racial taxonomy developed by Josiah Nott and George Gliddon in *Types of Mankind* (Philadelphia: Lippincott, 1854). He also cited the work of Samuel Morton, Alexander von Humboldt, and Louis Agassiz. Arthur B. Stout, *Chinese Immigration and the Physiological Causes of the Decay of a Nation* (San Francisco: Agnew & Deffebach, 1862), reprinted in CSBH, *Biennial Report, 1870–71*, pp. 58–63.

65. CSBH, *Biennial Report, 1870–71*, p. 63.

66. Ibid., p. 47.

67. A. B. Stout, cited in Canada, Royal Commission on Chinese Immigration, *Report of the Royal Commission on Chinese Immigration: Report and Evidence*, p. 312.

68. In 1880, section 5069 was amended to prohibit issuance of a marriage license to a white person wishing to marry a "Mongolian" (at this point, such a marriage was not actually illegal, however). In 1905, the marriage statute was amended to make all marriages between Mongolians and whites "illegal and void." In 1933 the category "Malays" was added in order to include Filipinos under the statute. *Cal. Stats. Code, Amendments*, 1933, ch. 41, sec. 1, p. 3; *Civil Code of the State of California*, 1883, article 2, para. 69; *Cal. Stats. Code*, 1905, ch. 414, para. 2, 554.

69. The following mentioned instances of white women marrying or cohabiting with Chinese men: The Reverend A. W. Loomis in 1876 counted five cases of Chinese men living with white women. In 1885 the board of supervisors reported ten cases of "white women living and cohabiting with Chinamen in the relation of wives or mistresses" and presented an inventory of street addresses of white women living with Chinese men. Augustus Ward Loomis, "Chinese in California," [articles and letters to H.H. Bancroft], 1876, in Hubert Howe Bancroft Collection, MSS C-E 158, BL; Farwell, *The Chinese at Home and Abroad*, pp. 15–16; Coolidge, *Chinese Immigration*, p. 441.

70. Miscegenation was invalidated by the California Supreme Court decision in *Perez v. Lippold* in 1948. The California legislature lacked the will to repeal the invalidated marriage code to conform with the jurisprudence until 1969, when the invalidated statutes were repealed. *Cal. Stats. Code*, 1969, ch. 1608, para. 3, p. 3313; *California Civil Code, Annotated* (West 1982).

71. *The Workingman's Advocate*, October 9, 1869, October 11, 1873, and May 6, 1876, cited in Miller, *The Unwelcome Immigrant*, p. 198; H. S. West, comp., *The Chinese Invasion, Revealing the Habits, Manners, and Customs of the Chinese, Political, Social, and Religious, on the Pacific Coast, Coming in Contact with the Free and Enlightened Citizens of America* (San Francisco: Bacon and Company, 1873), pp. 68–70, 107.

72. U.S. Congress, Senate, *Report of the Joint Special Committee*, pp. 131, 132, 180, 182, 199–201, 202–5, 1100.

73. "Abstract of the Proceedings of the Board," included in CSBH, *Biennial Report*, 1892–94, p. 7.

74. SFBH, *Annual Report*, 1907–08, p. 11.

75. After the deportation, public health officials believed the leprosy crisis had been solved, and for two years they denied the existence of any more Chinese lepers in the city. In October 1878, under mounting political pressure, the city admitted fifteen new leprosy cases to the Smallpox Hospital in a period of three weeks.

76. Letter to John J. Reichenbach, Chairman of the Hospital Committee of the Board of Supervisors, from Dr. John W. Foye, Resident Physician, City

and County Small-pox Hospital [Twenty-sixth Street Smallpox Hospital], January 15, 1884, reprinted in Farwell, *The Chinese at Home and Abroad*, pp. 105–10; F. W. Hopkins, "Leprosy in Madeira and San Francisco—a Contrast," *Pacific Medical Journal* 38, no. 12 (December 1895): 743.

77. *New York Times*, September 28, 1878; Zachary Gussow, *Leprosy, Racism, and Public Health: Social Policy in Chronic Disease Control* (Boulder, Colo.: Westview Press, 1989), p. 128.

78. Lloyd, *Lights and Shades in San Francisco*, p. 264.

79. *Chinatown, San Francisco, California* (San Francisco: Bancroft Company, 1893), p. 6.

80. Miller, *The Unwelcome Immigrant*, p. 164; SFBH, *Annual Report*, 1878–79, p. 6; SFBH, *Annual Report*, 1883–84, p. 6; U.S. Congress, Senate, *Report of the Joint Special Committee*, p. 204; Henry Gibbons Sr., "On the Danger of Pestilence in California," included in CSBH, *Biennial Report*, 1878–79, pp. 89–90, reprinted in *PMSJ* 22, no. 6 (November 1879): 253; "Leprosy in California," *New York Times*, July 20, 1881, cited in Gussow, *Leprosy, Racism, and Public Health*, p. 128.

81. Dr. A. W. Saxe, "Hawaiian Leprosy," *Transactions of the Medical Society of the State of California* 14 (1883–84): 210–16; "Leprosy in Hawaii," *OMT* 4, no. 8 (August 1890): 441–45; Dr. L. F. Alvarez, "Leprosy in the Hawaiian Islands," *Pacific Medical Journal* 38, no. 1 (January 1895): 17–23; Dr. Winslow Anderson, "The Hawaiian Islanders and Leprosy," *Pacific Medical Journal* 39, no. 9 (September 1896): 551–58.

82. "Society Proceedings—Sacramento Society for Medical Improvement, Annual Meeting, March 20, 1894," *OMT* 8, no. 5 (May 1894): 322–24; Letter to Reichenbach from Foye, reprinted in Farwell, *The Chinese at Home and Abroad*, pp. 105–10; F. B. Sutliff, "A Safe View Regarding the Contagion of Leprosy," *OMT* 9, no. 4 (April 1895): 194–98; Albert S. Ashmead, "Is Leprosy Contagious or Not?" *Pacific Medical Journal* 40, no. 12 (December 1897): 747; "Dermatology, Syphilis, and Venereal Disease," *OMT* 12, no. 2 (February 1908): 91–92; "Leprosy in the United States," *Pacific Medical Journal* 45, no. 8 (August 1902): 487–88.

83. "Society Proceedings—Sacramento Society for Medical Improvement, Annual Meeting, March 20, 1894," pp. 322–24; Sutliff, "A Safe View Regarding the Contagion of Leprosy," pp. 194–98.

84. Testimony of John Meares, in U.S. Congress, Senate, *Report of the Joint Special Committee*, cited in Canada, Royal Commission on Chinese Immigration, *Report of the Royal Commission on Chinese Immigration: Report and Evidence*, p. 198; and testimony of Fred Gibles, in U.S. Congress, Senate, *Report of the Joint Special Committee*, p. 203.

85. Henry R. Brown, "Summary of Leprosy Cases, February 16, 1894," included in SFBH, *Annual Report*, pp. 84–92, reprinted in *Pacific Medical Journal* 37, no. 10 (October 1894): 614–25.

86. SFBH, *Annual Report*, 1883–84, p. 6.

87. Ibid.

88. Farwell, *The Chinese at Home and Abroad*, p. 111.

89. Reddy, "Homes, Houses, Non-Identity," pp. 355–79; Gordon Brent

Ingram, Anne-Marie Bouthillette, and Yolanda Ritter, eds., *Queers in Space: Communities, Public Places, Sites of Resistance* (Seattle: Bay Press, 1997), p. 10.

## CHAPTER 4. WHITE WOMEN, HYGIENE, AND THE STRUGGLE FOR RESPECTABLE DOMESTICITY

1. Martha H. Verbrugge, *Able-Bodied Womanhood: Personal Health and Social Change in Nineteenth Century Boston* (New York: Oxford University Press, 1988), p. 4.

2. Rosemary Maragoly George, "Recycling: Long Routes to and from Domestic Fixes," in *Burning Down the House: Recycling Domesticity* (Boulder, Colo.: Westview Press, 1998), p. 3.

3. Kathryn K. Sklar, *Catherine Beecher: A Study in American Domesticity* (New Haven: Yale University Press, 1973); Anita Clair Fellman and Michael Fellman, *Making Sense of Self: Medical Advice Literature in Late Nineteenth Century America* (Philadelphia: University of Pennsylvania Press, 1981).

4. Kaplan, "Manifest Domesticity"; Rafael, "Colonial Domesticity," pp. 639–66; Joan Jacobs Brumberg, "The Ethnological Mirror: American Evangelical Women and Their Heathen Sisters, 1870–1910," in *Women and the Structure of Society,* ed. Barbara J. Harris and JoAnn McNamara (Durham, N.C.: Duke University Press, 1984), pp. 108–28; Patricia Hill, *The World Their Household: American Woman's Foreign Mission Movement and Cultural Transformation, 1870–1920* (Ann Arbor: University of Michigan Press, 1985).

5. Paul Boyer, *Urban Masses and Moral Order in America, 1820–1920* (Cambridge: Harvard University Press, 1978); Gwendolyn Wright, *Moralism and the Model Home: Domestic Architecture and Cultural Conflict in Chicago, 1873–1913* (Chicago: University of Chicago Press, 1980); Stephanie Coontz, *The Way We Never Were: The American Family and the Nostalgia Trap* (New York: Basic Books, 1992); Valverde, *The Age of Light, Soap, and Water;* Leonore Davidoff and Catherine Hall, *Family Fortunes: Men and Women of the English Middle Class, 1780–1850* (Chicago: University of Chicago Press, 1987); John Comaroff and Jean Comaroff, "Homemade Hegemony," in *Ethnography and the Historical Imagination* (Boulder, Colo.: Westview Press, 1992).

6. Sawtelle, "The Plague Spot," p. 11.

7. Sawtelle, "The Foul Contagious Disease," pp. 1, 4; Mosse, *Nationalism and Sexuality.*

8. Sawtelle, "The Foul Contagious Disease," pp. 1–3, 6–8.

9. *Medico-Literary Journal* 1, no. 6 (May 1879): 20; *Medico-Literary Journal* 1, no. 1 (September 1878): 6.

10. Sklar, *Catherine Beecher;* Fellman and Fellman, *Making Sense of Self;* Verbrugge, *Able-Bodied Womanhood.*

11. Letter from Jeffrey Christensen, Ann Arbor, September 4, 1979, in File on California Women, Special Collections on Women in Medicine, Medical College of Pennsylvania Archives; *Medico-Literary Journal* 1, no. 1 (September 1878): 25–26; *Medico-Literary Journal* 1, no. 9 (May 1879): 20; *Medico-Literary Journal* 4, no. 2 (October 1881): 18–21.

12. Sawtelle, "The Foul Contagious Disease," pp. 1, 8.

13. *Medico-Literary Journal* 1, no. 4 (December 1878): 10.

14. Ibid., pp. 4–7.

15. Sawtelle, "The Foul Contagious Disease," p. 4.

16. Ibid., p. 2.

17. Ibid.

18. Ibid., p. 7.

19. Robert J. C. Young, *Colonial Desire: Hybridity in Theory, Culture, and Race* (London: Routledge, 1990); Bederman, *Manliness and Civilization*; Nancy Leys Stepan, *In the Hour of Eugenics: Race, Gender, and Nation in Latin America* (Ithaca: Cornell University Press, 1991).

20. Sawtelle, "The Foul Contagious Disease," p. 6.

21. Sawtelle closely modeled her plans on the proposal forwarded by the U.S. Navy's medical director, Dr. A. L. Gibson, in his report to the American Public Health Association, "State Sanitation," *Medico-Literary Journal* 2, no. 6 (February 1880): 3–8.

22. Neil Larry Shumsky, "The Municipal Clinic of San Francisco: A Study of Medical Structure," *Bulletin of the History of Medicine* 52 (1978): 542–49; Julius Rosenstirn, *The Municipal Clinic of San Francisco* (New York: William Wood, 1913); Pillors, "The Criminality of Prostitution in the United States."

23. Prince Morrow, *Social Diseases and Marriage: Social Prophylaxis* (Philadelphia: Lea Brothers, 1904).

24. Statutes of California (1939), pp. 1716–18. This testing was ruled constitutional by the California Supreme Court in the case that invalidated miscegenation statutes, *Perez v. Sharp*, 32 Cal. 2d 711 (1948). *California Jurisprudence*, vol. 32, 2nd ed. (San Francisco: Bancroft-Whitney, 1956), pp. 340–41.

25. Ryan, *Women in Public*, pp. 120–27.

26. Peggy Pascoe, *Relations of Rescue: The Search for Female Moral Authority in the American West, 1874–1939* (New York: Oxford University Press, 1991), pp. 1–69, esp. 13–17.

27. Women's Foreign Missionary Society of the Presbyterian Church, Occidental Branch (WFMS-OB hereafter), *Annual Report* (San Francisco: C. W. Gordon, 1878), p. 8.

28. WFMS-OB, *Annual Report, 1883*, cited in Pascoe, *Relations of Rescue*, p. 41.

29. Mrs. I. M. Condit, "A Day in Chinatown," included in WFMS-OB, *Annual Report, 1878*, p. 21. Emma Cable also invokes the "Zenanas of India" to direct attention to the similar and equally pressing problems in San Francisco's Chinatown. Cable, "Report on House to House Visitation," included in WFMS-OB, *Annual Report, 1889*, p. 52.

30. Brumberg, "The Ethnological Mirror," pp. 108–28; Hill, *The World Their Household*.

31. Emma R. Cable, "Missionary Work among Heathen Women," included in WFMS-OB, *Annual Report, 1881*, p. 40.

32. Ibid.

33. Emma R. Cable, "House to House Visitation," included in WFMS-OB, *Annual Report, 1888*, pp. 44–46.

34. Mrs. J. M. Stewart and Mrs. J. K. Van Slyhe, "Secretary's Report," included in WFMS-OB, *Annual Report*, 1880, p. 11. Condit, "House to House Visitation," included in WFMS-OB, *Annual Report*, 1881, p. 37.

35. Missionaries described their work as an "endeavor to enforce the maxim of Wesley": "Cleanliness is next to Godliness." M. Culbertson, "Report," included in WFMS-OB, *Annual Report*, 1884, p. 26.

36. Emma R. Cable, "House to House Visitation" included in WFMS-OB, *Annual Report*, 1883, p. 56.

37. Cable, "House to House Visitation," 1888, p. 44; Condit, "Annual Report of House to House Visitation, 1884–85," included in WFMS-OB, *Annual Report*, 1885, p. 45.

38. Condit, "House to House Visitation," 1881, p. 37.

39. Emma R. Cable, "House to House Visitation," included in WFMS-OB, *Annual Report*, 1887, p. 57.

40. Ibid., 1890, p. 39.

41. Condit, "Report of House to House Visitations among Christian Families," included in WFMS-OB, *Annual Report*, 1880, p. 36.

42. Condit, "A Day in Chinatown," pp. 18–19.

43. Condit, "Report of House to House Visitations among Christian Families," p. 36.

44. Condit, "Annual Report of House to House Visitation, 1884–85," p. 39.

45. Annie B. Laughlin, "Three Chinese Women of San Francisco," *Woman's Work for Woman* 24, no. 8 (August 1909): 174.

46. Mrs. E. Y. Garrette, "Report of the Evangelistic House to House Work in Chinatown," included in WFMS-OB, *Annual Report*, 1905, p. 55.

47. Ibid., 1903, pp. 42–43.

48. Mary H. Field, "Two Homes," *Woman's Work for Woman* 15, no. 8 (August 1900): 212.

49. Ibid., pp. 212–14.

50. Ibid.

51. Gail Caskey Winkler and Roger W. Moss, "How the Bathroom Got White Tiles . . . and Other Victorian Tales," *Historic Preservation* 36, no. 1 (1984): 33, 35; Tomes, *The Gospel of Germs*, pp. 84–87.

52. Ruth Frankenberg, *White Women, Race Matters: The Social Construction of Whiteness* (Minneapolis: University of Minnesota Press, 1993); Roediger, *The Wages of Whiteness*; R. Dyer, "White," pp. 44–64; Ware, *Beyond the Pale*; Morrison, *Playing in the Dark*.

53. Robert T. Handy, *A Christian America: Protestant Hopes and Historical Realities* (New York: Oxford University Press, 1984), p. 123.

54. Wesley Woo, "Protestant Work among the Chinese in the San Francisco Bay Area, 1850–1920" (Ph.D. diss., Graduate Theology Union, Berkeley, 1983), p. 93.

55. Charles Nash, cited in ibid., p. 94.

56. Horace Greeley, "Chinese Emigration to California," *New York Tribune*, September 29, 1854, cited in Miller, *The Unwelcome Immigrant*, pp. 169–70.

57. Kaplan, "Manifest Domesticity"; Lisa Lowe, "The International within

National: American Studies and Asian American Critique," *Cultural Critique* (fall 1998): 29–47.

58. Richard L. Bushman and Claudia L. Bushman, "The Early History of Cleanliness in America," *Journal of American History* 74 (March 1988): 1225–66; Tomes, *The Gospel of Germs;* Suellen Hoy, *Chasing Dirt: The American Pursuit of Cleanliness* (New York: Oxford University Press, 1995); Martha H. Verbrugge, "The Gospel and Science of Health: Hygienic Ideology in America, 1830–1920," *Reviews in American History* 11, no. 4 (December 1983): 507.

59. See chapter 8. See also Yung, *Unbound Feet.*

## CHAPTER 5. PLAGUE AND MANAGING THE COMMERCIAL CITY

1. The name of the first suspected plague victim varies in the historical record. In the public health reports, he is usually referred to as Wing Chung Ging, his formal name as offered by his brother; the newspapers, however, used the name Chick Gin, a nickname with a slightly different romanization of the Chinese. Several historians have chosen a variation of the nickname, but I have chosen to use his formal name. *San Francisco Examiner,* March 7, 1900; *San Francisco Chronicle,* March 8, 1900; W. H. Kellogg, "The Plague-Report of Cases," *OMT* (July 1900): 197.

2. The historians Silvio Onesti, Philip Kalisch, and Charles McClain have all provided detailed description and analysis of the stark debate on the news and editorial pages of the local newspapers. The *San Francisco Examiner* and the *Sacramento Record-Union* endorsed the existence of bubonic plague and the actions taken by the federal and local health officials, while the *San Francisco Chronicle, San Francisco Call,* and *San Francisco Bulletin* remained skeptical and were vociferous critics of the Board of Health and the U.S. Public Health Service, particularly in the period of the most controversial actions, between March and July 1900. Silvio J. Onesti Jr., "Plague, Press, and Politics," *Stanford Medical Bulletin* 13, no. 1 (February 1955): 1–10; Philip A. Kalisch, "The Black Death in Chinatown: Plague and Politics in San Francisco, 1900–04," *Arizona and the West* 14 (1972): 113–36; McClain, "Of Medicine, Race, and American Law: The Bubonic Plague Outbreak of 1900," *Law and Social Inquiry* 13, no. 3 (1988): pp. 447–513.

3. Bubonic plague, commerce, and quarantine have an entangled history that stretches back to the fourteenth-century "black plague" pandemic, when Italian port cities first imposed systematic quarantine to isolate "plague ships." The term *quarantine* derived from the Italian word for *forty days,* one of the arbitrary periods during which ships arriving from regions of contagious diseases were held at a distance from the people of a seaport. Although historians disagree about the exact date of the establishment of "modern" quarantine, most agree that the development of systematic quarantine procedures first occurred in the coastal Italian city-states during the fourteenth century. J. Gerlitt, "The Development of Quarantine," *Ciba Symposia* 2, no. 6 (1950): 566–80; G. Rosen, *A History of American Public Health,* pp. 63–69; W. T. Wythe, "On Quarantine," *Transactions of the Medical Society of the State of California* 1 (1870–71): 151–57; Kraut, *Silent Travelers,* pp. 24–30.

4. Delaporte, *Disease and Civilization,* p. 190; Prashad, "Native Dirt/Imperial Ordure," pp. 243–60; Martin S. Pernick, "Politics, Parties, and Pestilence: Epidemic Yellow Fever in Philadelphia and the Rise of the First Party System," in *Sickness and Health in America: Readings in the History of Medicine and Public Health,* ed. Judith Waltzer Leavitt and Ronald L. Numbers (Madison: University of Wisconsin Press, 1985), pp. 356–71.

5. David F. Musto, "Quarantine and the Problem of AIDS," *Milbank Quarterly* 64, suppl. 1 (1986): 97–117.

6. Fraser, "Rethinking the Public Sphere," pp. 1–32; Negt and Kluge, *Public Sphere and Experience;* Holt, "Afterword: Mapping the Black Public Sphere," pp. 325–26. In *The Public City,* Phil Ethington develops a historical formulation regarding the late-nineteenth-century public sphere in San Francisco.

7. Gyan Prakash, "Subaltern Studies as Postcolonial Criticism," *American Historical Review* 99, no. 5 (December 1994): 1475–90; Ranajit Guha, *Elementary Aspects of Peasant Insurgency* (Dehli: Oxford University Press, 1982); Guha, "The Prose of Counter-Insurgency," in *Subaltern Studies: Writings on South Asian History and Society,* vol. 2 (Oxford University Press, 1982), pp. 3–26; David Arnold, *Colonizing the Body: State Medicine and Epidemic Disease in Nineteenth-Century India* (Berkeley and Los Angeles: University of California Press, 1993); Daston, "Historical Epistemology," pp. 282–89; Michel Foucault, "Two Lectures," in *Power/Knowledge,* trans. Colin Gordon (New York: Pantheon Books, 1980), pp. 81–83; Nicholas B. Dirks, Geoff Eley, and Sherry B. Ortner, introduction to *Culture/Power/History* (Princeton: Princeton University Press, 1994), pp. 3–46.

8. Henry B. Hemenway, *American Public Health Protection* (Indianapolis: Bobbs-Merrill, 1916), pp. 65–68; F. E. Freemantle, *A Traveler's Study of Health and Empire,* 2nd ed. (London: Heath and Cranton, 1917), pp. 293–314; Vernon B. Link, *A History of Plague in the United States of America,* Public Health Monograph No. 26, Publication No. 392 (Washington, D.C.: Government Printing Office, 1955); Victor H. Haas, "When Bubonic Plague Came to Chinatown," pt. 1, *American Journal of Tropical Medicine and Hygiene* 8, no. 2 (March 1959): 141–47; Loren George Lipson, "Plague in San Francisco in 1900: The United States Marine Hospital Service Commission to Study the Existence of Plague in San Francisco," *Annals of Internal Medicine* 77 (1972): 303–10; Onesti, "Plague, Press, and Politics," pp. 1–10; Kalisch, "The Black Death in Chinatown," pp. 113–36; Mullan, *Plagues and Politics;* Bess Furman, *A Profile of the United States Public Health Service, 1798–1948* (Washington, D.C.: Government Printing Office, 1973), pp. 231–34, 244–55.

9. Trauner, "The Chinese as Medical Scapegoats in San Francisco," pp. 70–87; Kraut, *Silent Travelers,* pp. 78–96; Power, "Media Dependency," pp. 89–110.

10. McClain, "Of Medicine, Race, and American Law," pp. 447–513.

11. As Linda Singer has noted, the logic of an epidemic ensured the discursive proliferation of danger in order to implement regulatory intervention. Singer, *Erotic Welfare,* p. 29.

12. The U.S. public health agency had several identities during this period. In the late nineteenth century it was the U.S. Marine Hospital Service, but in

1912 it was renamed the U.S. Public Health and Marine Hospital Service, which was shortened that same year to the U.S. Public Health Service. For the purpose of clarity, I will use PHS to identify this federal agency.

13. Lipson, "Plague in San Francisco in 1900," pp. 303–10; Leonard Fabian Hirst, *The Conquest of Plague: A Study of the Evolution of Epidemiology* (Oxford: Clarendon Press, 1953), pp. 101–6; Walter Wyman, *The Bubonic Plague,* Public Health Service Bulletin No. 7 (Washington, D.C.: Government Printing Office, 1900), pp. 6–7.

14. Faced with spreading infection, heavy mortality, and rapid depopulation of colonial Indian port cities, British administrators in India took drastic measures to suppress the plague and curtail its spread. The death toll in India was devastating, exceeding 12 million recorded deaths from 1896 to 1930. Arnold, *Colonizing the Body,* pp. 200–239.

15. More than a dozen disease-causing organisms were identified in the last decades of the nineteenth century: leprosy (1880), malaria (1880), tuberculosis (1882), cholera (1883), streptococcus (1883), diphtheria (1884), typhoid (1884), tetanus (1884), pneumococcus (1886), plague (1894), botulism (1894), and dysentery (1898). See G. Rosen, *A History of Public Health,* p. 314.

16. George Rosen, *Preventive Medicine in the United States, 1900–1975: Trends and Interpretations* (New York: Science History Publications, 1975), pp. 20–25; G. Rosen, *A History of Public Health,* pp. 319–36; Arthur M. Silverstein, *A History of Immunology* (San Diego: Academic Press, 1989); Anne Marie Moulin, *Le Dernier Langage de la Medicine: Histoire de lmmunologie de Pasteur au SIDA* (Paris: Presses Universitaires de France, 1991), pp. 67–97; Howard Taylor Ricketts, *Infection, Immunity, and Serum Therapy* (Chicago: American Medical Association, 1906).

17. J. Taylor, "Haffkine's Plague Vaccine," *Indian Medical Research Memoirs,* memoir no. 27 (1933): pp. 3–7; Arnold, *Colonizing the Body.*

18. Mullan, *Plagues and Politics,* pp. 7, 35; Furman, *A Profile of the United States Public Health Service, 1798–1948,* pp. 199–229.

19. Letter to Walter Wyman, Washington, D.C., from Stuart Eldridge, Office of Sanitary Inspector, U.S. Marine Hospital, Yokohama, March 8, 1899, in Record Group (RG hereafter) 90, Box 554, National Archives (Washington, D.C.) (NA hereafter); Telegram to Kinyoun from Wyman, November 18, 1899, in RG 90, Box 15, Vol. 2, National Archives (San Bruno) (NASB hereafter); Letter to the Surgeon General from James C. Perry, Hong Kong, January 2, 1900, in RG 90, Box 553, NA; Letter to Edward Souchon, President, Louisiana State Board of Health, New Orleans, from J. N. Thomas, Quarantine Inspector, New Orleans, December 17, 1899, in RG 90, Box 558, NA; Letter to the Surgeon General from Souchon, New Orleans, January 27, 1900, in RG 90, Box 558, NA.

20. U.S. Marine Hospital Service, *Annual Report of the Supervising Surgeon General* (Washington, D.C.: General Printing Office, 1895–96), p. 547; Letters to Wyman from Eldridge, Office of Sanitary Inspector, Yokohama, March 8 and 24, 1899, in RG 90, Box 544, NA.

21. Letters to Wyman from Eldridge, Office of Sanitary Inspector, Yoko-

hama, June 8 and June 28, 1899, in RG 90, Box 544, NA; Telegram to the Surgeon General from Kinyoun, June 26, 1899, in RG 90, Box 552, NA.

22. G. Rosen, *Preventive Medicine in the United States,* pp. 20–25; Mullan, *Plagues and Politics,* pp. 35–39.

23. Telegram to the Surgeon General from Kinyoun, San Francisco, July 1, 1899, in RG 90, Box 552, NA; "Plague Ship Nippon Maru Arrives Flying a Yellow Flag and Goes into Quarantine," *San Francisco Chronicle,* June 28, 1899; "It Was Not Plague," *San Francisco Chronicle,* July 8, 1899; Letter to Kinyoun from W. B. Coffey and J. Henry Barbat, Committee of the San Francisco Board of Health, San Francisco, July 10, 1899, in RG 90, Box 558, NA.

24. Letter to the Surgeon General from Kinyoun, July 24, 1899, in RG 90, Box 552, NA.

25. Letter to Wyman from Eldridge, Yokohama, July 11, 1899; Letter to Wyman from Eldridge, November 24, 1899. Both letters are in RG 90, Box 554, NA.

26. Letter to the Surgeon General from Perry, Hong Kong, January 2, 1900, in RG 90, Box 553, NA. Circular Letter of the Sanitary Inspector for the United States, Yokohama, December 14, 1899, in RG 90, Box 554, NA; Letter to the Surgeon General from Eldridge, Yokohama, November 24, 1899, in RG 90, Box 554, NA.

27. "Normal Conditions Again," *Honolulu Bulletin,* December 19, 1899; "Island Steamers Depart," "Tabu Pau in Chinatown," "Strong Measure Coming," and "Major Wood's Opinion," *Hawaiian Star,* December 19, 1899; "The Patrol Stops," *Pacific Commercial Advertiser,* December 20, 1899; Judy Hammond, "Chinatown in Honolulu," *San Francisco Examiner,* September 12, 1993.

28. Telegrams to the Surgeon General from Kinyoun, Angel Island, January 20, February 1, February 10, and February 23, 1900, in RG 90, Box 552, NA; Transcript of Telephone Message to the Surgeon General from Quartermaster at Honolulu, Major Ruhlen, February 15, 1900, in RG 90, Box 561, NA.

29. Letter to the Surgeon General from D. A. Carmichael, Honolulu, February 18, 1900, in RG 90, Box 553, NA.

30. Letter to the Surgeon General from M. J. Rosenau, Angel Island, July 26, 1897, in RG 90, Box 555, NA.

31. Telegram to Kinyoun, Angel Island, from Wyman, February 10, 1900, in RG 90, Box 16, Vol. 3, NASB; Telegram to the Surgeon General from Kinyoun, January 20, 1900, in RG 90, Box 552, NA; Telegrams to Kinyoun from Wyman, January 6 and 18, 1900, in RG 90, Box 15, Vol. 2, NASB.

32. Wyman, *The Bubonic Plague,* see esp. pp. 10–17. The pamphlet was an expanded version of an article that appeared in U.S. Marine Hospital Service, *Annual Report of the Supervising Surgeon General* (Washington, D.C.: General Printing Office, 1896–97).

33. Letter to the Surgeon General from Charles E. Decker, Medical Officer in Command, San Diego, January 19, 1900, in RG 90, Box 554, NA. Decker contracted tuberculosis while serving as a PHS medical officer; he died in 1903.

34. Letters to the Surgeon General from Decker, San Diego, January 19, January 23, January 31, and February 2, 1900, in RG 90, Box 554, NA.

35. Telegram to James A. Gassaway from Wyman, March 8, 1900, in RG 90, Box 16, Folder 3, NASB, reprinted in U.S. Marine Hospital Service, *Annual Report of the Supervising Surgeon General* (Washington, D.C.: General Printing Office, 1900–01), p. 531; *San Francisco Examiner,* March 8, 1900, cited in McClain, "Of Medicine, Race, and American Law," p. 460.

36. Singer, *Erotic Welfare,* pp. 29–30.

37. The turn of the century was an era of highly developed print capitalism, which complicates how historians can conceptually think of the "elite." The profuse array of newspapers, pamphlets, and journals often has been mistakenly perceived as "popular," as distinct from "elite" sources. This assumption confuses sharp and contentious debate with the expression of equally sharp social differences. As with any historical period, those who dominated political structures and economic and cultural production at the cusp of the twentieth century were not monolithic and homogenous in their ideas, expressions, and politics. I understand citywide daily newspapers, because of the access to economic power such an undertaking requires, to be "elite" sources, even when they are meant for "popular" consumption.

38. The historian Sucheng Chan has made summaries in English of the *Chung Sai Yat Po* available to Charles McClain, who has incorporated a number of these texts in his study "Of Medicine, Race, and American Law." For the history of the newspaper and its editor, Ng Poon Chew, see Shehong Chen, "Being Chinese, Becoming Chinese American: The Transformation of Chinese Identity in the United States, 1910–1928" (Ph.D. diss., University of Utah, June 1997), pp. 22, 25–27.

39. Chen, "Being Chinese, Becoming Chinese American"; Liu Boji, *A History of the Chinese in United States* (Taipei: Liming, 1976); Him Mark Lai, *From Chinese to Chinese Americans* (Hong Kong: Joint Publishing, 1992); L. Eve Armentrout Ma, "Chinatown Organizations and the Anti-Chinese Movement, 1883–1914," in *Entry Denied: Exclusion and the Chinese Community in America, 1882–1943,* ed. Sucheng Chan (Philadelphia: Temple University Press, 1991), pp. 147–69.

40. W. H. Kellogg, "The Plague—Report of Cases," *OMT* 14, no. 7 (July 1900): 197–202; Dr. J. J. Kinyoun, "Report of Inoculation Experiments," *OMT* 14, no. 7 (July 1900): 202–7; "Plague Fake Is Exploded," *San Francisco Chronicle,* March 9, 1900.

41. *Chung Sai Yat Po,* March 8, 1900, cited in McClain, "Of Medicine, Race, and American Law," p. 455.

42. *San Francisco Examiner,* March 13, 1900, cited in ibid., pp. 461–62. Telegram to Wyman from Gassaway, March 14, 1900, in RG 90, Box 16, Folder 3, NASB, reprinted in U.S. Marine Hospital Service, *Annual Report of the Supervising Surgeon General* (Washington, D.C.: General Printing Office, 1899–1900), pp. 532–33.

43. *San Francisco Chronicle,* March 24 and 27, 1900, cited in McClain, "Of Medicine, Race, and American Law," pp. 460–64.

44. See McClain, "Of Medicine, Race, and American Law," pp. 462–64, for a fuller narrative.

45. Inspectors were posted at common points of exit from the city and at the borders of Arizona, Nevada, and Oregon. Telegrams to Kinyoun from Wyman, May 15, 18, and 19, 1900, in RG 90, Box 29, Vols. 1 and 2, NASB.

46. U.S. Marine Hospital Service, *Department Circular 93* (May 22, 1900), cited in McClain, "Of Medicine, Race, and American Law," p. 471.

47. "What We Should Do about Inoculation," *Chung Sai Yat Po,* May 18, 1900, cited in McClain, "Of Medicine, Race, and American Law," pp. 471–72.

48. "The Background of the Vaccination," *Chung Sai Yat Po,* May 19, 1900, cited in McClain, "Of Medicine, Race, and American Law," p. 472.

49. Telegram to Chinese Minister from CCBA, May 18, 1900, and Telegram to Chinese Minister from Consul General Ho, May 18, 1900, cited in McClain, "Of Medicine, Race, and American Law," pp. 472–73, fn. 101.

50. Translation of poster, San Francisco Health Department, May 18, 1900, in RG 90, Box 29, Vols. 1 and 2, NASB.

51. California Academy of Medicine, "Society Proceedings, May 1900 Meeting," *OMT* 14, no. 7 (July 1900): 226.

52. Ibid., p. 227.

53. My methodological understanding of analyzing rumors is drawn from the theoretical work of David Arnold, "Touching the Body: Perspectives on the Indian Plague, 1896–1900," in *Subaltern Studies V: Writings on South Asian History and Society,* ed. Ranajit Guha (Delhi: Oxford University Press, 1987), pp. 68–77.

54. In communication to Wyman, Kinyoun speculated that a number of unscrupulous white physicians in Chinatown circulated among the Chinese and warned them that Haffkine prophylactic was extremely dangerous and had killed people when used elsewhere. Telegram to Wyman from Kinyoun, June 11, 1900, cited in Kalisch, "The Black Death in Chinatown," p. 123.

55. Guha, "The Prose of Counter-Insurgency," pp. 2–3; Prakash, "Subaltern Studies as Postcolonial Criticism," p. 1479.

56. *Chung Sai Yat Po,* May 23, 1900, cited in McClain, "Of Medicine, Race, and American Law," p. 473, fn. 103. See also Carol Benedict, *Bubonic Plague in Nineteenth Century China* (Stanford: Stanford University Press, 1997).

57. *Sacramento Record-Union,* May 20, 1900, cited in McClain, "Of Medicine, Race, and American Law," p. 473.

58. Shih-Shan Henry Tsai, *China and the Overseas Chinese in the United States, 1868–1911* (Fayetteville: University of Arkansas Press, 1983), p. 129; K. Scott Wong, "Cultural Defenders and Brokers: Chinese Responses to the Anti-Chinese Movement," in *Claiming America: Constructing Chinese American Identities during the Exclusion Era,* ed. K. Scott Wong and Sucheng Chan (Philadelphia: Temple University Press, 1998), pp. 3–41.

59. Two telegrams to Kinyoun from Wyman, both dated May 19, 1900, in RG 90, Box 29, Vol. 1, NASB.

60. "A Notice Given by the Wicked Health Officers," *Chung Sai Yat*

*Po,* May 21, 1900, cited in McClain, "Of Medicine, Race, and American Law," p. 474.

61. *Sacramento Record-Union,* May 22, 1900, cited in McClain, "Of Medicine, Race, and American Law," p. 474.

62. "Zhao and Shen's Case Is a Warning to Us," *Chung Sai Yat Po,* May 23, 1900, cited in McClain, "Of Medicine, Race, and American Law," p. 475.

63. Letter to Kinyoun from Wyman, May 23, 1900, in RG 90, Box 29, Vols. 1 and 2, NASB.

64. McClain, *In Search of Equality,* pp. 277–83.

65. For a more detailed discussion of the Wong Wai case and Morrow's decision, see McClain, *In Search of Equality,* pp. 475, 482; *Wong Wai v. Williamson,* 103 U.S. 4–9 (1900), cited in McClain, "Of Medicine, Race, and American Law," pp. 480–81.

66. "Plague Fake Put Through," *San Francisco Chronicle,* May 30, 1900.

67. *Sacramento Record-Union* cited in McClain, "Of Medicine, Race, and American Law," p. 487.

68. The Board of Health's appropriations had already been depleted, and private funds were necessary to tide the agency over until the beginning of the new fiscal year on July 1. "San Francisco Merchants in Mass-Meeting Aid the Health Board in Quarantine," *San Francisco Examiner,* June 2, 1900.

69. "Providing for Wants of a Quarantined Chinese Confided to a Committee of Leading Citizens" and "The Chinese in Quarantine," *San Francisco Examiner,* June 3, 1900.

70. Erica Y. Z. Pan, *The Impact of the 1906 Earthquake on San Francisco's Chinatown* (New York: Peter Lang, 1995).

71. "Chinese Wreck Mongol Morgue," *San Francisco Examiner,* June 12, 1900.

72. Ibid.; "Chinese Looting Shops and Rooms," *San Francisco Examiner,* June 13, 1900.

73. "Suspicious Mongols Mob an Inoffensive Watchman," *San Francisco Examiner,* June 3, 1900.

74. "Chinese Wreck Mongol Morgue."

75. "Merchants Provide Funds," *San Francisco Examiner,* June 8, 1900; "Quarantined Mongolians Grow Rabid," *San Francisco Examiner,* June 11, 1900; "Chinese Wreck Mongol Morgue."

76. "Chinese Looting Shops and Rooms."

77. "Quarantined Mongolians Grow Rabid."

78. The *San Francisco Examiner* stated, "Female practitioners were mentioned as especially objectionable," but no explanation was given. See also "Chinese Wreck Mongol Morgue."

79. "Board of Health Awaits Decision of the Court, Chinese Mob Merchant Who Was Inoculated," *San Francisco Examiner,* June 7, 1900.

80. "Quarantined Mongolians Grow Rabid."

81. "Released the Cook," *San Francisco Examiner,* June 13, 1900.

82. *Jew Ho v. Williamson* Case File, Answer to the Complainant's Bill of Complaint, pp. 14–16, 22, in RG 21, Series 6, Box 746, Folder 12940, NASB;

"State Executive's Findings," June 13, 1900, in RG 21, Series 6, Box 746, Folder 12940, NASB. For a more detailed summary of the case, oral arguments, and decision, see McClain, "Of Medicine, Race, and American Law," pp. 496–504.

83. *Jew Ho v. Williamson,* 103 U.S. 17–24 (1900); *San Francisco Examiner,* June 16, 1900, cited in McClain, "Of Medicine, Race, and American Law," pp. 502–3.

84. *Chung Sai Yat Po,* June 22, 1900, cited and cover reprinted in Kalisch, "The Black Death in Chinatown," p. 125.

85. Affidavits of Dr. B. C. Atterbury, Dr. Minnie Power, Dr. John Stephen, and Dr. Ernst S. Pillsbury in *Jew Ho v. Williamson* Case File, in RG 21, Series 6, Box 746, Folder 12940, NASB.

86. Risse, "A Long Pull, a Strong Pull, and All Together," pp. 263–64.

87. Arnold, *Colonizing the Body,* p. 211.

88. The commission consisted of three eminent biological scientists and educators: Professors Simon Flexner of the University of Pennsylvania, F. G. Novy of the University of Michigan, and Lwellys Barker of the University of Chicago.

89. A few months later, Kinyoun resigned from the PHS. "The Plague Situation," *OMT* 15 (March 1901): 135; Philip A. Kalisch, "The Black Death in Chinatown: Plague and Politics in San Francisco, 1900–1904," *Arizona and the West* 14 (1972): 128–30.

90. Telegram to Wyman from Joseph D. Sayers, March 21, 1901; Telegram to M. J. White from Wyman, March 21, 1901; Telegram to Wyman from M. J. White, San Francisco, April 2, 1901; Letter to Mr. Chew Wo, Secretary, Chinese Six Companies, San Francisco, from M. J. White, April 4, 1901; Letters to Wyman from M. J. White, April 10 and 30, 1901. All of the preceding are in RG 90, Box 550, NA.

91. Letter to Wyman, Washington, D.C., from M. J. White, San Francisco, September 14, 1901, RG 90, Box 550, NA; Kalisch, "Black Death in Chinatown," pp. 132–34.

92. Letter to Wyman from A. H. Glennan, February 4, 1903, and "Resolutions of the Mercantile Joint Committee," both in RG 90, Box 551, NA; Confidential Letter to Wyman from Glennan, January 30, 1903, in RG 90, Box 541, NA; L. M. King, "The Record of the Merchants' Association in Regard to the Bubonic Plague in San Francisco," *Merchants' Association Review* 7, no. 79 (March 1903), in RG 90, Box 541, NA. For background on these organizations and their interests in municipal government, see Issel and Cherny, *San Francisco, 1865–1932;* McDonald, *Parameters of Urban Fiscal Policy,* pp. 222–31.

93. Telegram (copy) to Wyman, Washington, D.C., from Glennan, San Francisco, February 3, 1903; Letter (copy) to Glennan from Yee Fun, Secretary, CCBA, February 7, 1903; Letter (copy) to the San Francisco Board of Health from Frank J. Symmes, Joint Mercantile Committee, March 16, 1903. All of the preceding are in RG 90, Box 551, NA. Rupert Blue made monthly statements regarding inspection of the "Chinese and Japanese District," in RG 90, Box 541, NA; Furman, *A Profile of the United States Public Health Service, 1798–1948,* p. 253.

94. Four registration books kept by Inspector James R. Dunn, who had jurisdiction over Jackson Street and vicinity, have been deposited in the Holt-Atherton Collection, University of the Pacific, Stockton, California; see Ms. 130, San Francisco Chinatown Residential Inspection Records, ca. 1904, in this collection.

95. Letter to Wyman, Washington, D.C., from Rupert Blue, San Francisco, June 8, 1903; Letter to Wyman, Washington, D.C., from Blue, San Francisco, October 3, 1903. Both letters are in RG 90, Box 541, NA.

96. Lucy E. Sayler, *Laws Harsh as Tigers: Chinese Immigrants and the Shaping of Modern Immigration Law* (Chapel Hill: University of North Carolina Press, 1994); Mae Ngai, "Illegal Aliens and Alien Citizens: United States Immigration Policy and Racial Formation, 1924–1945" (Ph.D. diss., Columbia University, 1998).

97. Letters to the Health Officers of Oakland, Berkeley, Alameda, Sacramento, Davisville, Stockton, Fresno, Bakersfield, Watsonville, San Jose, and Los Angeles from M. Gardner (Representative of the State Board of Health), A. P. O'Brien (Health Officer, San Francisco), and Glennan, ca. February 1903; Letter (copy) to Union Pacific Railroad from J. N. Hall, Colorado State Board of Health, Denver, January 4, 1903; Letters to Wyman from Glennan, November 23, November 30, December 8, December 27, 1902, and February 23, 1903. All of the preceding are located in RG 90, Box 551, NA. Confidential Letter to Wyman from Glennan, January 30, 1903, in RG 90, Box 541, NA.

98. Memorandum prepared by Dr. D. M. Currie under the direction of Glennan, ca. January 1903, in RG 90, Box 551, NA; Letters to Wyman from Blue, September 25 and October 14, 1901, in RG 90, Box 541, NA; Letter to Wyman from White, October 29, 1902, in RG 90, Box 549, NA.

99. Letters to Wyman from Blue, July 23, August 17, and October 3, 1903, in RG 90, Box 541, NA.

100. Letters to Wyman from Blue, February 10 and 23, 1904; Minutes of the Meeting, April 30, 1904; Letters to Wyman from Blue, March 2, March 18, and October 8, 1904; Letters to Wyman from Blue, April 4 and August 18, 1904; Public Health Commission of California, Minutes of Meetings, April 15 and 30, 1904. All of the preceding are in RG 90, Box 542, NA.

101. Letters to Wyman from Blue, March 10 and 18, 1904, in RG 90, Box 542, NA; "Plague in San Francisco, 1903–04," in RG 90, Box 542, NA; Dr. William C. Hassler, "Methods Employed in the Eradicating of an Infectious Disease in the Chinese Quarter of San Francisco," *California State Journal of Medicine* 3, no. 12 (December 1905): 389–91.

102. Deverell, "Plague in Los Angeles: Ethnicity and Typicality," pp. 172–200.

103. Young, *San Francisco,* 2:937.

104. "Chinatown Purified," *Pacific Medical Journal* 49, nos. 5–6 (May-June 1906): 271; "The Purification of San Francisco," *Blackwood's Edinburgh Magazine* (New York) (June 1906): 832–43.

105. John Francis Dyer, "Rebuilding Chinatown," *World Today* 8 (May 1906): 553–54; Charles Keeler, "Municipal Art in American Cities: San

Francisco," *Craftsman* 8 (August 1905): 597; *San Francisco Chronicle*, May 3, 10, 11, 14, and 17 and June 16, 1906; Judd Kahn, *Imperial San Francisco: Politics and Planning in an American City, 1897–1906* (Lincoln: University of Nebraska Press, 1979), pp. 202–5; Pan, *The Impact of the 1906 Earthquake*, p. 72.

106. *San Francisco Chronicle*, May 15, 1906; Kahn, *Imperial San Francisco*; Pan, *The Impact of the 1906 Earthquake*, pp. 90–94.

107. "Sub-Committee on Building Laws and General Architecture and Engineering Plans of the Committee of Forty," *San Francisco Examiner*, May 21, 1906; "Bubonic Plague in San Francisco," *Pacific Medical Journal* 50, no. 10 (October 1907): 609.

108. *Chung Sai Yat Po*, October 16, 1906; *San Francisco Bulletin*, October 17, 1906; *Journal of Progress*, October 20, 1906; "Chinatown," *Heritage Newsletter* 14, no. 1 (April 1986): 1–4; Christopher Lee Yip, "San Francisco's Chinatown: An Architectural and Urban History" (Ph.D. diss., University of California at Berkeley, 1985); Frank Morton Todd, *The Chamber of Commerce Handbook for San Francisco* (San Francisco: San Francisco Chamber of Commerce, 1914), pp. 66–67; Kahn, *Imperial San Francisco*, p. 205.

109. Alexander McLeod, *Pigtails and Gold Dust: A Panorama of Chinese Life in Early California* (Caldwell, Idaho: Caxton Printers, 1948), p. 8.

110. Excerpt from *Collier's Weekly*, October 10, 1908, cited in the *Proceedings of the Asiatic Exclusion League*, ca. October 1908, p. 323, in the Asiatic Exclusion League Papers, San Francisco Labor Archive and Research Center, San Francisco State University.

111. Augustin C. Keane, "San Francisco's Plague War," *American Monthly Review of Reviews* 38, no. 5 (November 1908): 562; "Bubonic Plague in San Francisco," p. 613.

112. "Bubonic Plague in San Francisco," pp. 608–12; Report, November 11, 1907, in RG 90, Box 543, NA; Letter to the Surgeon General from W. C. Hobdy, February 28, 1908, in RG 90, Box 5, Vol. 34, NASB.

113. "Plague Situation in San Francisco," *Pacific Medical Journal* 51, no. 2 (February 1908): 71–73; W. A. Briggs, "The Permanent Eradication of the Plague," *California State Journal of Medicine* 6, no. 2 (February 1908): 40–43; Dr. B. J. Lloyd, "The Rat and His Parasites: His Role in the Spread of Disease, with Special Reference to Bubonic Plague," *California State Journal of Medicine* 6, no. 1 (January 1908): 4–10; Dr. C. F. Buckley, "The Rat and the Flea," *Pacific Medical Journal* 51, no. 3 (March 1908): 159–64.

114. Frank Morton Todd, *Eradicating Plague from San Francisco: Report of the Citizens' Health Committee and an Account of Its Work* (San Francisco: Murdock and Company, 1909), p. 30.

115. Dorothy Porter, "'Enemies of the Race': Biologism, Environmentalism, and Public Health in Edwardian England," *Victorian Studies* 34, no. 2 (winter 1991): 158–71; Judith Waltzer Leavitt, "'Typhoid Mary' Strikes Back: Bacteriological Theory and Practice in Early Twentieth Century Public Health," *ISIS: International Review Devoted to the History of Science and Its Cultural Influence* 83, no. 4 (1992): pp. 608–29.

116. Walter Wyman, *Bubonic Plague,* Treasury Department Document No. 2165 (Washington, D.C.: Government Printing Office, 1900), p. 12.

117. "Bubonic Plague in San Francisco," p. 609; Dr. N. K. Foster, Secretary of the California State Board of Health, Diary, entry for November 9, 1907, p. 73, Thomas Muldrup Logan Papers, C-R 114, BL.

118. Todd, *Eradicating Plague from San Francisco,* p. 38.

119. *San Francisco Chronicle,* April 1, 1909; *San Francisco Examiner,* April 1, 1909; Furman, *A Profile of the United States Public Health Service, 1798–1948,* p. 255.

## CHAPTER 6. WHITE LABOR AND THE AMERICAN STANDARD OF LIVING

1. See SFBH, *Annual Report,* 1880–81, p. 6; and "Memorial on Chinatown by an Investigating Committee of the Anti-Chinese Council, WPC," in WPC, *Chinatown Declared a Nuisance!* p. 13. For analysis see chapters 1 and 2.

2. Dana Frank, *Buy American: The Untold Story of Economic Nationalism* (Boston: Beacon Press, 1999); Frank, *Purchasing Power: Consumer Organizing, Gender, and the Seattle Labor Movement, 1919–1929* (New York: Cambridge University Press, 1994); Lawrence B. Glickman, *A Living Wage: American Workers and the Making of Consumer Society* (Ithaca: Cornell University Press, 1997), pp. 36–38.

3. Saxton, *The Indispensable Enemy.*

4. *Daily Alta California,* September 14, November 2, and November 18, 1859; Ira B. Cross, *A History of the Labor Movement in California* (Berkeley and Los Angeles: University of California Press, 1935), pp. 78–79.

5. There are differences in the documentation of the origins of the union label. Many contemporary labor leaders and, subsequently, historians have identified its originators as the Chinese cigar makers of 1874, but Ira Cross and Jules Tygiel have traced the origins of the union label to the 1869 San Francisco Carpenters Trade Union. However, it was the San Francisco cigar makers and shoemakers who, in 1874, deployed the label as a "seal of white labor." Cross, *A History of the Labor Movement,* pp. 136–38; Tygiel, "Workingmen in San Francisco, 1880–1901" (Ph.D. diss., University of California at Los Angeles, 1977), p. 70.

6. *Cigar Maker's Official Journal* (October 1878): 1; Ernest Radcliffe Spedden, *The Trade Union Label* (Baltimore: Johns Hopkins Press, 1910), pp. 10–11. *The Trade Union Label* was originally a 1909 Ph.D. dissertation that Spedden wrote for a degree at Johns Hopkins University.

7. Roediger, *The Wages of Whiteness;* Saxton, *The Rise and Fall of the White Republic.*

8. William Woltz, "From the Pacific Coast," *Cigar Maker's Official Journal* (October 10, 1878), cited in Glickman, *A Living Wage,* p. 109, fn. 3.

9. As Sucheng Chan has detailed, the Chinese laborers who came to North America had bought their tickets on credit and were not contract workers. See S. Chan, *This Bittersweet Soil.*

10. Saxton, *The Indispensable Enemy.*

11. See chapter 3.

12. Constitutional Convention of California, *Debates and Proceedings of the Constitutional Convention of California,* 1:637–39. O'Donnell's rhetoric shifted often from the identification of a finite number of lepers among the Chinese population to the equation of all Chinese immigrants with lepers: "In Chinatown . . . there are 79,000 of those lepers living. I call them lepers because they are nothing else. . . . They live like hogs/and die like dogs" (p. 639).

13. Stallybrass and White, *The Politics and Poetics of Transgression;* W. Anderson, "Excremental Colonialism, Public Health, and the Poetics of Pollution," pp. 640–69; David Sibley, *Geographies of Exclusion* (London: Routledge, 1997).

14. "Memorial on Chinatown by an Investigating Committee of the Anti-Chinese Council, WPC," pp. 12–13.

15. Mosse, *Nationalism and Sexuality;* Bederman, *Manliness and Civilization;* Stoler, *Race and the Education of Desire.*

16. *San Francisco Bulletin,* March 24, 1880; Cross, *A History of the Labor Movement in California,* pp. 124–26.

17. Despite the most flamboyant anti-Chinese rhetoric of the city health officer, Dr. Meares, the Board of Health's powers had always been constrained to placing targeted, individual sanctions on buildings and persons. The more general campaign of Chinese expulsion advocated by the Workingmen's Party and implicit in the Board of Health's declaration necessitated extralegal action and official complicity. This strategic necessity was evident in the "driving out" campaigns conducted against Chinese in small towns and cities across the western states during this period. For a catalogue of the range of expulsions, see Sandmeyer, *The Anti-Chinese Movement;* S. Chan, *Asian Americans;* Takaki, *Strangers from a Different Shore.*

18. Neil Larry Shumsky, *The Evolution of Political Protest and the Workingmen's Party of California* (Columbus: Ohio State University Press, 1991); Tygiel, "Workingmen in San Francisco."

19. Saxton, *The Indispensable Enemy,* pp. 214–15; Dr. Tony Hyman, "'Look for the Union Label': A Guide to Union Labels for Collectors," *Antique Trader Weekly* (March 11, 1987): 68–71; Patricia A. Cooper, *Once a Cigarmaker: Men, Women, and Work Culture in American Cigar Factories, 1900–1919* (Urbana: University of Illinois Press, 1987), pp. 10–40.

20. *Cigar Maker's Official Journal* (October 1880): 7, cited in Spedden, *The Trade Union Label,* pp. 14–15.

21. See CMIU no. 228, "Protect Home Industry" certificate, 1887, in Certificate Collection, California Historical Society, San Francisco. These changes made the label adaptable to trade union struggles across the nation, such as the 1877 cigar makers' strike in New York against tenement house production. Boris, *Home to Work;* Cooper, *Once a Cigarmaker.*

22. Spedden, *The Trade Union Label,* pp. 19–22; Albert Choppé, *Le Label* (Paris: Giard, 1908), pp. 221–337.

23. "Chinese Exclusion," *Labor Clarion (LC* hereafter) 1, no. 1 (February 28,

1902): 6–9; "Mayor Schmitz on Chinese Exclusion," *LC* 1, no. 5 (March 28, 1902): 1.

24. "American Labor vs. Chinese Coolies," *LC* 1, no. 18 (June 28, 1902): 1, 9.

25. "A Union Label Talk," *LC* 1, no. 19 (July 4, 1902): 1; "How the Label Originated," *LC* 5, no. 45 (January 11, 1907): 15; "Evolution of the Union Label," *LC* 6, no. 16 (June 7, 1907): 10–11; John Graham Brooks, "Short History of the Label," *LC* 8, no. 5 (March 19, 1909): 3–4; "Origin of the Union Label," *LC* 9, no. 38 (November 4, 1910): 9.

26. Roediger, *The Wages of Whiteness*; Saxton, *The Rise and Fall of the White Republic*; Frank, *Buy American*.

27. "A Union Label Talk," *LC* 1, no. 19 (July 4, 1902): 1.

28. Brooks, "Short History of the Label," pp. 3–4; "The Cigarmakers 'Blue Label,'" *LC* 6, no. 35 (October 18, 1907): 7.

29. Although William Bonsor's explicit use of "white man's standard" was infrequent, "white" was implicit in the definition of "American," as it was continually contrasted with the "Asiatic" race as well as defined against black, Latino, and the southern and eastern European races within the United States. William T. Bonsor, "Dangers of Asiatic Competition," *LC* 13, no. 30 (September 4, 1914): 40.

30. American Federation of Labor, *Some Reasons for Chinese Exclusion*. Also published as U.S. Congress, Senate, 57th Cong., 1st sess., 1901–02, S. Doc. 137; and serialized in the *Labor Clarion*: "Meat vs. Rice—Part I," *LC* 7, no. 16 (June 5, 1908): 1, 6, 7; "Meat vs. Rice—Part II," *LC* 7, no. 17 (June 12, 1908): 1, 6, 7; "Meat vs. Rice—Part III," *LC* 7, no. 19 (June 26, 1908): 1, 6; and "Meat vs. Rice—Part IV," *LC* 7, no. 20 (July 3, 1908): 1, 6, 7. Finally, the Asiatic Exclusion League in San Francisco published an abridged and edited version titled *Meat vs. Rice* (San Francisco: Asiatic Exclusion League, 1908). For background information see Saxton, *The Indispensable Enemy*, pp. 270–73; Frank, *Buy American*.

31. Senator James G. Blaine, speech on February 14, 1879, to the U.S. Senate, cited in Samuel Gompers and Herman Gutstadt, "Meat vs. Rice—Part III," *LC* 7, no. 19 (June 26, 1908): 1, 6.

32. For more on the meanings and codes of masculinity for the nineteenth-century working class, see Ava Baron, "Gender and Labor History: Learning from the Past, Looking to the Future," in *Work Engendered: Toward a New History of American Labor*, ed. Ava Baron (Ithaca: Cornell University Press, 1991), pp. 1–46; Baron, "Questions of Gender: Deskilling and Demasculinzation in the U.S. Printing Industry, 1830–1915," *Gender and History* 1, no. 2 (summer 1989): 178–99; Keith McClelland, "Some Thoughts on Masculinity and the 'Respectable Artisan' in Britain, 1850–1880," *Gender and History* 1, no. 2 (summer 1989): 164–77.

33. Boris, *Home to Work*. For then-contemporary publicity of these movements, see "Union Label Prize Essays," *LC* 3, no. 20 (July 8, 1904): 2–3. Articles about sweatshops and industrial sanitary reform frequently appeared in the *Labor Clarion*; see, for example, Charles H. Leichtliter, "Horrors of the

Sweatshops," *LC* 5, no. 36 (November 9, 1906): 1, 8, 9; "Chicago Factory Inspector," *LC* 5, nos. 50–52 (February 15, 1907): 8; "The Sweatshop and the White Plague," *LC* 6, no. 17 (June 14, 1907): 7; "Industrial Hygiene and How to Secure It," *LC* 8, no. 46 (December 31, 1909): 3, 6, 7; "Expert Medical Opinion," *LC* 10, no. 6 (March 24, 1911): 3.

34. "The Broom-Making Industry," *LC* 1, no. 36 (October 31, 1902): 1. For further reporting and endorsements of white, union broom makers, see "The Union Label Broom Agitation," *LC* 1, no. 40 (November 28, 1902): 9.

35. "Progress of the Union Label," *LC* 3, no. 28 (September 2, 1904): 12.

36. "The Woman as Factor in Label Agitation," *LC* 7, no. 52 (February 12, 1909): 9. See also "Progress of the Union Label," *LC* 3, no. 28 (September 2, 1904): 12.

37. "The Woman as Factor in Label Agitation," p. 9. See also "Progress of the Union Label," p. 12.

38. Advertisement, *LC* 2, no. 13 (May 22, 1903): 7; "Cigar Makers Label Agitation," *LC* 3, no. 19 (July 3, 1903): 8; "High Praise for Union Cigars," *LC* 2, no. 45 (January 1, 1904): 11; "Label Counterfeiters Convicted," *LC* 2, no. 50 (February 5, 1904): 9.

39. "Union Label Sentences," *LC* 6, no. 32 (September 27, 1907): 7.

40. "Union Label a Safeguard," *LC* 6, no. 47 (January 10, 1908): 11. For other examples of advertising, see advertisement, *LC* 1, no. 25 (August 15, 1902): 13; advertisement, *LC* 2, no. 41 (December 4, 1903): 12–13; "Why You Should Wear Clothes with This Label," *LC* 11, no. 3 (March 1, 1912): 10.

41. "Union Label a Safeguard," p. 11; advertisement, *LC* 1, no. 25 (August 15, 1902): 13; advertisement, *LC* 2, no. 41 (December 4, 1903): 12–13.

42. "Why You Should Wear Clothes with This Label," p. 10.

43. The International Ladies Garment Workers Union (ILGWU), the San Francisco local, demanded the exclusion of Asians from the organization. A year later the union's governing constitution was amended to bar Chinese and Japanese locals. In 1902 an amendment passed to prohibit Asian membership altogether. *The International Ladies Garment Workers Union, 1900–1990,* exhibit catalog (San Francisco: San Francisco Labor Archive and Research Center, 1992), p. 11, San Francisco Labor Archive and Research Center, San Francisco State University; see also Jack Hardy, *The Clothing Workers: A Study of the Conditions and Struggles in the Needle Trades* (New York: International Publishers, 1935); Louis L. Lorwin [Louis Levine], *The Women's Garment Workers* (New York: B. W. Heubsch, 1924; reprint, New York: Arno and the New York Times, 1969); Benjamin Stolberg, *Tailor's Progress: The Story of a Famous Union and the Men Who Made It* (New York: Doubleday, Doran, and Company, 1944).

44. Daisy A. Houck, "United Garment Workers Union," *LC* 26, no. 31 (September 2, 1927): 37–39.

45. For an exploration of venereal disease scares, female prostitution, and political and police activity in the late nineteenth and early twentieth centuries, see Ruth Rosen, *The Lost Sisterhood: Prostitution in America, 1900–1918* (Baltimore: Johns Hopkins University Press, 1982); Barbara M. Hobson, *Uneasy*

*Virtue: The Politics of Prostitution and the American Reform Tradition* (New York: Basic Books, 1987); Timothy J. Gilfoyle, *City of Eros: New York City Prostitution and the Commercialization of Sex, 1790–1920* (New York: Norton, 1992); Mark Connelly, *The Response to Prostitution in the Progressive Era* (Chapel Hill: University of North Carolina Press, 1980); Elizabeth Fee, "Sin versus Science: Venereal Disease in Twentieth Century Baltimore," in *AIDS: The Burdens of History,* ed. Elizabeth Fee and Daniel M. Fox (Berkeley and Los Angeles: University of California Press, 1988); Pillors, "The Criminality of Prostitution in the United States."

46. Nancy Tomes, "The Private Side of Public Health: Sanitary Science, Domestic Hygiene, and the Germ Theory, 1870–1900," *Bulletin of the History of Medicine* 64 (1990): 509–39; Regina Morantz, "Making Women Modern: Middle-Class Women and Health Reform in Nineteenth-Century America," *Journal of Social History* 10 (1977): 490–507; S. Hoy, *Chasing Dirt.*

47. "Union Label Prize Essays," p. 1.

48. "Woman's Union Label League," *LC* 4, no. 11 (May 5, 1905): 11; "Women's Union Label League," *LC* 4, no. 22 (July 21, 1905): 6; "Women's Union Label League," *LC* 4, no. 23 (July 28, 1905): 5.

49. "Support of the Union Label," *LC* 4, no. 11 (May 5, 1905): 13.

50. "Woman's International Union Label League," *LC* 4, no. 50 (February 2, 1906): 11.

51. "Union Label Agitation," *LC* 4, no. 35 (October 20, 1905): 8.

52. "Union Label Calendar," *LC* 4, no. 39 (November 17, 1905): 8; "The Label Calendar," *LC* 7, no. 1 (February 21, 1908): 8; "Label Committee's Report," *LC* 7, no. 10 (April 24, 1908): 2–3; "Mailers' Union, No. 18, Issues Post Cards, Beautifully Illustrated, Bearing Label Doctrine," *LC* 8, no. 23 (July 23, 1909): 3; "The Label Show," *LC* 12, no. 12 (May 2, 1913): 13.

53. Dana Frank, "Gender, Consumer Organizing, and the Seattle Labor Movement, 1919–1929," in *Work Engendered: Toward a New History of American Labor,* ed. Ava Baron (Ithaca: Cornell University Press, 1991): 273–95; Frank, *Purchasing Power.*

54. For context see Lillian Ruth Matthews, *Women in Trade Unions in San Francisco* (Berkeley and Los Angeles: University of California Press, 1913).

55. "Educate, Interest the Women," *LC* 4, no. 2 (March 3, 1905): 10; "Woman's Responsibility: The Success of the Labor Movement Depends on Her Loyalty to the Cause," *LC* 5, no. 3 (March 6, 1906): 7; Annie Fitzgerald, "Women and the Union Label," *LC* 6, no. 36 (October 25, 1907): 7.

56. Glickman, *A Living Wage,* pp. 36–38.

57. Susan Englander, *Class Conflict and Coalition in the California Women's Suffrage Movement, 1907–1912* (Lewiston, N.Y.: Edwin Mellen Press, 1992).

58. Susan W. Fitzgerald, "Women in the Home," *LC* 8, no. 32 (September 24, 1909): 8; "The Home and the New Woman," *LC* 8, no. 37 (October 29, 1909): 10; "For Women in Union and Home," *LC* 10, no. 17 (June 2, 1911): 15; "Woman and the Ballot," *LC* 11, no. 7 (March 29, 1912): 3; "Humane Legislation League," *LC* 11, no. 9 (April 12, 1912); "Humane Legislation League,"

*LC* 11, no. 19 (June 21, 1912): 7; Alice Park, "What New Laws Do California Women Want?" *LC* 11, no. 29 (August 30, 1912): 44.

59. "Asiatic Exclusion League Notes," *LC* 9, no. 43 (December 9, 1910): 13; "Hookworm among Immigrants," *LC* 11, no. 19 (June 21, 1912): 3.

60. Earle William Gage, "Hindu Immigration," *LC* 6, no. 47 (January 10, 1908): 10–11; "Hookworm and Asiatic Exclusion," *LC* 9, no. 38 (November 11, 1910): 11; "Stop the Hindu Invasion," *LC* 9, no. 26 (August 12, 1910): 8; A. E. Yoell, "A Hindoo Question in California," *Proceedings of the Asiatic Exclusion League* (February 16, 1908): 174; Yoell, "Report on Hindus," *Proceedings of the Asiatic Exclusion League* (January 16, 1910): 491, in San Francisco Labor Archive and Research Center, San Francisco State University; Russell I. Wisler, "Why Japanese and Koreans Should Be Excluded," *LC* 4, no. 12 (May 12, 1905): 1, 8, 9; "Characteristics of Asiatics," *LC* 8, no. 28 (August 27, 1909): 8.

61. Naomi Rogers, "Germs with Legs: Flies, Disease, and the New Public Health," *Bulletin of the History of Medicine* 63, no. 4 (1989): 599–617; Tomes, "The Private Side of Public Health," pp. 409–539; Richard A. Meckel, *Save the Babies: American Public Health Reform and the Prevention of Infant Mortality, 1850–1920* (Baltimore: Johns Hopkins University Press, 1990).

62. "Steps in the Right Direction," *LC* 1, no. 18 (June 27, 1902): 8; "The Health Campaign," *LC* 6, no. 52 (February 14, 1908): 8; "The Right Man in the Right Place," *LC* 9, no. 25 (August 5, 1910): 9; "Activity of the State Board of Health," *LC* 9, no. 27 (August 19, 1910): 9; "Plan a Real Clean City," *LC* 9, no. 28 (August 26, 1910): 9; "Health Bulletin Discusses Vaccination," *LC* 9, no. 31 (September 16, 1910): 9; "The Work of Protecting Health," *LC* 9, no. 52 (September 23, 1910): 9; "Do Prisons Breed Crime and Disease?" *LC* 9, no. 46 (January 13, 1911): 7; "Vacation and Sanitation," *LC* 12, no. 12 (May 2, 1913): 7; "Wages War on Syphilis," *LC* 13, no. 31 (September 11, 1914): 13; "The Problem of a Clean City," *LC* 12, no. 33 (September 26, 1913): 7; "Disease and Poverty," *LC* 13, no. 42 (November 27, 1914): 13; "Vacations Bring Typhoid," *LC* 14, no. 24 (July 23, 1915): 7; "Poverty and Health," *LC* 15, no. 11 (April 21, 1916): 5; "Let's Stop Diphtheria," *LC* 15, no. 46 (December 22, 1916): 6; "The Wealthiest Most Healthy," *LC* 15, no. 47 (December 29, 1916): 11; "Influenza Prevalent," *LC* 17, no. 38 (October 25, 1918): 6; "The Plagues," *LC* 19, no. 47 (December 24, 1920): 14; "Skin Diseases," *LC* 19, no. 51 (January 21, 1921): 5; "Board of Health Answers Critics," *LC* 20, no. 7 (March 18, 1921): 11; "Man Made Diseases," *LC* 20, no. 12 (April 22, 1921); "The Red Plague," *LC* 20, no. 20 (June 17, 1921): 13; "Vaccination Is 2000 Years Old," *LC* 22, no. 9 (March 30, 1923): 4; "Mothers of San Francisco," *LC* 22, no. 14 (May 4, 1923): 13; "Can Leprosy Be Cured?" *LC* 23, no. 40 (October 31, 1924): 9; "Venereal Diseases," *LC* 24, no. 4 (February 27, 1925): 5; "Campaign for Hospital," *LC* 24, no. 8 (March 27, 1925): 4; "Ventilation," *LC* 26, no. 31 (September 2, 1927): 75–80.

63. "The Sanitarians of Labor," *LC* 11, no. 36 (October 18, 1912): 5; "Industrial Hygiene and How to Secure It," *LC* 8, no. 46 (December 31, 1909): 3, 6, 7; "Joseph H. O'Neill," *LC* 7, no. 16 (June 5, 1908): 8.

64. "The Menace of Manila Cigars," *LC* 8, no. 31 (September 17, 1909): 7.

65. See Angela Nugent, "Organizing Trade Unions to Combat Disease: The

Workers' Health Bureau, 1921–1928," *Labor History* 26 (summer 1985): 423–46; David Rosner and Gerald Markowitz, "Safety and Health as a Class Issue: The Worker's Health Bureau of America during the 1920s," in *Dying for Work,* ed. David Rosner and Gerald Markowitz (Bloomington: Indiana University Press, 1987), pp. 53–64.

## CHAPTER 7. MAKING MEDICAL BORDERS AT ANGEL ISLAND

1. A British medical officer, Dr. F. E. Freemantle, praised the U.S. system of monitoring disease as a model of "health-intelligence." Freemantle, *A Traveler's Study of Health and Empire,* pp. 315–30.

2. Kraut, *Silent Travelers;* Howard Markel, *Quarantine! East European Jewish Immigrants and the New York City Epidemics of 1892* (Baltimore: Johns Hopkins University Press, 1997).

3. Sucheng Chan, ed., *Entry Denied: Exclusion and the Chinese Community in America, 1882–1943* (Philadelphia: Temple University Press, 1994); Sayler, *Laws Harsh as Tigers;* Michael Hunt, "The Hierarchy of Race," *Ideology and U.S. Foreign Policy* (New Haven: Yale University Press, 1987), pp. 46–91; Lowe, *Immigrant Acts.*

4. More immigrants came through Ellis Island in New York in a single month than Angel Island in an entire year. Usually 750,000 "alien immigrants" were inspected annually at Ellis Island, while the numbers at Angel Island fluctuated from 10,000 to 60,000.

5. On how to think critically about the logic of science and the fixing of social difference, see Cindy Patton, *Inventing AIDS* (New York: Routledge, 1990), pp. 54–55; Nancy Leys Stepan and Sander L. Gilman, "Appropriating the Idioms of Science: Rejecting Scientific Racism," in *The "Racial" Economy of Science: Toward a Democratic Future,* ed. Sandra Harding (Bloomington: University of Indiana Press, 1993), pp. 170–93; Jennifer Terry and Jacqueline Urla, eds., *Deviant Bodies: Critical Perspectives on Difference in Science and Popular Culture* (Bloomington: University of Indiana Press, 1995).

6. Elizabeth Yew, "Medical Inspection of the Immigrant at Ellis Island, 1891–1924," *Bulletin of the New York Academy of Medicine* 56 (1980): 488–510; Amy Lauren Fairchild, "Science at the Borders: Immigrant Medical Inspection and the Defense of the Nation, 1891 to 1930" (Ph.D. diss., Columbia University, 1997), p. 14.

7. The community historians Him Mark Lai, Genny Lim, and Judy Yung, and the other participants in both the poetry project published as the book *Island: Poetry and History of Chinese Immigrants on Angel Island, 1910–1940,* ed. Him Mark Lai, Genny Lim, and Judy Yung (Seattle: University of Washington Press, 1980), and the Angel Island Oral History Project (AIOHP hereafter) have produced invaluable documentation of the Chinese American experience on Angel Island. I am especially grateful to Judy Yung for depositing the transcripts of the oral history interviews for public use at the Asian American Studies Library, University of California at Berkeley (AASL hereafter).

8. SFBH, *Annual Report, 1872–73*, pp. 12–13; C. M. Bates, "Health Officer's Report," 1869–70, p. 230.

9. Fairchild, "Science at the Borders," p. 8; Edward Morman, "Scientific Medicine Comes to Philadelphia: Public Health Transformed, 1854–1899" (Ph.D. diss., University of Pennsylvania, 1986); Kraut, *Silent Travelers.*

10. Michael Les Benedict, "Contagion and the Constitution: Quarantine Agitation from 1859 to 1866," *Journal of the History of Medicine and Allied Sciences* 25 (April 1970): 177–93; Margaret Humphreys, *Yellow Fever and the South* (New Brunswick: Rutgers University Press, 1992); Rosencrantz, *Public Health and the State;* E. P. Hutchinson, *Legislative History of American Immigration Policy, 1798–1965* (Philadelphia: University of Pennsylvania Press, 1981); "A Sensible View of State and National Quarantine Relations," *PMSJ* 23, no. 8 (August 1880): 114–15.

11. Mullan, *Plagues and Politics;* and "The Quarantine Station at San Francisco," *OMT* 3, no. 1 (January 1889): 34–36.

12. Federal law in 1891 put immigration under federal control and delineated the exclusion of certain classes of immigrants, including "idiots, insane persons, paupers, or persons likely to become a public charge, and persons suffering from a loathsome or a dangerous, contagious disease." Criteria for exclusion became more detailed and elaborate with successive laws passed in 1903, 1907, and 1917.

13. Letter to the San Francisco Board of Health from M. J. Rosenau, San Francisco Quarantine Station, Angel Island, May 2, 1896; Letter to the San Francisco Board of Health from William G. Stimpson, San Francisco Quarantine Station, Angel Island, December 18, 1896; Telegram (copy) to Surgeon General Wyman, Washington, D.C., from Stimpson, December 18, 1896; Letter to the San Francisco Board of Health from Stimpson, December 23, 1896. The preceding letters are found in RG 90, Box 665, Folder 16090, NA. Letter to the Medical Officer in Command, San Francisco Quarantine Station, Angel Island, from the Office of the Supervising Surgeon General, Washington, D.C., June 5, 1899, in RG 90, Box 15, Vol. 2, NASB.

14. Report of the Medical Officer in Command, San Francisco Quarantine Station, Angel Island, included in U.S. Marine Hospital Service, *Annual Report of the Supervising Surgeon General*, 1895–96, p. 548.

15. Letter to the Surgeon General, Washington, D.C., from Hugh Cummings, San Francisco Quarantine Station, Angel Island, December 29, 1904, in RG 90, Box 655, Folder 16090, NA.

16. Letter to the Surgeon General, Washington, D.C., from Cummings, San Francisco Quarantine Station, Angel Island, June 30, 1904, in RG 90, Box 1, Vol. 23, NASB; Letter to the Surgeon General, Washington, D.C., from F. E. Trotter, San Francisco Quarantine Station, Angel Island, August 3, 1909, in RG 90, Box 6, Vol. 38, NASB.

17. Letter to the Commissioner of Immigration, San Francisco, from M. W. Glover, Medical Officer in Command, May 5, 1910, copy in Department of Justice, "Investigation of the Immigration Service," San Francisco, 1910, pp. 584–85, in General Correspondence, RG 85, Box 184, File 53108/24, NA; U.S.

Marine Hospital Service, *Annual Report of the Surgeon General of the Public Health and Marine Hospital Service of the United States* (Washington, D.C.: General Printing Office, 1909–10), p. 172.

18. U.S. Marine Hospital Service, *Annual Report of the Surgeon General of the Public Health Service* (Washington, D.C.: General Printing Office, 1920–21), p. 232.

19. Letter to Medical Officer in Command, San Francisco Quarantine Station, Angel Island, from Wyman, Surgeon General, October 20, 1903, in RG 90, Box 17, Vol. 6, NASB.

20. Letter to Dr. William F. Snow, Secretary, California State Board of Health, Sacramento, from Trotter, San Francisco Quarantine Station, Angel Island, October 2, 1911, in RG 90, Box 7, Vol. 42, NASB; Letter to Assistant Surgeon R. H. Heterick, Quarantine Steamer *Argonaut,* Meiggs Wharf, San Francisco, from Trotter, in RG 90, Box 7, Vol. 43, NASB.

21. Yew, "Medical Inspection of the Immigrant at Ellis Island," pp. 488–510; Rosebud T. Solis-Cohen, "The Exclusion of Aliens from the United States for Physical Defects," *Bulletin of the History of Medicine* 21 (1947): 33–50.

22. The composite description of medical inspection was developed from PHS documents and interview testimony of several participants in the Angel Island Oral History Project, including Mr. Leung, interviewed in Chinese by Judy Yung and Him Mark Lai, San Francisco, December 28, 1975, Judy Yung Collection, Box 1, Folder 40, AIOHP, AASL; Mrs. Chew, interviewed in Chinese by Judy Yung, San Francisco, ca. 1977, Judy Yung Collection, Box 1, Folder 2, AIOHP, AASL; Mr. Lew, interviewed in Chinese by Judy Yung and Him Mark Lai, San Francisco, August 17, 1977, Judy Yung Collection, Box 1, Folder 29, AIOHP, AASL. See also W. C. Billings, "Oriental Immigration," *Journal of Heredity* 6 (1915): 467; U.S. Marine Hospital Service, *Annual Report of the Surgeon General of the Public Health Service* (Washington, D.C.: General Printing Office, 1921–22), p. 207. Report of the Medical Officer in Command, San Francisco Quarantine Station, Angel Island, included in U.S. Marine Hospital Service, *Annual Report of the Supervising Surgeon General,* 1895–96, p. 548.

23. Martin Pernick argues that early-twentieth-century public health and eugenics projects shared overlapping goals, programs, methods, and personnel, but advocated different solutions to ensure the overall fitness of the population. Martin Pernick, "Eugenics and Public Health in American History," *American Journal of Public Health* 87, no. 11 (November 1997), pp. 1767–72. For the history of physical examinations see Audrey B. Davis, "Life Insurance and the Physical Examination: A Chapter in the Rise of American Medical Technology," *Bulletin of the History of Medicine* 55 (1981), pp. 392–406; Stanley J. Reiser, "The Emergence of the Concept of Screening for Disease," *Millbank Memorial Fund Quarterly* 56:4 (1978), pp. 403–25.

24. Kraut, *Silent Travelers,* pp. 66–69. See also Fairchild, "Science at the Borders"; Alexandra Minn Stern, "Buildings, Boundaries, and Blood: Medicalization and Nation-Building on the U.S.–Mexico Border, 1910–1930," *Hispanic American Historical Review* 79, no. 1 (February 1999): 41–82.

25. Alan Kraut has argued that the unwillingness of the PHS officers to adjudicate final appeals by immigrants to the INS Board of Special Inquiry was in-

dicative of a general reluctance of PHS officers to "exceed their function as physicians making medical diagnoses and to involve themselves in the decision to debar particular immigrants." *Silent Travelers,* p. 69.

26. Letter to Trotter from Wyman, March 1, 1910, in RG 90, Box 20, Vol. 12, NASB; Letter to Wyman from Trotter, February 5, 1910, in RG 90, Box 6, Vol. 38, NASB; Letter to Trotter from T. M. Crawford, Chief Immigrant Inspector, Department of Commerce and Labor, Immigration Service, Angel Island, California, February 3, 1910, in RG 90, Box 6, Vol. 38, NASB.

27. The other was pulmonary tuberculosis. Among the category of "loathsome diseases" were favus, syphilis, gonorrhea, and leprosy. Other diseases enumerated were medical conditions such as hernia and varicose veins; the immigration authorities believed a sufferer of such a condition was "likely to be [a] public charge."

28. For statistical calculations and comparisons between immigration stations, see U.S. Marine Hospital Service, *Annual Report of the Supervising Surgeon General* (Washington, D.C.: Government Printing Office, 1891/92–1900/01), U.S. Marine Hospital Service, *Annual Report of the Surgeon General of the Public Health and Marine Hospital Service of the United States* (Washington, D.C.: Government Printing Office, 1901/02–1910/11), and U.S. Marine Hospital Service, *Annual Report of the Surgeon General of the Public Health Service* (Washington, D.C.: Government Printing Office, 1911/12–1923/24); U.S. Bureau of Immigration, *Annual Report of the Commissioner General of Immigration* (Washington, D.C.: Government Printing Office, 1899), 40; all cited in Kraut, *Silent Travelers,* pp. 66–67.

29. Letter to Cummings, San Francisco Quarantine Station, Angel Island, from W. J. Pettue, Assistant Surgeon General, April 23, 1903, in RG 90, Box 17, Vol. 5, NASB.

30. Letter to the Surgeon General from Glover, March 7, 1913, in RG 90, Box 8, Vol. B1, NASB.

31. Traiferro Clark and J. W. Schereschewsky, *Trachoma: Its Character and Effects,* Public Health Service Bulletin No. 19 (Washington, D.C.: Government Printing Office, 1910).

32. Letter to Trotter from Wyman, August 28, 1905, in RG 90, Box 18, Vol. 7, NASB.

33. Geiser advised PHS officers to distinguish between those individuals who have "fine" granules under their eyelids and those with "*thickening*" granules [italics in the original]. He recommended that "Orientals" suffering from fine granules should be permitted to land but those with thickening granules should be recommended for rejection. Geiser argued that "fine" granules were endemic. Under treatment this condition would disappear in "another race," but in "Orientals" it was "more or less permanent." Letter to the Surgeon General, Washington, D.C., from Victor G. Geiser, Chief Quarantine Officer in the Philippine Islands, Manila, April 21, 1905, in RG 90, Box 666, Folder 16090, NA.

34. Letter to the Surgeon General from Carl Remeus, Honolulu Quarantine Station, September 22, 1911, in RG 90, Box 269, Folder 3126, NA.

35. Stephen Jay Gould, *The Mismeasure of Man* (New York: W. W. Norton, 1981); J. S. Haller, *Outcasts from Evolution: Scientific Attitudes of Racial Infe-*

*riority, 1859–1900* (Urbana: University of Illinois Press, 1971); Stanton, *The Leopard's Spots;* Nancy Leys Stepan, *Idea of Race in Science: Great Britain 1880–1960* (Hampden, Conn.: Archon Books, 1982).

36. Letter to the Surgeon General from Remeus, Honolulu Quarantine Station, September 22, 1911; Letter to the Surgeon General from Glover, Immigration Service, Medical Division, Angel Island, June 26, 1911; Letter to the Surgeon General from Trotter, June 12, 1911. All three letters are in RG 90, Box 269, Folder 3126, NA.

37. Letter to the Surgeon General from Glover, March 7, 1913, in RG 90, Box 8, Vol. B1, NASB.

38. Letter to the Surgeon General, Washington, D.C., from L. E. Cofer, Assistant to the Surgeon General, Washington, D.C., October 27, 1909, in RG 90, Box 666, Folder 16090, NA.

39. Dr. M. W. Glover, *Annual Report, San Francisco, California, 1910– 1911 (Immigration Duty);* Glover, "Report of the Inspection of Aliens at San Francisco, California, for Fiscal Year Ending June 30, 1910." Both reports are in RG 90, Box 666, Folder 16090, NA.

40. McClain, "Of Medicine, Race, and American Law," pp. 447–513; Risse, "A Long Pull, a Strong Pull, and All Together," pp. 263–64.

41. Excerpt of the *California State Board of Health Special Bulletin,* cited in *Pang Hing v. White,* Petition for Writ of Certiorari to the U.S. Supreme Court, Jackson H. Ralson, Attorney, Brief in Support (1921), pp. 10–11, in BL.

42. Letter to the Surgeon General from Glover, Immigration Service, Medical Division, San Francisco, October 1, 1910, in RG 90, Box 666, Folder 16090, NA.

43. Priscilla Wald, "Cultures and Carriers," pp. 181–214; Judith Waltzer Leavitt, *Typhoid Mary: Captive to the Public's Health* (Boston: Beacon, 1996).

44. "Hookworm Infests Hindu Applicants: Dr. Glover's Discovery Will Raise Barrier against India's Natives," *San Francisco Bulletin,* September 29, 1910; "Uncle Sam to Stop Hindu Immigration: Hookworm Discovery at Angel Island Takes Alarming Aspect," *San Francisco Bulletin,* September 30, 1910.

45. William Osler, *Principles and Practices of Medicine,* 8th ed. (New York: D. Appleton, 1912), pp. 302–3, cited in Alan I. Marcus, "Physicians Open Up a Can of Worms: American Nationality and Hookworm in the United States, 1893–1909," *American Studies* 30, no. 2 (1989): 104.

46. U.S. Marine Hospital Service, *Annual Report of the Surgeon General of the Public Health and Marine Hospital Service of the United States* (Washington, D.C.: General Printing Office, 1907–08), pp. 52–54; J. W. Amesse, "America's Contribution to Tropical Medicine"; U.S. Marine Hospital Service, *Annual Report of the Surgeon General of the Public Health and Marine Hospital Service of the United States* (Washington, D.C.: General Printing Office, 1904–05), 264–68; Marcus, "Physicians Open Up a Can of Worms"; James H. Cassedy, "The 'Germ of Laziness' in the South, 1900–1915: Charles Wardell Stiles and the Progressive Paradox," *Bulletin of the History of Medicine* 45 (1971): 159– 69; Mary Boccaccio, "Ground Itch and Dew Poison: The Rockefeller Sanitary Commission, 1910–1914," *Journal of the History of Medicine and Allied Sciences* 27 (1972): 30–53; John Ettling, *The Germ of Laziness: Rockefeller Phil-*

*anthropy and Public Health in the New South* (Cambridge: Harvard University Press, 1981).

47. "Hookworm Infests Hindu Applicants."

48. The designation was less an explicit confusion about their religious identity and more a reference to their "national" origin—Hindustani.

49. "The 'Filth of Asia,'" *White Man* 1, no. 2 (August 1910).

50. "Asiatic Exclusion League Notes," *LC* 9, no. 43 (December 9, 1910): 13; "Hookworm among Immigrants."

51. Earle William Gage, "Hindu Immigration," *LC* 6, no. 47 (January 10, 1908): 10–11; "Hookworm and Asiatic Exclusion," *LC* 9, no. 38 (November 11, 1910): 11; "Stop the Hindu Invasion," *LC* 9, no. 26 (August 12, 1910): 8; Yoell, "A Hindoo Question in California"; Yoell, "Report on Hindus," pp. 174, 491, in San Francisco Labor Archive and Research Center, San Francisco State University; Russell I. Wisler, "Why Japanese and Koreans Should Be Excluded," *LC* 4, no. 12 (May 12, 1905): 1, 8, 9; "Characteristics of Asiatics," *LC* 8, no. 28 (August 27, 1909): 8.

52. Department of Justice, Investigation of the Immigration Service, San Francisco, 1910, General Correspondence, RG 85, Box 184, File 53108/24, NA.

53. When the S.S. *Asia* docked on October 1, 1910, with 111 Asian Indian men in steerage, Glover had the opportunity to order full-scale bacteriological examinations. The exams took more than a week to complete. "Uncle Sam to Stop Hindu Immigration"; Letter to the Surgeon General from Glover, San Francisco, October 1, 1910; Letter to the Surgeon General from Glover, October 14, 1910. All are located in RG 90, Box 666, Folder 16090, NA.

54. Glover, *Annual Report, San Francisco, California, 1910–1911 (Immigration Duty).*

55. Letter to the Surgeon General from Glover, October 14, 1910, in RG 90, Box 666, Folder 16090, NA; Glover, *Annual Report, San Francisco, California, 1910–1911 (Immigration Duty).*

56. Letter to the Surgeon General from Glover, Immigration Service, Medical Division, San Francisco, October 1, 1910, in RG 90, Box 666, Folder 16090, NA.

57. Tropical medicine as a field developed in the United States with the establishment of an American empire that included the newly colonized territories of the Philippines, Guam, and Puerto Rico. The experiments with tropical medicine also literally connected the U.S. South and Southwest and the monitoring of U.S. borders with the imperial possessions in the Caribbean and the Pacific. Amesse, "America's Contribution to Tropical Medicine," pp. 264–68; Warwick Anderson, "Race, Disease, and Tropical Medicine," *Bulletin of the History of Medicine* 70 (1996): 94–118; Kelvin Santiago-Valles, "On the Historical Links between Coloniality and the Violent Production of the Native Body and the Manufacture of Pathology," *Centro* 7, no. 1 (1995): 108–18.

58. "Pointed Paragraphs," *Chinese Defender* 1, no. 3 (November 1910): 1.

59. U.S. Marine Hospital Service, *Annual Report of the Surgeon General of the Public Health Service* (Washington, D.C.: General Printing Office, 1913–14), pp. 220–21; U.S. Marine Hospital Service, *Annual Report of the Surgeon General of the Public Health Service* (Washington, D.C.: General Printing Of-

fice, 1925–26), p. 183; Chew, interviewed in Chinese by Judy Yung. In the 1910–11 fiscal year report on medical inspection of aliens on Angel Island, Dr. Glover reported that 65.6 percent of "Hindus" examined were infected with uncinariasis, or hookworm; 54.1 percent of the Japanese examined were infected; 29.4 percent of the Chinese; and 12 percent of the whites. U.S. Marine Hospital Service, *Annual Report of the Surgeon General of the Public Health and Marine Hospital Service of the United States* (Washington, D.C.: General Printing Office, 1910–11), p. 142; Glover, *Annual Report, San Francisco, California, 1910–1911 (Immigration Duty)*; Glover, "Report of the Inspection of Aliens at San Francisco, California, for Fiscal Year Ending June 30, 1910"; Letter to the Surgeon General, Washington, D.C., from Billings, Immigration Service, Medical Division, Angel Island, May 1, 1912, in RG 90, Box 666, Folder 16090, NA; Letter to the Surgeon General from Billings, Immigration Service, Angel Island, June 17, 1912, in RG 90, Box 666, Folder 16090, NA.

60. *San Francisco Chronicle*, November 29, 1910, cited in "The Chinese Immigrant's New Bugaboo," *Chinese Defender* 1, no. 4 (December 1910): 7–8.

61. For the rise of and ambivalence about bacteriology and laboratory medical practice, see Fairchild, "Science at the Borders"; Warwick Anderson, "Immunities of Empire: Race, Disease, and the New Tropical Medicine," *Bulletin of the History of Medicine* 70 (1996): 94–118; Warwick Anderson, Myles Jackson, and Barbara Gutmann Rosencrantz, "Toward an Unnatural History of Immunology," *Journal of the History of Biology* 27 (1994): 575–94; Bruno Latour, *The Pasteurization of France*, trans. Alan Sheridan and John Law (Cambridge: Harvard University Press, 1988); Risse, "A Long Pull, a Strong Pull, and All Together."

62. Letter to Carroll Cook, Esquire, Attorney for CCBA, San Francisco, from F. H. Jarned, Acting Commissioner-General [Bureau of Immigration], December 3, 1910, Nos. 53059/61 and 53108/63, in Ng Poon Chew Collection, Box 3, Folder 10, AASL.

63. Sometimes a chloroform–castor oil mixture and sodium bicarbonate were used, in which case usually only one or two treatments were necessary for a cure. U.S. Marine Hospital Service, *Annual Report of the Surgeon General of the Public Health and Marine Hospital Service of the United States*, 1910–11, p. 209; Ettling, *Germ of Laziness*, p. 228, n. 12.

64. Mrs. Chin, interviewed in Chinese by Judy Yung, San Francisco, December 28, 1975, Judy Yung Collection, Box 1, Folder 1, AIOHP, AASL.

65. Poem number 48 in *Island: Poetry and History of Chinese Immigrants on Angel Island, 1910–1940*, ed. Him Mark Lai, Genny Lim, and Judy Yung (Seattle: University of Washington Press, 1980), p. 100.

66. Poem number 49 in *Island: Poetry and History of Chinese Immigrants on Angel Island, 1910–1940*, ed. Him Mark Lai, Genny Lim, and Judy Yung (Seattle: University of Washington Press, 1980), p. 163. Mr. Tong interviewed in Chinese by Him Mark Lai and Judy Yung, San Francisco, January 18, 1976, Judy Yung Collection, Box 1, Folder 22, AIOHP, AASL. This version also appeared in Lai et al., *Island*, p. 108. A similar story was related by Mr. Chan, interviewed in Chinese and English by Judy Yung, San Francisco, June 6, 1990, Judy Yung Collection, Box 1, Folder 25, AIOHP, AASL.

67. As Cindy Patton has recognized in her study of the role that this science knowledge has played in the conceptualization and treatment of AIDS, "promoting science-logic over complex folk-logics steeped in rich metaphors and mores of a community makes people dependent on the medical bureaucracy instead of pursuing their own strategies for social change." Patton, *Inventing AIDS*, pp. 54–55.

68. Bacteriological facilities were available at Ellis Island in the middle of the second decade of the twentieth century, but bacteriological exams were never routinely conducted on all arriving immigrants. Rather, bacteriological testing was conducted only after an individual's physical appearance prompted the inspector's suspicion. After 1915 there was a rapid increase in tests nationwide. Fairchild, "Science at the Borders."

69. Ibid., pp. 226–28.

70. In November 1910, the Chinese consulate general employed a local white physician, Dr. G. H. Richardson, who had clinical experience in the Philippines, and the CCBA invited Dr. Herbert Gunn, associate professor of tropical medicine at San Francisco Polyclinic and Post Graduate Medical School. *San Francisco Chronicle*, November 29, 1910; Letter to Yee Ling, Secretary, Chinese Six Companies, San Francisco, from Richardson, Imperial Chinese Consulate General, San Francisco, November 26, 1910, Ng Poon Chew Collection, Box 3, Folder 10, AASL.

71. *San Francisco Chronicle*, November 29, 1910, cited in "The Chinese Immigrant's New Bugaboo," pp. 7–8.

72. Stallybrass and White, *The Politics and Poetics of Transgression*; W. Anderson, "Excremental Colonialism, Public Health, and the Poetics of Pollution," pp. 640–69.

73. Nesbitt's comments submitted to the *Congressional Record* on February 19, 1914, were reprinted in the *Labor Clarion*: "Oriental Dangers, " *LC* 13, no. 26 (August 7, 1914): 6. See also William T. Bonsor, "Dangers of Asiatic Immigration," *LC* 13, no. 30 (September 4, 1914): 40–41.

74. U.S. Marine Hospital Service, *Annual Report of the Surgeon General of the Public Health and Marine Hospital Service of the United States*, 1907–08, pp. 52–54; Amesse, "America's Contribution to Tropical Medicine," 264–68.

75. *Pang Hing v. White*, Petition for Writ of Certiorari to the U.S. Supreme Court, pp. 10–12.

76. *Hee Fuk Yuen v. White*, 273 U.S. 10 (1921); *Pang Hing v. White*, Petition for Writ of Certiorari to the U.S. Supreme Court, pp. 1–17.

77. *Pang Hing v. White*, Petition for Writ of Certiorari to the U.S. Supreme Court, pp. 8, 10–12.

78. A San Francisco attorney, McGee, was hired by the CCBA to land fifty-three merchants who had been barred from entry by a clonorchiasis diagnosis. In a 1923 case, Chung Fook pleaded for his wife, Lee Shee, to be allowed to enter the United States despite her diagnosis of clonorchiasis. Although Chung Fook was a U.S. citizen by birth, he was not eligible for the same privileges as a naturalized male citizen, whose wife and minor children could be admitted without detention or treatment in a hospital. The courts ruled that the provision did not apply to a citizen's wife who, by her Chinese nationality, was ineligible for

naturalized citizenship. This case redoubled the jeopardy of Chinese Americans, who were already subject to the vagaries of Chinese exclusion law. *Chung Fook v. White,* 287 U.S. 533 (1923); *Chung Fook v. White,* Certiorari to the Circuit Court of Appeals for the Ninth Circuit, 264 U.S. 443 (1924).

79. Mr. Gintjee, a representative of the CCBA, secured the top floor of the Oriental Hotel on Stockton Street as a temporary hospital. John L. McNab presented the plan to Surgeon General Hugh Cummings, who was responsive, and who began to negotiate on issues such as PHS surgeons' participation and precautions for the disposal of excrement. Negotiations fell apart when the CCBA became embroiled in a legal dispute with another attorney over landing the fifty-three merchants who had been excluded from entry because of clonorchiasis. The litigation lasted five years, but in the interim five Chinese patients were successfully treated in Boston, demonstrating that the disease was curable. Wong Yu Fong, comp., *Historical Review of Clonorchiasis* (Berkeley: Fred A. Borland, [ca. 1928]): see especially Wong Yu Fong, "History of the Investigations on Clonorchiasis," pp. 16–17; John L. McNab, "Brief Report of Clonorchiasis Activities," pp. 13–15; Letter (copy) to Assistant Secretary E. J. Henning, Bureau of Immigration, and Cummings, Surgeon General, Bureau of Public Health Service, Washington, D.C., December 7, 1921, pp. 18–19; Letters (copies) to the Chinese Six Companies, San Francisco, from John L. McNab, September 14 and December 3, 1926, pp. 22–25.

80. His observations of the prevalence of clonorchiasis among Chinese immigrants relied on the findings of earlier surveys. As in the case of the classification of other parasite diseases, bacteriological investigations had been responsible for the identification of the liver fluke. In California, several areas of research contributed to the association of clonorchiasis with the Chinese population: the investigation of Dr. M. J. White of the PHS, who reported liver flukes found during autopsies of Chinese plague victims in 1900–02; Dr. Herbert Gunn's study of cloronochiasis as an Oriental disease; Dr. W. W. Cort's study of the health of Chinese in the San Joaquin Delta, sponsored by the California State Board of Health; and the records of the San Francisco Immigration Station. M. J. White, "The Anatomical Characters of Opisthorchis Sinensis and the Statistics of Its Occurrence in the United States," *Military Surgeon* (1906); Rupert Blue, "Prevention of Oriental Diseases" (address before the American Academy of Medicine, New York, 1915); Herbert Gunn, "Clonorchis Sinensis in Orientals Arriving in the United States," *Journal of the American Medical Association* 67, no. 25 (1916): 1935; W. W. Cort, "Oriental and Tropical Parasitic Diseases," Special Bulletin No. 28, California State Board of Health, May 1918.

81. Fong, comp., *Historical Review of Clonorchiasis:* see especially Wong Yu Fong, "History of the Investigations on Clonorchiasis," pp. 16–17; Letter (copy) to W. Y. Fong, Secretary, Chinese Six Companies, from Roger O'Donnell, Washington, D.C., November 3, 1927, p. 52; N. E. Wayson, "An Investigation to Determine Whether Clonorchiasis May Be Disseminated on the Pacific Slope," *American Journal of Tropical Medicine* 3, no. 6 (November 1923): 74–81; A. W. Mellon, Secretary of the Treasury, "Amendment No. 1 to the Public Health Service Regulations Governing the Medical Inspection of Aliens," October 24, 1927.

82. Kraut, *Silent Travelers*, pp. 65, 276.

83. Letters to W. Y. Fong from the Surgeon General, November 18 and 27, 1927, cited in Fong, comp., *Historical Review of Clonorchiasis*, pp. 62, 65.

84. Wong Yu Fong, comp., acknowledgments in *Historical Review of Clonorchiasis*, pp. 72–73.

85. "Imprisonment in the Wooden Building," *Chinese World* (March 16, 1910), reprinted in Him Mark Lai, Genny Lim, and Judy Yung, eds. *Island: Poetry and History of Chinese Immigrants on Angel Island, 1910–1940* (Seattle: University of Washington Press, 1980), pp. 139–40.

86. Letter to Supervising Architect, Washington, D.C., from Trotter, San Francisco Quarantine Station, Angel Island, March 31, 1910, in RG 90, Series 6, Box 39, NASB; Letter to the Surgeon General from Trotter, April 4, 1910, in RG 90, Series 6, Box 39, NASB; Estimate of Repairs for Fiscal 1913 by Glover, in RG 90, Series 8, Box 1, NASB; Letter to the Surgeon General from Glover, September 3, 1913, in RG 90, Series 8, Box 2, NASB; "Angel Island Quarantine Station, San Francisco," Jan 14, 1924, in RG 90, Series 12, Box 14, NASB.

87. Charles E. Rosenberg, "Disease and Social Order in America: Perceptions and Expectations," *Milbank Quarterly* 64, suppl. 1 (1986): 35; Charles E. Rosenberg, "Illness, Society, and History," in *Framing Disease: Studies in Cultural History,* ed. Charles E. Rosenberg and Janet Golden (New Brunswick: Rutgers University Press, 1992), pp. xiv–xv.

## CHAPTER 8. HEALTHY SPACES, HEALTHY CONDUCT

1. William C. Hassler, "Typhoid Fever Epidemic Occurring during the Summer of 1928," *American Journal of Public Health* 20, no. 2 (February 1930): 137–46; "A Triumph for Public Health" (editorial), *American Journal of Public Health* 23, no. 7 (July 1933): 704–5; W. H. Kellogg, "The Plague Situation," *American Journal of Public Health* 25, no. 3 (March 1935): 319–22; J. C. Geiger, "Poliomyelitis in San Francisco, 1948," *American Journal of Public Health* 39, no. 12 (December 1949): 1567–70.

2. Martin S. Pernick, "Eugenics and Public Health in American History," *American Journal of Public Health* 87, no. 11 (November 1997): 1767–72; Osborne, "Security and Vitality"; Poovey, *Making a Social Body;* Robert Crawford, "The Boundaries of the Self and the Unhealthy Other," pp. 1347–65.

3. Fung, "Burdens of Representation, Burdens of Responsibility," pp. 291–99; Ting, "Bachelor Society," pp. 271–79.

4. Aiwha Ong, "Cultural Citizenship as Subject Making: New Immigrants Negotiate Racial and Cultural Boundaries," *Current Anthropology* 37, no. 5 (December 1996): 737–62; Renato Rosaldo, "Cultural Citizenship," *Cultural Anthropology* 7 (1994); Kaplan, "Manifest Domesticity."

5. Gwendolyn Wright, *Building the Dream: A Social History of Housing in America* (Cambridge: MIT Press, 1981), p. xv; David Armstrong, "Public Health Spaces and the Fabrication of Identity," *Sociology* 27, no. 3 (August 1993): 393–410.

6. Linda Gordon, "Putting Children First: Women, Maternalism, and Wel-

fare in Twentieth Century America" (manuscript, University of Wisconsin at Madison, Institute for the Research of Poverty Discussion Papers, January 1993); Kathryn Kish Sklar, "The Historical Foundations of Women's Power in the Creation of the American Welfare State, 1830–1930," in *Mothers of a New World: Maternalist Politics and the Origins of Welfare States,* ed. Seth Koven and Sonya Michel (New York: Routledge, 1993), pp. 43–93; Gwendolyn Mink, "The Lady and the Tramp: Gender, Race, and the Origins of the American Welfare State," in *Women, the State, and Welfare,* ed. Linda Gordon (Madison: University of Wisconsin Press, 1990); Theda Skocpol, *Protecting Soldiers and Mothers: The Political Origins of Social Policy in the United States* (Cambridge: Harvard University Press, 1992).

7. Yung, *Unbound Feet;* Sucheng Chan, "The Exclusion of Chinese Women, 1870–1943," in *Entry Denied: Exclusion and the Chinese Community in America, 1882–1943,* ed. Sucheng Chan (Philadelphia: Temple University Press, 1991), pp. 94–146; Takaki, *Strangers from a Different Shore;* S. Chan, *Asian Americans,* pp. 104–7; Eliot Mears, *Resident Orientals on the American Pacific Coast,* p. 408.

8. Yung, *Unbound Feet,* p. 57; Nancy Cott, "Marriage and Women's Citizenship in the United States, 1830–1934," *American Historical Review* 103, no. 5 (December 1998): 1440–74; Mae Ngai, "The Architecture of Race in American Immigration Law: A Reexamination of the Immigration Act of 1924," *Journal of American History* 86, no. 1 (June 1999): 67–92.

9. California State Emergency Relief Administration, "Survey of Social Work Needs of the Chinese Population of San Francisco, California," 1935, pp. 6–8, in BL; Geiger, *The Health of the Chinese in an American City,* pp. 7–10.

10. Yung, *Unbound Feet,* pp. 77–79; S. Chan, "The Exclusion of Chinese Women," pp. 94–146.

11. Sanborn Fire Insurance Map for San Francisco, 1913; U.S. Bureau of the Census, *Thirteenth Census of the United States, Taken in the Year 1910,* Washington, D.C., 1910; *San Francisco Architectural Heritage Newsletter* 14, no. 1, Chinatown supplement (April 1986): 1–4; Yung, *Unbound Feet.*

12. *Chung Sai Yat Po,* July 10, November 2, and December 25, 1912, and August 5, 1913; Chen, "Being Chinese, Becoming Chinese American"; "The Chinese Community and the Chinese YMCA," *Bulletin, Chinese Branch of the YMCA of San Francisco* 1, no. 5 (September 1919): 3, in Donaldina Cameron Collection, San Francisco Theological Union, San Anselmo (SFTU hereafter); A. K. Wong, "A Sanitary Survey of San Francisco Chinatown," July 1930, typescript report, unpaginated, in Special Collections, Lane Medical Library, Stanford University.

13. "The Chinese Community and the Chinese YMCA," p. 3; A. K. Wong, "A Sanitary Survey of San Francisco Chinatown."

14. *Chung Sai Yat Po,* September 28, 1929; *Chinese Press,* January 30, 1941, cited in Yung, *Unbound Feet,* pp. 94–98, 273.

15. I borrow the term "monogamous morality" from Nancy Cott, comment on Nayan Shah, "Paradoxes of Inclusion and Exclusion in American Modernity: Formations of the Modern Self, Domicile, and Domesticity" (paper presented to the conference "Project to Internationalize the Study of American History,"

Joint Project of New York University and the Organization of American Historians, Villa La Pietra, Florence, Italy, July 4–7, 1999).

16. California State Emergency Relief Administration, *Survey of Social Work Needs of the Chinese Population of San Francisco, California*, pp. 3–4.

17. Ibid.; "Social Needs," *Chinese Digest* 1, no. 1 (November 15, 1935): 4; Yung, *Unbound Feet.*

18. Crawford, "The Boundaries of the Self and the Unhealthy Other"; Charles E. Rosenberg, *The Care of Strangers: The Rise of America's Hospital System* (New York: Basic Books, 1987).

19. Farquhar, *Knowing Practice;* Nathan Sivin, "Science and Medicine in Imperial China—the State of the Field," *Journal of Asian Studies* 47 (1988); Marta Hanson, "Inventing a Tradition in Chinese Medicine"; Sivin, "The History of Chinese Medicine," pp. 731–62.

20. *The Chinese Hospital of San Francisco,* pp. 1–3.

21. *Tung Wah* referred to the people of China's southeastern seaboard provinces and to the name of a famous hospital in Hong Kong.

22. A wide cross section of community groups mobilized to raise funds, including the CCBA, Chinese Chamber of Commerce, Chinese American Citizens Alliance, Chinese Christian Union, and Chinese YMCA. Dr. Collin P. Quock, *The Dawning* (San Francisco: Chinese Hospital Medical Staff Archives, 1978), pp. 1–2.

23. The construction plans received influential input from the national Hospital Betterment Services Committee of the League for the Conservation of Public Health. Quock, *The Dawning,* pp. 1–4; Invitation to the "Opening of the New Chinese Hospital," ca. April 1925, in Chinese Historical Society of San Francisco Collection, Box 3, Folder 11, AASL.

24. Among the hospital staff were Dr. James Hiquong Hall and Dr. Margaret Chung. Hall had graduated from Stanford Medical College in 1922 and Chung from the University of Southern California. Both had arrived in San Francisco to begin their practices, where they joined Dr. Joseph Lee, who had begun his practice in homeopathy soon after his graduation from the University of California in 1918. These physicians were joined by Dr. Rose Goong Wong, a 1924 graduate of the Women's Medical College in Pennsylvania, who specialized in obstetrics and gynecology and began her practice in San Francisco in 1927; Dr. D. K. Chang, a 1928 graduate of Stanford Medical School, who had immigrated to San Francisco from Hawaii in 1916 at the age of eighteen; Dr. Collin Dong, who graduated from Stanford in 1931 and shortly afterward began a practice in San Francisco; and Dr. Helen Tong Chinn, who graduated from Berkeley in 1933. Quock, *The Dawning;* Quock, comp., *Following the Dawn* (San Francisco: Chinese Hospital Medical Staff Archives, 1979); Judy Tzu-Chun Wu, "Mom Chung of the Fair-Haired Bastards: A Thematic Biography of Doctor Margaret Chung (1889–1959)" (Ph.D. diss., Stanford University, 1997).

25. Dr. Collin H. Dong, autobiographical statement, in Quock, *Following the Dawn,* pp. 32–40.

26. Dr. Helen Tong Chinn, autobiographical statement, in ibid., pp. 62–66.

27. Chinese patients also had other options available to them. By 1929 they could access a variety of charity clinics at more established hospitals, such as

Lane Medical Clinic, Telegraph Hill Health Center, Children's Hospital, and San Francisco City and County Hospital. D. K. Chang and H. D. Cheu, "A Sanitary Survey of San Francisco Chinatown," typescript report, June 1927, pp. 21–22; A. K. Wong, "A Sanitary Survey of San Francisco Chinatown."

28. Shehong Chen offers a detailed explanation of the 1925 legislative bill and the formation of the Association to Defend Chinese Medicine, based on articles in *Chinese World,* February 11, 1925, and March 25, 1925, cited in Chen, "Being Chinese, Becoming Chinese American," pp. 214–21; Haiming, "The Resilience of Ethnic Culture."

29. Chang and Cheu, "A Sanitary Survey of San Francisco Chinatown," p. 42.

30. "Functions in Public Health Nursing," *Public Health Nursing* (November 1936); *Know Your Public Health Nurse,* pamphlet; *The Influence of the Public Health Nurse with Allied Agencies,* pamphlet. All are located in California Nurses Association Papers, RG 4.1, Box 3, Public Health Nursing Folder, University of California at San Francisco Archives; Geiger, *Health of the Chinese in an American City,* p. 17; Chang and Cheu, "A Sanitary Survey of San Francisco Chinatown," pp. 40–42.

31. L. Gordon, "Putting Children First"; Sklar, "The Historical Foundations of Women's Power in the Creation of the American Welfare State," pp. 43–93; Mink, "The Lady and the Tramp"; Skocpol, *Protecting Soldiers and Mothers;* Anne Firor Scott, "Women's Voluntary Associations: From Charity to Reform," in *Lady Bountiful Revisited: Women, Philanthropy, and Power,* ed. Kathleen D. McCarthy (New Brunswick: Rutgers University Press, 1990), pp. 35–49.

32. Christmas letter of the Baby Hygiene Committee, December 1918; Letter to the Friends and Contributors of the Baby Hygiene Committee from Anne Van Winkle, ca. December 1920; "Chairman's Annual Report, May 1923–May 1924," Baby Hygiene Committee; Elise W. Graupner, 'The Infancy and Maternity Act as an Educational Factor," ca. 1927. All items are located in Baby Hygiene Committee Collection, Ms. 51, Box 4, Folder 34, California Historical Society, San Francisco (CHS hereafter).

33. Alisa Klaus, *Every Child a Lion: The Origins of the Infant Health Policy in the United States and France, 1890–1920* (Ithaca: Cornell University Press, 1993); Richard A. Meckel, *Save the Babies: American Public Health Reform and the Prevention of Infant Mortality, 1850–1929* (Baltimore: Johns Hopkins University Press, 1990); Molly Ladd-Taylor, *Mother Work: Women, Child Welfare, and the State, 1890–1930* (Urbana: University of Illinois Press, 1994).

34. Tadini Bacigalupi, "Report to the American Association of University Women Convention," April 1925, pp. 1–2; Mrs. A. E. Graupner, "Today's Babies Are Tomorrow's Citizens," Talk over Radio Station KYA, November 12, 1934, p. 6. Both items are in Baby Hygiene Committee Collection, Ms. 51, Box 4, Folder 34, CHS.

35. Alisa Klaus, "Depopulation and Race Suicide: Maternalism and Pronatalist Ideologies in France and the United States," in *Mothers of a New World: Maternalist Politics and the Origins of Welfare States,* ed. Seth Koven and Sonya Michel, 43–93 (New York: Routledge, 1993), pp. 188–212; Richard Meckel,

"Racialism and Infant Death: Late Nineteenth- and Early Twentieth-Century Socio-Medical Discourses on African American Infant Mortality," in *Migrants, Minorities, and Health: Historical and Contemporary Studies,* ed. Lara Marks and Michael Worboys (London: Routledge, 1997), pp. 70–92.

36. Graupner, "Today's Babies Are Tomorrow's Citizens."

37. Infant mortality rates fluctuated from year to year. For instance, the mortality rate in 1929 was 71 per 1,000 live births among the Chinese, compared to the citywide rate of 49 per 1,000; and in 1936 it was 84 per 1,000 live births among the Chinese, and 42 per 1,000 live births citywide. Geiger, *The Health of the Chinese in an American City,* p. 25.

38. Yung, *Unbound Feet,* pp. 97–98; Klaus, *Every Child a Lion,* pp. 144–54.

39. Annie Soo, "The Life and Career of Minnie Fong Lee," *Chinese America: History and Perspectives* (San Francisco) (1991): 67–74. Lee had graduated from the San Francisco School of Nursing in the mid-1920s; she later took public health courses at the University of California at Berkeley. She worked as a night nurse at the Chinese Hospital and took the public health nurse examination. Lee was disqualified because she was too short. Under political pressure from both Chinese community organizations and white medical professionals, the Public Health Department offered a special examination and created the category of Chinese visiting nurse to circumvent height restrictions.

40. Recreation Project, California, *Survey of San Francisco, California, by Districts (Recreation)* (San Francisco: Works Progress Administration, June 1937), p. 28; Geiger, *The Health of the Chinese in an American City,* pp. 16–17; Chang and Cheu, "A Sanitary Survey of San Francisco Chinatown," p. 42; H. T. Chinn, autobiographical statement, in Quock, comp., *Following the Dawn,* pp. 62–66; Dr. J. C. Geiger, *Child Welfare Centers* (San Francisco: San Francisco Department of Public Health, August 1935), in Baby Hygiene Committee Collection, Ms. 51, Box 11, Folder 101, CHS; Dorothy Walker, untitled article, unidentified newspaper, August 11, 1942, in Chinese Historical Society of San Francisco Collection, Box 3, Folder 111, AASL; Barbara Bedecarre, "Chinatown Goes to Yee Sung: Patients Ask Advice of the White Woman Doctor," unidentified San Francisco newspaper, July 1, 1948, in Chinese Historical Society of San Francisco Collection, Box 3, Folder 111, AASL; Ethel Lum, "Child Welfare Conferences," *Chinese Digest* 1, no. 7 (December 27, 1935): 10.

41. Letter to Health Officer from Eleanor Stockton, Director, Bureau of Field Nursing, Department of Public Health, April 5, 1927, in Baby Hygiene Committee Collection, Ms. 51, Box 2, Folder 19, CHS; "Report of the Chairman, 1927–1928," in Baby Hygiene Committee Collection, Ms. 51, Box 4, Folder 34, CHS; Bacigalupi, "Report to American Association of University Women Convention," p. 3; Sue Willard, R.N., "Post Natal Reports, 1933–34," in Baby Hygiene Committee Collection, Ms. 51, Box 4, Folder 36, CHS; Ethel Lum, "Chinese during the Depression," *Chinese Digest* 1, no. 2 (November 22, 1935): 10; Geiger, *The Health of the Chinese in an American City,* pp. 5–6; Recreation Project, *Survey of San Francisco, California, by Districts (Recreation),* pp. 19–20; Quock, *The Dawning,* pp. 7–8; San Francisco Department of Public Health, *A Study of Maternity Cases Cared for by the Division of Field*

*Nursing of the San Francisco Department of Public Health during the Period from 1931 to 1938* (San Francisco, 1939).

42. Thomas W. Chinn, *Bridging the Pacific: San Francisco's Chinatown and Its People* (San Francisco: Chinese Historical Society, 1989), pp. 35–36.

43. Bacigalupi, "Report to American Association of University Women Convention," p. 3; Mrs. Walker, Publicity for Community Chest, ca. 1927; in Baby Hygiene Committee Collection, Ms. 51, Box 4, Folder 39, CHS.

44. Geiger, *The Health of the Chinese in an American City,* p. 15.

45. Bacigalupi, "Report to American Association of University Women Convention," pp. 1–2; Graupner, "Today's Babies Are Tomorrow's Citizens," p. 6. For the national political and legislative context, see G. Rosen, *A History of Public Health,* pp. 351–64; Molly Ladd-Taylor, "'My Work Came Out of Agony and Grief': Mothers and the Making of the Sheppard-Towner Act," in *Mothers of a New World: Maternalist Politics and the Origins of Welfare States,* ed. Seth Koven and Sonya Michel (New York: Routledge, 1993), pp. 321–42.

46. Cruikshank, *The Will to Empower.* On the question of the social, see Denise Riley, *"Am I That Name?"* p. 49; Jacques Donzelot, *The Policing of Families* (New York: Pantheon, 1990); Paul Hirst, "The Genesis of the Social," *Politics and Power* 3 (1981): 67–82; Graham Burchell, "Liberal Government and the Techniques of the Self," in *Foucault and Political Reason: Liberalism, Neo-Liberalism, and Rationalities of Government,* ed. Andrew Barry, Thomas Osborne, and Nikolas Rose (Chicago: University of Chicago Press, 1996).

47. Geneva S. Orcutt, "Report of the State Board of Charities on the Babies' Aid," ca. January 1921, pp. 1–3, in Babies' Aid Records, Ms. 94, Box 1, Folder 2, CHS.

48. Grace M. King, Field Nurse, State Board of Charities and Corrections, "Presbyterian Chinese Mission Home," November and December 1919, p. 12, in Mrs. Rawlins Cadwallader Papers, SFTU; Letter to Edna Voss, Board of National Missions, New York, from Mabel Weed, California Department of Social Welfare, February 9, 1928, in RG 101, Social Welfare File, Presbyterian Office of History, Philadelphia (POH hereafter); Letter to Voss, New York from Donaldina Cameron, San Francisco, May 20, 1929, in RG 101, Chinese Baby Home File, POH; Letter to Voss, New York, from Lynn T. White, San Anselmo, California, January 16, 1930, in RG 101, Chinese Baby Home File, POH; Letters to Voss, New York, from Cameron, June 20 and August 18, 1930, in RG 101, Chinese Baby Home File, POH.

49. In 1925, Presbyterian missionaries opened the Ming Quong Home, a lavish facility for school-age girls, in Oakland, to replace the Tooker School for Chinese Girls, which had opened in 1915. Together with Chung Mei, an orphanage for Chinese boys established in Berkeley by the Baptist Home Mission in 1922, Ming Quong provided institutional residences for orphaned and destitute Chinese children aged five to eighteen. Grace M. King, Field Nurse, State Board of Charities and Corrections, "Study of Tooker School For Chinese Girls," November and December 1919, pp. 2–4, in Mrs. Rawlins Cadwallader Papers, SFTU; Pascoe, *Relations of Rescue,* p. 205; Charles R. Shepard, *The Story of Chung Mei, Being the Authentic History of the Chung Mei Home for*

*Chinese Boys up to Its Fifteenth Anniversary, October 1938* (Philadelphia: Judson Press, 1938).

50. Letter to Voss, Board of National Missions, New York, from Weed, California Department of Social Welfare, February 9, 1928, in RG 101, Social Welfare File, POH.

51. Ethel Lum, "Mei Lun Yuen," *Chinese Digest* 2, no. 3 (January 17, 1936): 12, 14; Letter to Voss, New York, from Cameron, San Francisco, May 20, 1929, and August 18, 1930, in RG 101, Chinese Baby Home File, POH; Letter to Cameron from William Hassler, Health Officer, June 2, 1931, in RG 101, Chinese Baby Home File, POH; Letter to Voss from Cameron, June 6, 1931, in RG 101, Chinese Baby Home File, POH; Letter to Courtenay H. Fenn, Presbyterian Church Board of Foreign Missions, New York, from Dr. Martha Tracy, Dean, Women's Medical College of Pennsylvania, Philadelphia, October 15, 1928, in Special Collections on Women in Medicine, Medical College of Pennsylvania Archives, Philadelphia; "Dr. Bessie Jeong Heads Baby Cottage," *920 Newsletter* 1, no. 5 (March 1935): 3; Donaldina Cameron Biographical File, POH.

52. Letter to Ray Smith, Community Chest, from Mrs. Henry L. Baer, President, Babies' Aid, January 4, 1935, in Babies' Aid Records, Ms. 94 Box 1, Folder 7, CHS.

53. Samuel Lee, the case supervisor of the Chinatown District for the California State Relief Administration, reported an average of eight Chinese children per month who needed the protection of the Mei Lun Yuen. Many of these children were vulnerable because of the hospitalization or death of their mothers and were eligible for assistance because of their fathers' full-time employment by the State Relief Administration. Letter to Smith, Community Chest, from Baer, President, Babies' Aid, January 4, 1935, in Babies' Aid Records, Ms. 94, Box 1, Folder 7, CHS; San Francisco Community Chest, "Report of the Research Committee of the Directing Committee Concerning the Mei Lun Yuen Chinese Baby Cottage," typescript, February 13, 1936, pp. 12–14, in Babies' Aid Records, Ms. 94, Box 1, Folder 8, CHS.

54. Letter to Smith, Community Chest, from Baer, President, Babies' Aid, January 4, 1935, in Babies' Aid Records, Ms. 94, Box 1, Folder 7, CHS; San Francisco Community Chest, "Report of the Research Committee of the Directing Committee Concerning the Mei Lun Yuen Chinese Baby Cottage," pp. 12–14.

55. Letter to Smith, Community Chest, from Baer, President, Babies' Aid, January 4, 1935, in Babies' Aid Records, Ms. 94, Box 1, Folder 7, CHS.

56. Lum, "Mei Lun Yuen," p. 14.

57. Presbyterian Mission Home, *Mei Lun Yuen*, pamphlet, ca. 1934, in Babies' Aid Records, Ms. 94, Box 1, Folder 8, CHS; San Francisco Community Chest, "Report of the Research Committee of the Directing Committee Concerning the Mei Lun Yuen Chinese Baby Cottage," pp. 1–5; Letter to Smith, Community Chest, from Baer, President, Babies' Aid, January 4, 1935, in Babies' Aid Records, Ms. 94, Box 1, Folder 7, CHS; Babies' Aid Minutes, May 1934 and September 27, 1934, in Babies' Aid Records, Ms. 94, Box 1, Folder 9, CHS; "Mei Lun Yuen Board Seeks Funds," *920 Newsletter* 1, no. 5 (March 1935): 3, in Donaldina Cameron Biographical File, POH; Letter to Daniel E.

Koshland, Chairman Executive Committee, Community Chest, from Baer, President, Babies' Aid, June 23, 1936, in Babies' Aid Records, Ms. 94, Box 1, Folder 7, CHS; Lum, "Mei Lun Yuen," pp. 12, 14.

58. San Francisco Community Chest, "Report of the Research Committee of the Directing Committee Concerning the Mei Lun Yuen Chinese Baby Cottage," pp. 3–4, 12–13, 19; "Dr. Bessie Jeong Heads Baby Cottage," p. 3; Letter to Smith, Community Chest, from Baer, President, Babies' Aid, January 4, 1935, in Babies' Aid Records, Ms. 94, Box 1, Folder 7, CHS.

59. In June 1935, Mrs. Morrison Hawkins, Babies' Aid president, publicly addressed fears of depreciating property values by claiming that the other cottages operated by Babies' Aid had improved their neighborhoods by replacing barren, "weed-grown fields" with a "lovely garden." By addressing "institutional" qualms, Hawkins publicly skirted the issue of race. She believed that the cottage's billing as "exclusively Oriental" had provoked these prejudices, and decided that Babies' Aid would, in the future, deflate that claim. Letter to Smith, Executive Director, Community Chest, from Miriam L. Feldelym, June 15, 1935; Letter to Hawkins, President, Babies' Aid, from Smith, July 16, 1935; Letter to Smith from Hawkins, June 16, 1935; Letter to Feldelym from Hawkins, July 27, 1935. All of the preceding letters are in Babies' Aid Records, Ms. 94, Box 1, Folder 7, CHS.

60. San Francisco Community Chest, "Report of the Research Committee of the Directing Committee Concerning the Mei Lun Yuen Chinese Baby Cottage," pp. 9, 13; Minutes of Babies' Aid, May 21, October 22, and November 19, 1936, and February 25, 1937, in Babies' Aid Records, Ms. 94, Box 1, Folder 9, CHS.

61. Letter to Baer from Geiger, Director of Public Health, November 18, 1938; Letter to Baer from Geneva S. Orcutt, Supervisor, Division of Boarding Homes and Institutions for Children and Aged, California State Department of Social Welfare, April 5, 1939; Letter to Board of Directors, Babies' Aid, from T. Y. Tang, President, Mei Lun Yuen, May 27, 1939. All the preceding letters are in Babies' Aid Records, Ms. 94, Box 1, Folder 7, CHS.

62. Letter to Miss A. D. Donaldson, California State Department of Social Welfare, from President, Babies' Aid, December 13, 1939, in Babies' Aid Records, Ms. 94, Box 1, Folder 7, CHS; "A Private Enterprise. Chinese Mother 'Adopts' Six Homeless Youngsters," *San Francisco News,* January 25, 1940, in Chinese Historical Society of San Francisco Collection, Box 3, Folder 93, AASL.

63. The CSERA staff was supervised by T. Y. Chen. They conducted public health surveys and collected health statistics in order to develop a needs assessment. The needs assessment was a social-work tool that could be effectively used in progressive grassroots community politics to make claims of "need" on public welfare administrations and enlist government and charitable intervention. California State Emergency Relief Administration, *Survey of Social Work Needs of the Chinese Population,* p. 1; Donald E. Johnson et al., eds., *Needs Assessment: Theory and Methods* (Ames: Iowa State University Press, 1987).

64. California State Emergency Relief Administration, *Survey of Social Work Needs of the Chinese Population,* p. 10.

65. Ibid., pp. 3–4; "Social Needs," *Chinese Digest* 1, no. 1 (November 15, 1935): 4.

66. "Social Needs," pp. 3, 11.

## CHAPTER 9. REFORMING CHINATOWN

1. Ivan Light, "From Vice District to Tourist Attraction: The Moral Career of American Chinatowns, 1880–1940," *Pacific Historical Review* 43, no. 3 (1974): 367–94; Chen, "Being Chinese, Becoming Chinese American"; Yip, "San Francisco's Chinatown"; Pan, *The Impact of the 1906 Earthquake on San Francisco's Chinatown;* Yung, *Unbound Feet.*

2. Geiger, *The Health of the Chinese in an American City,* p. 7; "The Health of the Chinese in San Francisco," *San Francisco Tuberculosis Association Bulletin* (April-May 1925): 2–3.

3. A. Ong, "Cultural Citizenship as Subject Making," pp. 737–62; Rosaldo, "Cultural Citizenship"; Turner, "Contemporary Problems in the Theory of Citizenship"; Warwick Anderson, "Leprosy and Citizenship," *Positions: East Asian Critique* 6, no. 3 (winter 1998): 707–30.

4. Yung, *Unbound Feet;* California State Emergency Relief Administration, *Survey of Social Work Needs of the Chinese Population;* California State Emergency Relief Administration, "A Study of the Prevalent Diseases among the Chinese," typescript, ca. 1935, in University of California at Berkeley, Institute of Government Studies Collection, C-R 131, BL; San Francisco Department of Public Health, "A Study of 2739 Cases of Tuberculosis Reported to the San Francisco Department of Public Health 1934, 1935, and 1936," October 1937, BL.

5. Barbara Bates, *Bargaining for Life: A Social History of Tuberculosis, 1876–1938* (Philadelphia: University of Pennsylvania Press, 1992); Sheila Rothman, *Living in the Shadow of Death: Tuberculosis and the Social Experience of Illness in American History* (New York: Basic Books, 1994); Barron H. Lerner, *Contagion and Confinement: Controlling Tuberculosis along Skid Row* (Baltimore: Johns Hopkins University Press, 1998).

6. Geiger, "The Health of the Chinese in an American City," pp. 6–7; Lim P. Lee, "White Plague: Chinatown's Poor Housing Is Breeder of Tuberculosis," *Chinese Press,* February 21, 1941; "Free Chest X-Rays Planned for November," *Chinese Press,* September 30, 1949; "YMCA to Bring Free TB X-Ray Test Unit," *Chinese Press,* September 9, 1949; "Free TB Tests," *Chinese Press,* October 21, 1949; "X-Rays Start Oct. 31," *Chinese Press,* October 28, 1949; "2600 Free X-Rays Made in S.F. Survey," *Chinese Press,* November 18, 1949.

7. "Why the Digest," *Chinese Digest* 1, no. 1 (November 15, 1935): 8; Thomas Chinn, *Bridging the Pacific.*

8. "Firetraps Must Go!" *Chinese Digest* 1, no. 1 (November 15, 1935): 8; Lim P. Lee, "San Francisco Chinatown's Social Problems," *Chinese Digest* 4, no. 1 (January 1938): 10.

9. "Why the Digest"; "Firetraps Must Go!" p. 8.

10. "Miscellaneous Accounts," ca. 1926, p. 2, in Survey of Race Relations

Collection (SRR hereafter), Box 26, Folder 149, Hoover Library (HL hereafter); Tony S. Woo, Interview, May 7, 1976; Clemen Lowe, Interview, December 5, 1976; Jane Lee, Interview, March 28, 1974. All of the preceding interviews are located in Combined Asian American Resources Oral History Project (CAAROHP hereafter), BL.

11. San Jose Realty Board, *The Oriental and Property Values in San Jose, a Problem in City Planning and Expansion* (San Jose: San Jose Realty Board, October 17, 1924), pp. 2–3, in SRR, Box 37, Folder B-407, HL.

12. Lola E. Brown, "Sketch of Mrs. K.," ca. 1926, in SRR, Box 35, Folder 77, HL; Jane Lee, Interview, March 28, 1974.

13. "More on Housing," *Chinese Digest* 3, no. 8 (August 1937): 8.

14. Robert Moor Fisher, *Twenty Years of Public Housing: Economic Aspects of the Federal Program* (New York: Harper, 1959), pp. 8–12, 92–125; Gail Radford, *Modern Housing for America: Policy Struggles in the New Deal Era* (Chicago: University of Chicago Press, 1997); Thomas J. Sugrue, *Origins of the Urban Crisis: Race and Inequality in Postwar Detroit* (Princeton: Princeton University Press, 1996); Robert B. Fairbanks, *Making Better Citizens: Housing Reform and Strategy in Cincinnati, 1890–1960* (Urbana: University of Illinois Press, 1988); Lim P. Lee, "Chinatown's Housing Problem Due for Airing," *Chinese Digest* 3, no. 6 (June 1937): 5.

15. Chinatown Crier, "Housing Program Coming," *Chinese Digest* 4, no. 11 (November 1938): 2.

16. The report was produced by the School for Social Studies, a local progressive adult education program, but the authors of the study are unknown. It is not clear whether they were affiliated with any Chinese American individuals or associations. School for Social Studies, *Living Conditions in Chinatown* (San Francisco: School for Social Studies, [ca. 1939]), in San Francisco Labor Archive and Research Center, San Francisco State University.

17. Eleanor Roosevelt, "My Day," *San Francisco News,* July 6, 1939.

18. "San Francisco Chinatown Living Conditions Held Worse Than Any in World," unidentified newspaper, July 7, 1939, in Chinese Historical Society of San Francisco Collection, Box 3, Folder 77, AASL.

19. "'Chinatown Is Squalid Slum' Comparable with Worst in the World," *San Francisco News,* July 6, 1939; "S.F. Chinatown Called Slum in Social Survey," *San Francisco Chronicle,* July 7, 1939.

20. Arthur Caylor, "Behind the News," *San Francisco News,* July 8, 1939; "'Chinatown Is Squalid Slum'"; School for Social Studies, *Living Conditions in Chinatown,* p. 11.

21. School for Social Studies, *Living Conditions in Chinatown,* pp. 11–12; Ruth M. W. Chue and Lena A. Way, "Comments on Housing Action in Chinatown" (term paper for Social Welfare 190, University of California at Berkeley, May 1940), in Catherine Bauer Wurster Papers, 74/163 C, Box 6, Folder "Calif.—SF—Chinatown," BL.

22. "Chinatown Fights Back at Charge It's Largely a Slum," *San Francisco News,* July 8, 1939.

23. "Housing Has Its Enemies; Where Are Its Friends?" (editorial), *People's Daily World,* July 11, 1939; School for Social Studies, *Living Conditions in*

*Chinatown*, p. 6. See also Chue and Way, "Comments on Housing Action in Chinatown," p. 5.

24. Bill Simons, "Districts: Chinese Junior C. of C. Praised," unidentified San Francisco newspaper, July 7, 1940, in Chinese Historical Society of San Francisco Collection, Box 3, Folder 93, AASL; "Chinatown Slums: Clearance Move Is On," *San Francisco Chronicle*, November 15, 1939.

25. "Chinatown Slums: Clearance Move Is On"; "Chinatown's Slum Attacked. Junior C of C Starts New Drive," *San Francisco News*, November 15, 1939. The link between congested housing and delinquency was first made in the 1930 Community Chest study "Social Work Needs of the Chinese People," cited in Chue and Way, "Comments on Housing Action in Chinatown," p. 9.

26. School for Social Studies, *Living Conditions in Chinatown*, pp. 2–3; San Francisco Housing Authority, *The 1939 Real Property Survey of San Francisco, California* (San Francisco, 1939), p. 9; Chue and Way, "Comments on Housing Action in Chinatown," p. 13.

27. Samuel D. Lee and William Hoy, "The Need for Better Housing in Chinatown," *Chinese Digest* 4, no. 12 (December 1938): 7, 19.

28. Sarah Ellis, "Social and Philanthropic Work among Orientals," in *Oriental Mission Work on the Pacific Coast of the United States of America: Addresses and Findings of Conferences in Los Angeles and San Francisco, California, October 13, 14, 15, 1920* (New York: Home Missions Council, 1920), p. 30, in RG 81, Box 1, "Oriental Work" Folder, POH; "The Health of the Chinese in San Francisco," *San Francisco Tuberculosis Association Bulletin* (April–May 1925): 1–2, in University of California at San Francisco Archives; "Annual Report of the Committee on Housing, 1937–1938," (April 1938), in League of Women Voters Collection, Ms. 1270, Series 4, Box 17, Folder 77B, CHS.

29. Works Progress Administration and San Francisco Housing Authority, *The 1939 Real Property Survey*, p. 35; School for Social Studies, *Living Conditions in Chinatown*, pp. 17–18.

30. "Chinatown's Slum: It's Called the World's Worst Housing Area," *San Francisco Chronicle*, November 26, 1939; "Chinatown Slums: Clearance Move Is On"; Circular Letter to Civic and Improvement Clubs of San Francisco from Arthur J. Dolan Jr., President, San Francisco Junior Chamber of Commerce, November 10, 1939, Chinese Historical Society of San Francisco Collection, Box 3, Folder 79, AASL; "Chinatown Housing: Which Shall It Be?" poster, ca. 1939, Chinese Historical Society of San Francisco Collection, Box 3, Folder 79, AASL; "'Oriental' Chinatown Due," *Chinese Digest* 2, no. 21 (May 22, 1936): 8; "Housing Project," *Chinese Digest* 4, no. 3 (March 1938): 3.

31. San Francisco Junior Chamber of Commerce, *Speakers Manual: Chinatown Housing Program* (San Francisco: San Francisco Junior Chamber of Commerce, October 20, 1939), in Chinese Historical Society of San Francisco Collection, Box 3, Folder 79, AASL; Circular Letter to Civic and Improvement Clubs of San Francisco from Dolan.

32. "Chinatown Housing: Which Shall It Be?" The information was drawn from San Francisco Junior Chamber of Commerce, "Report on San Francisco's Chinatown Housing," in Catherine Bauer Wurster Papers, Banc MSS 74/163 C, Box 6, Folder "Calif.—SF—Chinatown," BL.

33. California State Emergency Relief Administration, *Survey of Social Work Needs of the Chinese Population,* pp. 9–10.

34. "Aid Is Pledged on Chinatown Slums," *San Francisco Chronicle,* March 5, 1940; Circular Letter to Civic and Improvement Clubs of San Francisco from Dolan.

35. "8 S.F. Housing Projects Are Authorized," *San Francisco News,* December 14, 1939. Many civic groups responded favorably to the campaign. Letter to Nathan Straus, Administrator, United States Housing Authority, from Mrs. Charles B. Porter, President, San Francisco Center of the California League of Women Voters, November 30, 1939, in California League of Women Voters Collection, Ms. 1270, Series 4, Box 17, Folder 77B, CHS; San Francisco Public Welfare Council Minutes, p. 10, in San Francisco Public Welfare Council Collection, Ms. 1886, CHS.

36. Letter to Porter, President, San Francisco Center of the California League of Women Voters, from Winters Haydock, Director, Region VII, Pacific Coast Region, United States Housing Authority, December 22, 1939, in California League of Women Voters Collection, Ms. 1270, Series 4, Box 17, Folder 77B, CHS; "Chinatown Housing Plea Cites Tuberculosis," *San Francisco News,* February 29, 1940; "Rossi Doubts Legality," *San Francisco News,* February 15, 1940.

37. *Chinese Digest* 6, no. 1 (January 1940): 1.

38. Lim P. Lee, "Public Cost of Tuberculosis Care of Chinese in San Francisco" (talk before the Board of Supervisors, San Francisco, February 1940), cited in Chue and Way, "Comments on Housing Action in Chinatown," p. 6; "Chinatown Housing Plea Cites Tuberculosis"; San Francisco Housing Authority, *Annual Report,* April 18, 1940, p. 17, in Chinese Historical Society of San Francisco Collection, Box 3, Folder 79, AASL.

39. "San Francisco Housing Project Has Three-Way Appeal," *San Francisco Chronicle,* March 1, 1940; "Cheap at the Price," *San Francisco News,* March 1, 1940; "Chinatown Housing Plan. $75,000 Appropriation before Supervisors," *San Francisco News,* March 2, 1940.

40. "San Francisco's New Designs for Living: City Realizes Its Big Responsibility in Chinatown," *San Francisco News,* March 23, 1940; San Francisco Housing Association, *Holly Courts: Special Bulletin* (San Francisco, [ca. June 1940]), in Chinese Historical Society of San Francisco Collection, Box 3, Folder 79, AASL; "Chinatown Housing," *Woman's Home Companion* 68, no. 5 (May 1941): 2.

41. San Francisco Federation of Taxpayers, "Report of Low Cost Housing in San Francisco," March 6, 1941, p. 3, in American Civil Liberties Union, Northern California Collection (ACLU-NC hereafter), Ms. 3580, Folder 566, CHS.

42. Chue and Way, "Comments on Housing Action in Chinatown"; Letter to Eugene Block, Jewish Survey Committee of San Francisco, from Ernest Besig, Director, ACLU Northern California, January 16, 1942, in ACLU-NC, Ms. 3580, Series 2, Box 28, Folder 581, CHS; Letter to Mrs. Leon Sloss Jr., San Francisco Center, from Londa S. Fletcher, October 6, 1941, in League of Women Voters Collection, Ms. 1270, Series 4, Box 17, Folder 77B, CHS; San Francisco

Housing Authority, "Resolution Declaring Policy of Selection of Tenants Re: All Projects," in ACLU-NC, Ms. 3580, Series 2, Box 27, Folder 566, CHS.

43. "Racial Occupancy Patterns of Public Housing Projects," San Francisco Field Office, September 30, 1950, in Catherine Bauer Wurster Papers, Banc MSS 74/163 C, Box 25, Race Relations Folder #5, BL; *Digest of the Real Property Survey* (San Francisco: Works Progress Administration, 1941), in ACLU-NC, Ms. 3580, Series 2, Box 27, Folder 566, CHS; "Report of the Western Addition Housing Council," January 2, 1942, in ACLU-NC, Ms. 3580, Folder 581, CHS; Albert S. Broussard, *Black San Francisco: The Struggle for Racial Equality in the West, 1900–1954* (Lawrence: University of Kansas Press, 1993), pp. 176–77.

44. Thomas J. Sugrue, *The Origins of the Urban Crisis: Race and Inequality in Postwar Detroit* (Princeton: Princeton University Press, 1996), pp. 73–81; John Bauman, *Public Housing, Race, and Renewal: Urban Planning in Philadelphia, 1920–1974* (Philadelphia: Temple University Press, 1987); Dominic J. Capeci Jr., *Race Relations in Wartime Detroit: The Sojourner Truth Housing Controversy of 1942* (Philadelphia: Temple University Press, 1984); Arnold R. Hirsch, *Making the Second Ghetto: Race and Housing in Chicago, 1940–1960* (New York: Cambridge University Press, 1983).

45. Richard O. Davies, *Housing Reform during the Truman Administration* (Columbia: University of Missouri Press, 1966); Harry Press, "Chinatown to Get Low-Rent Housing Soon. Construction Will Be of Reinforced Concrete," *San Francisco News,* October 12, 1949.

46. "Evict Forty Families for Proposed Housing Project," *Chinese Press,* November 25, 1949; "Boom! Ping Yuen Site Demolition Underway," *Chinese Press,* December 9, 1949; "Chinatown Housing Plans Set; Legislation Pending," *Chinese Press,* May 27, 1949; "Housing Site Demolition Starts," *Chinese Press,* September 9, 1949; "Ping Yuen Authorities Reject Merchants' Request," *Chinese Press,* September 16, 1949; "Housing Ground-Breaking Nov. 1," *Chinese Press,* October 14, 1949.

47. Christopher Yip, "San Francisco's Chinatown: An Architectural and Urban History" (Ph.D. diss., University of California at Berkeley, 1985), pp. 312–16.

48. "Plans for Ping Yuen Housing Units Ready," *San Francisco Examiner,* July 1, 1949; "Real History of Ping Yuen," *Chinese Press,* October 19, 1951.

49. "Real History of Ping Yuen"; "The Strength of Dreams" (editorial), *Chinese Press,* October 19, 1951; "Ping Yuen Housing Is . . . Culmination of a Dream," *Chinese Press,* October 19, 1951.

50. Godfrey Lehman, "For Chinese Only," *Frontier: Voice of the New West for the Council for Civic Unity of San Francisco* (February 1952), in Charles Leong Collection, Box 5, Folder 22, AASL.

51. Letter to Langdon W. Post, USHA-Region VII, San Francisco, from Albert J. Evers, SFHA, San Francisco, January 6, 1942, in ACLU-NC, Ms. 3580, Folder 581, CHS; "The Jim Crow Issue in S.F. Public Housing," *Among These Rights: Newsletter of the Council for Civic Unity of San Francisco* (ca. 1950): 2, in ACLU-NC, Ms. 3580, Series 2, Box 27, Folder 581, CHS; Letter to John W. Beard, SFHA, from Selah Chamberlain, San Francisco Planning and Housing

Association, December 23, 1949, in League of Women Voters Collection, Ms. 1270, Series 4, Box 17, Folder 77B, CHS.

52. Letter to Mrs. Wong and Charles Leong from Edward Howden, Council for Civic Unity of San Francisco, ca. 1949, Charles Leong Collection, Box 4, Folder 2, AASL; "The Jim Crow Issue in S.F. Public Housing," p. 2.

53. *San Francisco News,* March 20, 1950, cited in Connie Young Yu, "A History of San Francisco Chinatown Housing," *Amerasia* 8, no. 1 (1981): 105.

54. "The Henry Wongs—Ping Yuen's First Family," *San Francisco Chronicle,* October 18, 1951.

55. "New Face for S.F. Chinatown" (editorial), *San Francisco Chronicle,* October 20, 1951.

56. "100,000 Firecrackers vs. Evil Spirits," *San Francisco Chronicle,* October 21, 1951; "Ping Yuen Apartment Show Date Extended," *Chinese Press,* October 26, 1951.

57. "Evict Forty Families for Proposed Housing Project"; "Boom! Ping Yuen Site Demolition Underway"; "Chinatown Housing Plans Set; Legislation Pending"; "Housing Site Demolition Starts."

58. Yu, "A History of San Francisco Chinatown Housing," pp. 106–9.

59. "'Great Wall' Crumbling," *San Francisco News,* October 24, 1950, in Chinese Historical Society of San Francisco Collection, Box 3, Folder 81, AASL.

60. Jane Lee, Interview, March 28, 1974, p. 2.

61. Letter to Mrs. James Lawry from Alfred Ghiradelli, November 19, 1946, in Cow Hollow Improvement Club Records, Ms. 3191, Box 1, Folder 3, CHS.

62. Letter to Besig from Dr. Rodney Beard, ca. April 19, 1944, in ACLU-NC, Ms. 3580, Series 2, Box 27, Folder 566, CHS.

63. "Judge Upholds Race Restriction on Nob Hill," *San Francisco Chronicle,* June 29, 1946; Ben Woo, Interview, December 2, 1976, in CAAROHP, BL.

64. Edward Howden, Council for Civic Unity, *Community Action Stops Restrictive Covenant Suit. Council for Civic Unity of San Francisco Heads Successful Fight in Portola Heights Covenant Case* (San Francisco: Council for Civic Unity, June 26, 1946), in ACLU-NC, Ms. 3580, Series 2, Box 27, Folder 566, CHS.

65. "Real Estate Racial Fight on Peninsula," *San Francisco Chronicle,* July 12, 1947.

66. Ngai Ho Hong, "White Peninsula," *San Francisco Chronicle,* July 21, 1947.

67. "Real Estate Racial Fight on Peninsula."

## CONCLUSION: NORMS AS A WAY OF LIFE

1. My thanks to Leora Auslander for this formulation, which is based on a conversation we had in October 1991.

2. In the 1960s, 1970s, and beyond, Chinese American activists would continue to struggle to bring the onerous conditions of Chinatown housing and health to public attention. Chinese American access to government resources and charitable assistance continued to be uneven and unequal, occasioning protests, needs assessments, and renewed pressure on elected officials. Omatsu,

"The 'Four Prisons' and the Movements of Liberation," pp. 19–70; Ling-chi Wang, "Politics of Assimilation and Repression: History of the Chinese in the United States, 1940 to 1970" (manuscript, Asian American Studies Library, University of California at Berkeley).

3. Loo, *Chinatown: Most Time, Hard Time*.

4. Lisa Lowe, "The International within the National: American Studies and Asian American Critique," *Cultural Critique* (fall 1998): 29–47; Daniel Rodgers, "Exceptionalism," in *Imagined Histories: American Historians Interpret the Past*, ed. Anthony Moho and Gordon S. Wood (Princeton: Princeton University Press, 1998), pp. 21–40; Amy Kaplan, "Left Alone with America: The Absence of Empire in the Study of American Culture," in *Cultures of U.S. Imperialism*, ed. Amy Kaplan and Donald E. Pease (Durham, N.C.: Duke University Press, 1993), pp. 3–22.

5. Glickman, *A Living Wage*; Frank, *Buy American*; Coontz, *The Way We Never Were*; Peffer, *If They Don't Bring Their Women*; Cruikshank, *The Will To Empower*; Martin V. Melosi, *The Sanitary City: Urban Infrastructure in America from Colonial Times to the Present* (Baltimore: Johns Hopkins University Press, 2000); Mink, *The Wages of Motherhood*.

6. Allan Berube, "Don't Save Us from Our Sexuality," *Coming Up!* (April 1984). A similar strategy using "nuisance" law was reintroduced in a bill under consideration in the California State Legislature in 1997. "'Nuisance Bill' Approaches First Committee Meeting," *S.F. Frontiers* 15, no. 25 (April 10, 1997).

7. Steven Epstein, *Impure Science: AIDS, Activism, and the Politics of Knowledge* (Berkeley and Los Angeles: University of California Press, 1996); Patton, *Inventing AIDS*; Paula A. Triechler, *How to Have Theory in an Epidemic: Cultural Chronicles of AIDS* (Durham, N.C.: Duke University Press, 1999); Jeffrey Weeks, *Making Sexual History* (London: Polity Press, 2000); Simon Watney, *Practices of Freedom: Selected Writings on HIV/AIDS* (Durham, N.C.: Duke University Press, 1994); Fee and Fox, eds., *AIDS*.

8. Weeks, *Invented Moralities*.

9. Nikolas Rose, "The Death of the Social? Re-figuring the Territory of Government," *Economy and Society* 25, no. 3 (August 1996): 327–56; A. Ong, "Cultural Citizenship as Subject Making."

10. Bonnie Honig, "Immigrant America? How Foreignness Solves Democracy's Problems," *Social Text*, no. 56 (fall 1998): 1–27.

# Bibliography

PRIMARY SOURCES

MANUSCRIPT MATERIALS

*Asian American Studies Library, University of California at Berkeley*

Chinese Historical Society of San Francisco Collection.
Leong, Charles, Collection.
Ng Poon Chew Collection.
Yung, Judy, Collection.

*Bancroft Library, University of California at Berkeley*

Angel Island Immigration Station Collection. 78/122 C.
Asian American Oral History Composite. 78/123.
Bancroft, Hubert Howe, Collection, MSS C-E 158.
California State Emergency Relief Administration, "Survey of Social Work Needs
   of the Chinese Population of San Francisco, California," 1935.
Combined Asian American Resources Oral History Project Interviews, 1974–
   76. 80/31 C.
Griffith, Alice. Manuscript Collection. 70/102 C.
Jones, Lucy. Diary, 1874–75. C-F 205.
Logan, Thomas Muldrup. Papers. C-R 114.
Manion, John J. Papers, 1926–46. C-B 816.
Mason-McDuffie Collection. BANC MSS 89/12C.
Miscellaneous Papers Relating to the Chinese in California, 1894–1926.
   C-R 153.
Morris, George B. "The Chinaman as He Is." Manuscript. 71/206 C.

Phelan, James DuVal. Correspondence and Papers. C-B 800.
Scott, Mel. Papers. 70/73C.
University of California at Berkeley, Institute of Government Studies Collection.
    C-R 131.
Wurster, Catherine Bauer. Papers. 74/163.


*California Historical Society, San Francisco*

American Civil Liberties Union, Northern California Collection. Ms. 3580.
Babies' Aid Records. Ms. 94.
Baby Hygiene Committee Collection. American Association of University
    Women Records. Ms. 51.
Certificate Collection.
Cow Hollow Improvement Club Records. Ms. 3191.
League of Women Voters Collection. Ms. 1270.
San Francisco Chamber of Commerce Collection. Ms. 871.
San Francisco Public Welfare Council Collection. Ms. 1866.


*California State Library, Sacramento*

Chinese Pamphlets Collection.


*Chinese Hospital Archives, San Francisco*

Chinese Hospital Medical Staff Archives.


*Herbert Hoover Library, Stanford University*

Survey of Race Relations Collection.


*Lane Medical Library, Stanford University*

Stanford Medical School, Department of Public Health, Sanitary Surveys.


*Medical College of Pennsylvania Archives, Philadelphia*

Special Collections on Women in Medicine.


*National Archives (San Bruno, California)*

U.S. Bureau of Immigration, San Francisco. Chinese Case Files. Record
    Group 85.
U.S. District Court, Northern District of California, San Francisco. Record
    Group 21.
U.S. Public Health Service, Quarantine Station, Angel Island. Record
    Group 90.

*National Archives (Washington, D.C.)*

U.S. Bureau of Immigration, Department of the Treasury. Record Group 85.
U.S. Congress. Legislative Records Petitions, House and Senate Committees on Foreign Affairs. Record Group 46.
U.S. Public Health Service. Record Group 90.

*Presbyterian Office of History, Philadelphia*

Presbyterian Board of National Missions. Files of the Department of Education and Medical Work, 1878–1966. Record Group 101.

*San Francisco Labor Archive and Research Center,*
*San Francisco State University*

Asiatic Exclusion League Papers, 1906–09.

*San Francisco Theological Union, San Anselmo*

Mrs. Rawlins Cadwallader Papers.

*University of California at San Francisco Archives*

California Nurses Association Papers.
*San Francisco Tuberculosis Association Bulletin,* April-May 1925.

*University of the Pacific, Stockton, California*

Holt-Atherton Collection.

BOOKS, REPORTS, AND ARTICLES

Abel-Musgrave, Curt. *The Cholera in San Francisco: A Contribution to the History of Corruption in California.* San Francisco: San Francisco News Company, 1885.
American Federation of Labor. Some Reasons for Chinese Exclusion: Meat vs. Rice, American Manhood against Asiatic Cooliesism. Which Shall Survive? Washington: American Federation of Labor, 1901.
Asiatic Exclusion League of North America. Proceedings of the First International Convention of the Asiatic Exclusion League of North America. San Francisco: Allied Printing, 1908.
Bode, William W. *Lights and Shadows of Chinatown.* San Francisco: Crocker, 1896.
Buel, J. W. *Metropolitan Life Unveiled; or, the Mysteries and Miseries of America's Great Cities.* St. Louis: Historical Publishing Company, 1882.
California Legislature. Special Committee on Chinese Immigration. *Chinese Immigration: Its Social, Moral, and Political Effect.* Sacramento, 1876.

California Special Health Commission. *Representative of the Special Health Commission Appointed by the Governor to Confer with Federal Authorities at Washington Respecting the Alleged Existence of Bubonic Plague in California.* Sacramento, 1901.

California State Board of Health. *Biennial Report of the State Board of Health of California.* Sacramento, 1871–1910.

Canada. Royal Commission on Chinese Immigration. *Report of the Royal Commission on Chinese Immigration: Report and Evidence.* Ottawa: Royal Commission on Chinese Immigration, 1885.

*Chinatown, San Francisco, California.* San Francisco: Bancroft Company, 1893.

Chinese Consolidated Benevolent Association. *Memorial of the Six Chinese Companies: Address to the Senate and House of Representatives.* San Francisco: Alta Print, 1877.

*The Chinese Hospital of San Francisco.* Oakland: Carruth and Carruth, 1899.

Clark, Traiferro, and J. W. Schereschewsky. *Trachoma: Its Character and Effects.* Public Health Service Bulletin No. 19. Washington, D.C.: Government Printing Office, 1910.

Clarke, Alfred. *Report of Alfred Clarke, Special Counsel for the City and County of San Francisco, in the Laundry Order Litigation.* San Francisco: W. M. Hinton and Co., 1885.

Condit, Ira M. *The Chinaman as We See Him, and Fifty Years of Work for Him.* Chicago: F. H. Revell, 1900.

Constitutional Convention of California. *Debates and Proceedings of the Constitutional Convention of California, 1878–79.* Sacramento, 1880.

Densmore, G. B. *The Chinese in California: Description of Chinese Life in San Francisco. Their Habits, Morals, and Manners.* San Francisco: Pettit and Russ, 1880.

Dyer, John Francis. "Rebuilding Chinatown." *World Today* 8 (May 1906): 553–54.

Farwell, Willard B. *The Chinese at Home and Abroad, Together with the Report of the Special Committee of the Board of Supervisors of San Francisco on the Condition of the Chinese Quarter and the Chinese in San Francisco, July 1885.* San Francisco: Bancroft, 1885.

Fitch, George H. "A Night in Chinatown." *Cosmopolitan* 2, no. 6 (February 1887): 356.

Freemantle, F. E. *A Traveler's Study of Health and Empire.* 2nd ed. London: Heath and Cranton, 1917.

Gibson, Dr. A. L. "State Sanitation." *Medico-Literary Journal* 2, no. 6 (February 1880): 3–8.

Gibson, Otis. *The Chinese in America.* Cincinnati: Hitchcock, 1877.

Hall, Hastings S. *Health and Disease—How to Obtain One and Avoid the Other.* San Francisco: Towne and Bacon, 1867.

Hemenway, Henry B. *American Public Health Protection.* Indianapolis: Bobbs-Merrill, 1916.

Henshaw, Sarah E. "Chinese Housekeepers and Chinese Servants." *Scribner's Monthly* 12 (1876): 736.

Hinman, George Warren. *The Oriental in America*. New York: Missionary Education Movement of the United States and Canada, 1913.

Hoff, John J. *Report of the City Surveyor*. San Francisco: O'Meara and Painter, 1856.

Holder, Charles Frederick. "Chinese Slavery in America." *North American Review* 165 (September 1897): 288–94.

Hoy, William. *The Chinese Six Companies*. San Francisco: Chinese Consolidated Benevolent Association, 1942.

Humphreys, William P. *Report on the System of Sewerage for the City of San Francisco*. San Francisco: n.p., 1876.

Kane, H. H. *Opium Smoking in America and China: A Study of Its Prevalence and Effects, Immediate and Remote, on the Individual and the Nation*. New York: G. P. Putnam's Sons, 1882.

Keeler, Charles. "Municipal Art in American Cities: San Francisco." *Craftsman* 8 (August 1905): 597.

Kipling, Rudyard. *Rudyard Kipling's Letters from San Francisco*. San Francisco: Colt Press, 1949.

Lloyd, B. E. *Lights and Shades in San Francisco*. San Francisco: A. L. Bancroft and Co., 1876.

Loomis, Augustus Ward. "The Medical Art in the Chinese Quarter." *Overland Monthly* 2, no. 6 (1869): 496–506.

Manson, Marsden. *System of Sewerage for the City and County of San Francisco*. San Francisco: Bosqui Engraving and Printing, 1893.

Morrow, Prince. *Social Diseases and Marriage: Social Prophylaxis*. Philadelphia: Lea Brothers, 1904.

National Board of Health. *Annual Report*. Washington, D.C.: Government Printing Office, 1882.

Ng, Poon Chew. *The Treatment of the Exempt Classes of Chinese in the United States*. San Francisco: Ng Poon Chew, 1908.

Powderly, Terence V. "Exclude Anarchist and Chinaman!" *Collier's Weekly* (December 14, 1901).

———. "The Immigration Menace to National Health." *North American Review* 175 (1902): 53–60.

Raymond, Walter J. *Horrors of the Mongolian Settlement, San Francisco, California: Enslaved and Degraded Race of Paupers, Opium Eaters, and Lepers*. Boston: Cashman, Keating, and Company, 1886.

Recreation Project. California. *Survey of San Francisco, California, by Districts (Recreation)*. San Francisco: Works Progress Administration, June 1937.

Ricketts, Howard Taylor. *Infection, Immunity, and Serum Therapy*. Chicago: American Medical Association, 1906.

San Francisco Board of Health. *Annual Report of the Board of Health of the City and County of San Francisco*. San Francisco, 1869–1917.

———. *Health and Quarantine Laws for the City and Harbor of San Francisco Relating to the Public Health*. San Francisco, 1870–1889.

San Francisco Board of Supervisors. *General Orders of the Board of Supervisors*. San Francisco, 1890.

———. *Official Map of "Chinatown" in San Francisco*. San Francisco: Bosqui Engraving and Printing, 1885.

———. *Report of the Special Committee of the Board of Supervisors of San Francisco on the Condition of the Chinese Quarter and the Chinese in San Francisco, July 1885*. San Francisco, 1885.

———. *San Francisco Municipal Report*. San Francisco, 1855–1910.

San Francisco Common Council. *Ordinances and Joint Resolutions of the City of San Francisco*. San Francisco: Mason and Valentine, 1854.

San Francisco Department of Public Health. *A Study of Maternity Cases Cared for by the Division of Field Nursing of the San Francisco Department of Public Health during the Period from 1931 to 1938*. San Francisco, 1939.

San Francisco Housing Authority. *Annual Report*. San Francisco, 1939–50.

———. *The 1939 Real Property Survey of San Francisco, California*. San Francisco, 1939.

Sawtelle, Dr. M. P. "The Foul Contagious Disease: A Phase of the Chinese Question." *Medico-Literary Journal* 1, no. 3 (November 1878): 8.

School for Social Studies. *Living Conditions in Chinatown*. San Francisco: School for Social Studies, ca. 1939.

Shepard, Charles R. *The Story of Chung Mei, Being the Authentic History of the Chung Mei Home for Chinese Boys up to Its Fifteenth Anniversary, October 1938*. Philadelphia: Judson Press, 1938.

Sigma Xi. *Report of the Committee of the Society of Sigma Xi on the Plague Conditions in Berkeley, San Francisco, and Oakland*. Berkeley: n.p., 1908.

Soule, Frank H., et al. *Annals of San Francisco and History of California*. 1855; reprint, Palo Alto: Lewis Osborne, 1966.

Stout, Arthur B. *Chinese Immigration and the Physiological Causes of the Decay of a Nation*. San Francisco: Agnew & Deffebach, 1862.

Talbot, Eugene Solomon. *Degeneracy: Its Causes, Signs, Results*. New York: Charles Scribner's Sons, 1898.

Tisdale, William. "Chinese Physicians in California." *Lippincott's Magazine*, no. 63 (March 1899): 411–16.

Todd, Frank Morton. *The Chamber of Commerce Handbook for San Francisco*. San Francisco: San Francisco Chamber of Commerce, 1914.

———. *Eradicating Plague from San Francisco: Report of the Citizen's Health Committee and an Account of Its Work*. San Francisco: Murdock and Co., 1909.

U.S. Bureau of the Census. *Thirteenth Census of the United States, Taken in the Year 1910*. Washington, D.C., 1910.

U.S. Congress. Senate. *Report of the Joint Special Committee to Investigate Chinese Immigration*. 44th Cong., 2d sess., 1877. S. Rept. 689.

U.S. Marine Hospital Service. *Annual Report of the Supervising Surgeon General*. Washington, D.C.: General Printing Office, 1891/92–1900/01.

———. *Annual Report of the Surgeon General of the Public Health and Marine Hospital Service of the United States*. Washington, D.C.: General Printing Office, 1904/05–1910/11.

———. *Annual Report of the Surgeon General of the Public Health Service*. Washington, D.C.: General Printing Office, 1913/14–1925/26.

U.S. Public Health and Marine Hospital Service. *Book of Instructions for the Medical Inspection of Immigrants.* Washington, D.C.: Government Printing Office, 1903.

U.S. Treasury Department. Commission for the Investigation of Plague in San Francisco. *Report of the Committee Appointed by the Secretary of the Treasury for the Investigation of Plague in San Francisco under Instructions from the Surgeon General, Marine Hospital Service.* Washington, D.C.: Government Printing Office, 1901.

Waring, George E., Jr., comp. *Report on the Social Statistics of Cities.* Washington, D.C.: Government Printing Office, 1887.

West, H. S., comp. *The Chinese Invasion, Revealing the Habits, Manners, and Customs of the Chinese, Political, Social, and Religious, on the Pacific Coast, Coming in Contact with the Free and Enlightened Citizens of America.* San Francisco: Bacon and Company, 1873.

Wheeler, Rev. O. C. *The Chinese in America: A National Question.* Oakland, Calif.: Times, 1880.

Williams, Allen S. *The Demon of the Orient and His Satellite Fiends of the Joint: Our Opium Smokers as They Are in Tartar Hells and American Paradises.* New York: Allen S. Williams, 1883.

Women's Foreign Missionary Society of the Presbyterian Church, Occidental Branch. *Annual Report.* San Francisco: C. W. Gordon, 1875–1900.

Woo, Wesley. "Protestant Work among the Chinese in the San Francisco Bay Area, 1850–1920." Ph.D. diss., Graduate Theology Union, Berkeley, 1983.

Workingmen's Party of California, Anti-Chinese Council. *Chinatown Declared a Nuisance!* San Francisco: Workingmen's Party of California, 1880.

Wyman, Walter. *The Bubonic Plague.* Public Health Service Bulletin No. 7. Washington, D.C.: Government Printing Office, 1900.

———. *Bubonic Plague.* Treasury Department Document No. 2165. Washington, D.C.: Government Printing Office, 1900.

Young, John P. *San Francisco: A History of the Pacific Coast Metropolis.* 2 vol. San Francisco: S. J. Clarke Publishing Company, 1912.

NEWSPAPERS

*Chinese Defender*
*Chinese Press*
*Chung Sai Yat Po*
*Daily Alta California*
*Labor Clarion*
*People's Daily World*
*Sacramento Record-Union*
*San Francisco Bulletin*
*San Francisco Call*
*San Francisco Chronicle*
*San Francisco Evening Bulletin*
*San Francisco Examiner*
*San Francisco Morning Call*
*San Francisco News*

## PERIODICALS

*American Journal of Public Health*
*American Journal of Syphilography and Dermatology*
*American Journal of Tropical Medicine*
*American Monthly Review of Reviews*
*Antique Trader Weekly*
*Blackwood's Edinburgh Magazine*
*California Medical Gazette*
*California State Journal of Medicine*
*Chinese Digest*
*Chinese World*
*Cigar Maker's Official Journal*
*Collier's Weekly*
*Cosmopolitan*
*Craftsman*
*Harper's Weekly*
*Heritage Newsletter*
*Journal of Progress*
*Journal of the American Medical Association*
*Lippincott's Magazine*
*Medical and Surgical Reporter*
*Medico-Literary Journal*
*Military Surgeon*
*North American Review*
*Occidental Medical Times*
*Overland Monthly*
*Pacific Medical and Surgical Journal*
*Pacific Medical Journal*
*Public Health Nursing*
*San Francisco Tuberculosis Association Bulletin*
*Transactions of the American Medical Association*
*Transactions of the Medical Society of the State of California* (replaced in 1902
    by *California State Journal of Medicine*)
*Western Lancet*
*White Man*
*Woman's Home Companion*
*Woman's Work for Woman*
*World Today*


## SECONDARY SOURCES

Almaguer, Tomas. *Racial Fault Lines: The Historical Origins of White Suprem-
    acy in California.* Berkeley and Los Angeles: University of California Press,
    1994.

Anderson, Benedict. *Imagined Communities: Reflections on the Origins and Spread of Nationalism*. London: Verso, 1983.

Anderson, Kay J. "Engendering Race Research: Unsettling the Self-Other Dichotomy." In *Bodyspace: Destabilizing Geographies of Gender and Sexuality*, ed. Nancy Duncan, 197–211. New York: Routledge, 1996.

———. *Vancouver's Chinatown: Racial Discourse in Canada, 1875–1980*. Montreal: McGill-Queen's University Press, 1991.

Anderson, Margo J. *The American Census: A Social History*. New Haven: Yale University Press, 1988.

Anderson, Warwick. "Excremental Colonialism, Public Health, and the Poetics of Pollution." *Critical Inquiry* 21, no. 3 (spring 1995): 640–69.

———. "Immunities of Empire: Race, Disease, and the New Tropical Medicine." *Bulletin of the History of Medicine* 70, no. 1 (1996): 94–118.

———. "Leprosy and Citizenship." *Positions: East Asian Critique* 6, no. 3 (winter 1998): 707–30.

Anderson, Warwick, Myles Jackson, and Barbara Gutmann Rosencrantz. "Toward an Unnatural History of Immunology." *Journal of the History of Biology* 27 (1994): 575–94.

Andrews, Birdie J. "Tuberculosis and the Assimilation of Germ Theory in China, 1895–1937." *Journal of the History of Medicine and Allied Sciences* 52, no. 1 (January 1997): 114–57.

Armstrong, David. "Public Health Spaces and the Fabrication of Identity." *Sociology* 27, no. 3 (August 1993): 393–410.

Arnold, David. *Colonizing the Body: State Medicine and Epidemic Disease in Nineteenth-Century India*. Berkeley and Los Angeles: University of California Press, 1993.

———. "Touching the Body: Perspectives on the Indian Plague, 1896–1900." In *Subaltern Studies V: Writings on South Asian History and Society*, ed. Ranajit Guha. Delhi: Oxford University Press, 1987.

———, ed. *Imperial Medicine and Indigenous Societies*. Manchester: Manchester University Press, 1988.

Balibar, Etienne, and Immanuel Wallerstein. *Race, Nation, and Class: Ambiguous Identities*. London: Verso, 1991.

Barlow, Jeffrey. *China Doctor of John Day*. Portland, Ore.: Binford and Mort, 1979.

Barnhart, Jacqueline Baker. *The Fair but Frail: Prostitution in San Francisco, 1849–1900*. Reno: University of Nevada Press, 1986.

Baron, Ava. "Questions of Gender: Deskilling and Demasculinzation in the U.S. Printing Industry, 1830–1915." *Gender and History* 1, no. 2 (summer 1989): 178–99.

———, ed. *Work Engendered: Toward a New History of American Labor*. Ithaca: Cornell University Press, 1991.

Barth, Gunther. *Bitter Strength: A History of the Chinese in the United States, 1850–1870*. Cambridge: Harvard University Press, 1964.

Bates, Barbara. *Bargaining for Life: A Social History of Tuberculosis, 1876–1938*. Philadelphia: University of Pennsylvania Press, 1992.

Baudrillard, J. "Modernity." *Canadian Journal of Political and Social Theory* 11, no. 3 (1987): 63–72.

Bauman, John. *Public Housing, Race, and Renewal: Urban Planning in Philadelphia, 1920–1974.* Philadelphia: Temple University Press, 1987.

Bederman, Gail. *Manliness and Civilization: A Cultural History of Gender and Race in the United States, 1880–1917.* Chicago: University of Chicago Press, 1995.

Benedict, Carol. *Bubonic Plague in Nineteenth Century China.* Stanford: Stanford University Press, 1997.

Benedict, Michael Les. "Contagion and the Constitution: Quarantine Agitation from 1859 to 1866." *Journal of the History of Medicine and Allied Sciences* 25 (April 1970): 177–93.

Berlant, Lauren. "Intimacy." *Critical Inquiry* 24, no. 2 (winter 1998).

Berlant, Lauren, and Michael Warner. "Sex in Public." *Critical Inquiry* 24, no. 2 (winter 1998): 547–66.

Berthoff, Rowland. "Conventional Mentality: Free Blacks, Women, and Business Corporations as Unequal Persons, 1820–1870." *Journal of American History* 76 (December 1989): 753–84.

Berube, Allan. "Don't Save Us from Our Sexuality." *Coming Up!* (April 1984).

Bhabha, Homi. *The Location of Culture.* New York: Routledge, 1994.

———. "Race and the Humanities: The 'Ends' of Modernity." *Public Culture* 4, no. 2 (spring 1992): 81–85.

———. "Signs Taken for Wonders: Questions of Ambivalence and Authority under a Tree outside Delhi, May 1817." In *"Race," Writing, and Difference,* ed. Henry Louis Gates Jr., 163–84. Chicago: University of Chicago Press, 1986.

Blackmar, Elizabeth. "Accountability for Public Health: Regulating the Housing Market in Nineteenth Century New York City." In *Hives of Sickness,* ed. David Rosner, 42–64. New Brunswick: Rutgers University Press, 1995.

Boccaccio, Mary. "Ground Itch and Dew Poison: The Rockefeller Sanitary Commission, 1910–1914." *Journal of the History of Medicine and Allied Sciences* 27 (1972): 30–53.

Boji, Liu. *A History of the Chinese in United States.* Taipei: Liming, 1976.

Boris, Eileen. *Home to Work: Motherhood and the Politics of Industrial Homework in the United States.* New York: Cambridge University Press, 1994.

Bourdieu, Pierre. *Distinction: A Social Critique of the Judgement of Taste,* trans. Richard Nice. Cambridge: Harvard University Press, 1984.

———. "On the Family as a Realized Category." *Theory, Culture, Society* 13, no. 3 (1996): 19–26.

Boyer, Paul. *Urban Masses and Moral Order in America, 1820–1920.* Cambridge: Harvard University Press, 1978.

Broussard, Albert S. *Black San Francisco: The Struggle for Racial Equality in the West, 1900–1954.* Lawrence: University of Kansas Press, 1993.

Brumberg, Joan Jacobs. "The Ethnological Mirror: American Evangelical Women and Their Heathen Sisters, 1870–1910." In *Women and the Structure of Society,* ed. Barbara J. Harris and JoAnn McNamara, 108–28. Durham, N.C.: Duke University Press, 1984.

Buell, Paul D. "Chinese Medicine on Gold Mountain: Tradition, Adaptation, and Change." In *Disease and Medical Care in the Mountain West: Essays on Region, History, and Practice,* ed. Martha L. Hildreth and Bruce T. Moran, 95–109. Reno: University of Nevada Press, 1998.

———. "Theory and Practice of Traditional Chinese Medicine." In *Chinese Medicine on the Golden Mountain: An Interpretive Guide,* ed. Henry G. Schwartz, 25–50. Seattle: Wing Luke Memorial Museum, 1984.

Buell, Paul D., and Christopher Muench. "A Chinese Apothecary in Frontier Idaho." *Annals of the Chinese Historical Society of the Pacific Northwest* 1 (1983): 39–48.

Burchell, Graham. "Liberal Government and the Techniques of the Self." In *Foucault and Political Reason: Liberalism, Neo-Liberalism, and Rationalities of Government,* ed. Andrew Barry, Thomas Osborne, and Nikolas Rose. Chicago: University of Chicago Press, 1996.

Burke, Timothy. *Lifebuoy Men, Lux Women: Commodification, Consumption, and Cleanliness in Modern Zimbabwe.* Durham, N.C.: Duke University Press, 1996.

Burnham, John C. "Medical Inspection of Prostitutes in America in the Nineteenth Century: The St. Louis Experiment and Its Sequel." *Bulletin of the History of Medicine* 45, no. 3 (May-June 1971): 203–18.

Bushman, Richard L., and Claudia L. Bushman. "The Early History of Cleanliness in America." *Journal of American History* 74 (March 1988): 1225–66.

Butler, Judith. "Imitation and Gender Insubordination." In *Inside/Out: Lesbian Theories/Gay Theories,* ed. Diana Fuss, 13–31. New York: Routledge, 1991.

Calavita, Kitty. *Inside the State: The Bracero Program, Immigration, and the INS.* New York: Routledge, 1992.

Capeci, Dominic J., Jr. *Race Relations in Wartime Detroit: The Sojourner Truth Housing Controversy of 1942.* Philadelphia: Temple University Press, 1984.

Cassedy, James H. *Demography in Early America: The Beginnings of the Statistical Mind, 1600–1899.* Cambridge: Harvard University Press, 1982.

———. "The 'Germ of Laziness' in the South, 1900–1915: Charles Wardell Stiles and the Progressive Paradox." *Bulletin of the History of Medicine* 45 (1971): 159–69.

Cell, John W. "Anglo-Indian Medical Theory and the Origins of Segregation in West Africa." *American Historical Review* 91 (1986): 321–55.

———. *The Highest Stage of White Supremacy: The Origins of Segregation in South Africa and the American South.* Cambridge: Cambridge University Press, 1982.

Chamberlain, J. Edward, and Sander Gilman, eds. *Degeneration: The Dark Side of Progress.* New York: Columbia University Press, 1985.

Chan, Chun-wai, and Jade K. Chang. "The Role of Chinese Medicine in New York City's Chinatown." *American Journal of Chinese Medicine* 4, no. 1 (1976): 31–45; no. 2 (1976): 129–46.

Chan, Sucheng. *Asian Americans: An Interpretive History.* Boston: Twayne, 1991.

———. *This Bittersweet Soil: The Chinese in California Agriculture, 1860–1910.* Berkeley and Los Angeles: University of California Press, 1986.

————, ed. *Entry Denied: Exclusion and the Chinese Community in America, 1882–1943*. Philadelphia: Temple University Press, 1991.

Chaudhrui, Napur. "Memsahibs and Motherhood in Nineteenth Century Colonial India." *Victorian Studies* 31, no. 4 (1988): 517–36.

Chen, Shehong. "Being Chinese, Becoming Chinese American: The Transformation of Chinese Identity in the United States, 1910–1928." Ph.D. diss., University of Utah, June 1997.

Chen, Yong. *Chinese San Francisco, 1850–1943: A Trans-Pacific Community*. Stanford: Stanford University Press, 2000.

Chinn, Thomas W. *Bridging the Pacific: San Francisco's Chinatown and Its People*. San Francisco: Chinese Historical Society of America, 1989.

Chinn, Thomas W., Him Mark Lai, and Philip P. Choy. *A History of the Chinese in California: A Syllabus*. San Francisco: Chinese Historical Society of America, 1969.

Choppé, Albert. *Le Label*. Paris: Giard, 1908.

Choy, Curtis. *Fall of the I-Hotel*. 58 minutes. San Francisco: NAATA/Crosscurrents, original version 1983; revised 1993. Documentary film.

Chung, Sue Fawn. "The Chinese American Citizens Alliance: An Effort in Assimilation, 1895–1965." *Chinese America: History and Perspectives* (San Francisco) (1988): 30–47.

Cohen, Margaret, and Christopher Prendergast, eds. *Spectacles of Realism: Body, Gender, and Genre*. Minneapolis: University of Minnesota Press, 1995.

Cohn, Bernard S., and Nicholas B. Dirks. "Beyond the Fringe: The Nation State, Colonialism, and the Technologies of Power." *Journal of Historical Sociology* 1, no. 2 (June 1988): 224–29.

Comaroff, Jean, and John Comaroff. *Ethnography and the Historical Imagination*. Boulder, Colo.: Westview Press, 1992.

Connelly, Mark. *The Response to Prostitution in the Progressive Era*. Chapel Hill: University of North Carolina Press, 1980.

Coolidge, Mary Roberts. *Chinese Immigration*. New York: Henry Holt and Co., 1909.

Coontz, Stephanie. *The Way We Never Were: The American Family and the Nostalgia Trap*. New York: Basic Books, 1992.

Cooper, Frederick, and Ann Stoler. *Tensions of Empire: Colonial Cultures in a Bourgeois World*. Berkeley and Los Angeles: University of California Press, 1997.

Cooper, Patricia A. *Once a Cigarmaker: Men, Women, and Work Culture in American Cigar Factories, 1900–1919*. Urbana: University of Illinois Press, 1987.

Coronil, Fernando. "Beyond Occidentalism: Towards Nonimperial Geohistorical Categories." *Cultural Anthropology* 11, no. 1 (February 1996): 51–87.

Cott, Nancy. "Marriage and Women's Citizenship in the United States, 1830–1934." *American Historical Review* 103, no. 5 (December 1998): 1440–74.

Courtney, William J. *San Francisco Anti-Chinese Ordinances, 1850–1900*. San Francisco: Rand E. Research Associates, 1974).

Courtright, David T. *Dark Paradise: Opiate Addiction in America before 1940*. Cambridge: Harvard University Press, 1982.

Craddock, Susan Leigh. "Diseases on the Margin: Morphologies of Tuberculosis and Smallpox in San Francisco, 1860–1940." Ph.D. diss., University of California at Berkeley, 1994.

———. "Sewers and Scapegoats: Spatial Metaphors of Smallpox in Nineteenth Century San Francisco." *Social Science and Medicine* 41, no. 7 (1995): 957–68.

Crawford, Robert. "The Boundaries of the Self and the Unhealthy Other: Reflections on Health, Culture, and AIDS." *Social Science Medicine* 38, no. 10 (1994): 1347–65.

Cross, Ira B. *A History of the Labor Movement in California.* Berkeley and Los Angeles: University of California Press, 1935.

Cruikshank, Barbara. *The Will to Empower: Democratic Citizens and Other Subjects.* Ithaca: Cornell University Press, 1999.

Daniels, Douglas Henry. *Pioneer Urbanites: A Social and Cultural History of Black San Francisco.* Berkeley and Los Angeles: University of California Press, 1990.

Daniels, Roger. *Asian American: Chinese and Japanese in the United States since 1850.* Seattle: University of Washington Press, 1988.

Daston, Lorraine. "Historical Epistemology." In *Questions of Evidence: Proof, Practice, and Persuasion across the Disciplines,* ed. James Chandler, Arnold I. Davidson, and Harry Harootunian, 282–89. Chicago: University of Chicago Press, 1994.

Davidoff, Leonore, and Catherine Hall. *Family Fortunes: Men and Women of the English Middle Class, 1780–1850.* Chicago: University of Chicago Press, 1987.

Davies, Richard O. *Housing Reform during the Truman Administration.* Columbia: University of Missouri Press, 1966.

Davis, Audrey B. "Life Insurance and the Physical Examination: A Chapter in the Rise of American Medical Technology." *Bulletin of the History of Medicine* 55 (1981): 92–406.

Deacon, Harriet. "Racial Segregation and Medical Discourse in Nineteenth Century Cape Town." *Journal of Southern African Studies* 22, no. 2 (June 1996): 287–308.

Delaporte, François. *Disease and Civilization: The Cholera in Paris,* trans. Arthur Goldhammer. Cambridge: MIT Press, 1986.

De Lauretis, Theresa. "The Technology of Gender." In *Technologies of Gender: Essays on Theory, Film, and Fiction.* Bloomington: University of Indiana Press, 1987.

De Lepervanche, M. "The Naturalness of Inequality." In *Ethnicity, Class, and Gender in Australia,* ed. G. Bottomley and M. De Lepervanche, 49–71. Sydney: Allen and Unwin.

Deverell, William. "Plague in Los Angeles: Ethnicity and Typicality." In *Over the Edge: Remapping the American West,* ed. Valerie Matsumoto and Blake Allmendinger, 172–200. Berkeley and Los Angeles: University of California Press, 1999.

Dirks, Nicholas B., Geoff Eley, and Sherry B. Ortner. Introduction to *Culture/Power/History.* Princeton: Princeton University Press, 1994.

Donzelot, Jacques. *The Policing of Families*. New York: Pantheon, 1990.

Douglas, Mary. *Purity and Danger: An Analysis of Concepts of Pollution and Taboo*. Baltimore: Penguin, 1970.

DuBois, Ellen Carol. "Outgrowing the Compact of the Fathers: Equal Rights, Woman Suffrage, and the United States Constitution, 1820–1878." *Journal of American History* 74 (December 1987): 836–62.

Duffy, John. *The Sanitarians: A History of American Public Health*. Chicago: University of Illinois Press, 1990.

Dunn, Frederick. "Traditional Asian Medicine and Cosmopolitan Medicine as Adaptive Systems." In *Asian Medical Systems: A Comparative Study,* ed. Charles Leslie, 133–58. Berkeley and Los Angeles: University of California Press, 1976.

Dyer, Richard. *White*. London: Routledge, 1998.

———. "White." *Screen*, no. 29 (autumn 1988): 44–64.

Einhorn, Robin. *Property Rules: Political Economy in Chicago, 1833–1872*. Chicago: University of Chicago Press, 1991.

Eley, Geoff. "German History and the Contradictions of Modernity: The Bourgeoisie, the State, and the Mastery of Reform." In *Society, Culture, and the State in Germany,* ed. Geoff Eley, 67–104. Ann Arbor: University of Michigan Press, 1996.

Elias, Norbert. *The Civilizing Process*. Vol. 1: *The History of Manners*. Trans. E. Jephcott. New York: Pantheon Press, 1978.

Engelstein, Laura. "Combined Underdevelopment: Discipline and the Law in Imperial and Soviet Russia." *American Historical Review* 98, no. 2 (April 1993): 338–53.

Englander, Susan. *Class Conflict and Coalition in the California Women's Suffrage Movement, 1907–1912*. Lewiston, N.Y.: Edwin Mellen Press, 1992.

Epstein, Steven. *Impure Science: AIDS, Activism, and the Politics of Knowledge*. Berkeley and Los Angeles: University of California Press, 1996.

Ethington, Philip J. *The Public City: The Political Construction of Urban Life in San Francisco, 1850–1900*. New York: Cambridge University Press, 1994.

Ettling, John. *The Germ of Laziness: Rockefeller Philanthropy and Public Health in the New South*. Cambridge: Harvard University Press, 1981.

Fairbanks, Robert B. *Making Better Citizens: Housing Reform and Strategy in Cincinnati, 1890–1960*. Urbana: University of Illinois Press, 1988.

Fairchild, Amy Lauren. "Science at the Borders: Immigrant Medical Inspection and the Defense of the Nation, 1891 to 1930." Ph.D. diss., Columbia University, 1997.

Fanon, Franz. *A Dying Colonialism*. New York: Grove Press, 1965.

———. "Medicine and Colonialism." In *The Cultural Crisis of Modern Medicine,* ed. John Ehrenreich. New York: Monthly Review Press, 1978.

Farquhar, Judith. *Knowing Practice: The Clinical Encounter of Chinese Medicine*. Boulder, Colo.: Westview Press, 1994.

Fay, Peter Ward. *Opium War, 1840–1842*. New York: W. W. Norton, 1976.

Fee, Elizabeth, and Daniel M. Fox, eds. *AIDS: The Burdens of History*. Berkeley and Los Angeles: University of California Press, 1988.

Feldberg, Georgina D. *Disease and Class: Tuberculosis and the Shaping of Modern North American Society.* New Brunswick, N.J.: Rutgers University Press, 1995.

Fellman, Anita Clair, and Michael Fellman. *Making Sense of Self: Medical Advice Literature in Late Nineteenth Century America.* Philadelphia: University of Pennsylvania Press, 1981.

Fields, Barbara. "Slavery, Race, and Ideology in the United States of America." *New Left Review* (May-June 1990): 95–118.

Fisher, Robert Moor. *Twenty Years of Public Housing: Economic Aspects of the Federal Program.* New York: Harper, 1959.

Flint, Barbara. "Zoning and Residential Segregation: A Social and Political History, 1910–1940." Ph.D. diss., University of Chicago, Department of History, 1977.

Fong, Wong Yu, comp. *Historical Review of Clonorchiasis.* Berkeley: Fred A. Borland, [ca. 1928].

Foucault, Michel. *The Archaeology of Knowledge and the Discourse on Language.* New York: Pantheon, 1972.

———. *Discipline and Punish: The Birth of the Prison.* New York: Vintage Books, 1977.

———. "Governmentality." In *The Foucault Effect: Studies in Governmentality,* ed. Graham Burchell, Colin Gordon, and Peter Miller. Chicago: University of Chicago Press, 1991.

———. *History of Sexuality.* Vol. 1: *An Introduction.* 1976. Reprint; New York: Vintage Books, 1990.

———. *Power/Knowledge: Selected Interviews and Other Writings, 1972–1977,* ed. Colin Gordon. New York: Pantheon, 1980.

———. "Two Lectures." In *Power/Knowledge.* Trans. Colin Gordon, pp. 166–82 (New York: Pantheon Books, 1980.

Frank, Dana. *Buy American: The Untold Story of Economic Nationalism.* Boston: Beacon Press, 1999.

———. *Purchasing Power: Consumer Organizing, Gender, and the Seattle Labor Movement, 1919–1929.* New York: Cambridge University Press, 1994.

Frankenberg, Ruth. *White Women, Race Matters: The Social Construction of Whiteness.* Minneapolis: University of Minnesota Press, 1993.

Fraser, Nancy. "Rethinking the Public Sphere: A Contribution to the Critique of Actually Existing Democracy." In *The Phantom Public Sphere,* ed. Bruce Robbins, 1–32. Minneapolis: University of Minnesota Press, 1993.

———. *Unruly Practices: Power, Discourse, and Gender in Contemporary Social Theory.* Minneapolis: University of Minnesota Press, 1989.

Freedman, Estelle, and John D'Emilio. *Intimate Matters: A History of Sexuality in America.* New York: Harper and Row, 1988.

Freund, Ernst. *The Police Power: Public Policy and Constitutional Rights.* Chicago: Callaghan and Company, 1904.

Fritz, Christian G. "A Nineteenth Century 'Habeas Corpus Mill': The Chinese before the Federal Courts in California." *American Journal of Legal History* 32 (1988): 347–72.

Fung, Richard. "Burdens of Representation, Burdens of Responsibility." In *Constructing Masculinity,* ed. Maurice Berger et al., 291–99. London: Routledge, 1995.

Furman, Bess. *A Profile of the Public Health Service, 1798–1948.* Washington, D.C.: Government Printing Office, 1973.

Galishoff, Stuart. "Drainage, Disease, Comfort, and Class: A History of Newark's Sewers." *Societas* 6, no. 2 (1976): 121–38.

———. "Germs Know No Color Line: Black Health and Public Policy in Atlanta, 1900–1918." *Journal of History of Medicine* 40 (1985): 22–41.

———. *Newark, the Nation's Unhealthiest City, 1832–1895.* New Brunswick: Rutgers University Press, 1988.

Gallagher, Catherine. "The Body versus the Social Body in the Works of Thomas Malthus and Henry Mayhew." *Representations* 14 (spring 1986): 83–106.

Gamble, Vanessa. *Germs Have No Color Line: Blacks and American Medicine, 1900–1940.* New York: Garland Press, 1989.

George, Rosemary Maragoly. "Recycling: Long Routes to and from Domestic Fixes." In *Burning Down the House: Recycling Domesticity,* ed. Rosemary Maragoly George. Boulder, Colo.: Westview Press, 1998.

Gerlitt, J. "The Development of Quarantine." *Ciba Symposia* 2, no. 6 (1950): 566–80.

Gidden, Anthony. *The Consequences of Modernity.* Stanford: Stanford University Press, 1990.

Giglierano, Geoffrey. "The City and the System: Developing a Municipal Service, 1800–1915." *Cincinnati Historical Society Bulletin* 35 (1977): 223–47.

Gilfoyle, Timothy J. *City of Eros: New York City Prostitution and the Commercialization of Sex, 1790–1920.* New York: Norton, 1992.

———. "The Urban Geography of Commercial Sex: Prostitution in New York City, 1790–1860." *Journal of Urban History* 13 (August 1987): 384–87.

Gilman, Sander L. "AIDS and Syphilis: The Iconography of Disease." In *AIDS: Cultural Analysis Cultural Activism,* ed. Douglas Crimp, 87–107. Cambridge: MIT Press, 1988.

———. "Black Bodies, White Bodies: Toward an Iconography of Female Sexuality in Late Nineteenth Century Art, Medicine, and Literature." *Critical Inquiry* 12, no. 1 (1985): 204–42.

———. *Difference and Pathology: Stereotypes of Sexuality, Race, and Madness.* Ithaca: Cornell University Press, 1985.

Gilroy, Paul. *"There Ain't No Black in the Union Jack": The Cultural Politics of Race and Nation.* Chicago: University of Chicago Press, 1991.

Ginzberg, Lori. "Social Movements." Paper presented to the conference "Project to Internationalize the Study of American History," Joint Project of New York University and the Organization of American Historians, Villa La Pietra, Florence, Italy, July 4–7, 1999, manuscript in author's possession.

Glenn, Evelyn Nakano, Grace Chang, and Linda Rennie Forcey. *Mothering: Ideology, Experience, and Agency.* New York: Routledge, 1994.

Glickman, Lawrence B. "Inventing the 'American Standard of Living': Gender, Race, and Working-Class Identity, 1880–1925." *Labor History* 34, no. 2–3 (1993): 221–35.

———. *A Living Wage: American Workers and the Making of Consumer Society.* Ithaca: Cornell University Press, 1997.

Goldberg, David Theo. *Racist Culture: Philosophy and the Politics of Meaning.* Cambridge, England: Blackwell, 1993.

———. "The Social Formation of Racist Discourse." In *Anatomy of Racism,* ed. David Theo Goldberg. Minneapolis: University of Minnesota Press, 1990.

Goldstein, Jan. "Framing Discipline with Law: Problems and Promises of the Liberal State." *American Historical Review* 98, no. 2 (April 1993): 364–75.

———. "The Wandering Jew and the Problem of the Psychiatric Anti-Semitism in Fin-de-Siècle France." *Journal of Contemporary History* 20, no. 4 (1985): 521–52.

Goodnow, Frank G. "Summary Abatement of Nuisances by Boards of Health." *Columbia Law Review* (1902): 203–22.

Gopinath, Gayatri. "Homo-Economics: Queer Sexualities in a Transnational Frame." In *Burning Down the House,* ed. Rosemary Maragoly George. Boulder, Colo.: Westview Press, 1998.

Gordon, Colin. "Governmental Rationality: An Introduction." In *The Foucault Effect: Studies in Governmentality,* ed. Graham Burchell, Colin Gordon, and Peter Miller, 19–20. Chicago: University of Chicago Press, 1991.

Gordon, Linda. "Putting Children First: Women, Maternalism, and Welfare in Twentieth Century America." Manuscript, University of Wisconsin at Madison, Institute for the Research of Poverty Discussion Papers, January 1993.

Gould, Stephen Jay. *The Mismeasure of Man.* New York: W. W. Norton, 1981.

———. "Science and Jewish Immigration." *Hen's Teeth and Horse's Toes.* New York: W. W. Norton, 1984.

Gronewold, Sue. *Beautiful Merchandise: Prostitution in China, 1860–1936.* New York: Haworth Press, 1982.

Guha, Ranajit. *Elementary Aspects of Peasant Insurgency.* Delhi: Oxford University Press, 1983.

———. "The Prose of Counter-Insurgency." In *Subaltern Studies: Writings on South Asian History and Society,* ed. Ranajit Guha, 2:3–26. Delhi: Oxford University Press, 1982.

Guillaumin, Colette. "The Idea of Race and Its Elevation to Autonomous, Scientific, and Legal Status." In *Sociological Theories: Race and Colonialism,* 37–68. Paris: UNESCO, 1980.

———. "Race and Nature: The System of Marks." *Feminist Issues* 8 (fall 1988): 25–44.

———. *Racism, Sexism, Power, and Ideology.* London: Routledge, 1995.

Gussow, Zachary. *Leprosy, Racism, and Public Health: Social Policy in Chronic Disease Control.* Boulder, Colo.: Westview Press, 1989.

Gyory, Andrew. *Closing the Gate: Race, Politics, and the Chinese Exclusion Act.* Chapel Hill: University of North Carolina Press, 1998.

Haas, Victor H. "When Bubonic Plague Came to Chinatown." Pt. 1. *American Journal of Tropical Medicine and Hygiene* 8, no. 2 (March 1959): 141–47.

Habermas, Jurgen. "Modernity, an Incomplete Project." In *The Anti-Aesthetic: Essays on Postmodern Culture,* ed. Hal Foster, 3–15. Seattle: Bay Press, 1983.

Hage, Ghassan. "The Spatial Imaginary of National Practices: Dwelling—Domesticating—Being—Exterminating." *Environment and Planning D: Society and Space* 14 (1996): 463–85.

Haiming, Liu. "The Resilience of Ethnic Culture: Chinese Herbalists in the American Medical Profession." *Journal of Asian American Studies* 1, no. 2 (June 1998).

Hall, Stuart. "Gramsci's Relevance for the Study of Race and Ethnicity." *Journal of Communicative Inquiry* 10, no. 2 (1986): 5–27.

———. "Race, Articulation, and Societies Structured in Dominance." In *Sociological Theories: Race and Colonialism*. Paris: UNESCO, 1980.

Hall, Stuart, et al., eds. *Modernity and Its Futures*. Hempstead, N.Y.: Open University, 1993.

Haller, J. S. *Outcasts from Evolution: Scientific Attitudes of Racial Inferiority, 1859–1900*. Urbana: University of Illinois Press, 1971.

Handy, Robert T. *A Christian America: Protestant Hopes and Historical Realities*. New York: Oxford University Press, 1984.

Hanson, Marta. "Inventing a Tradition in Chinese Medicine: From Universal Canon to Local Medical Knowledge in South China, 17th Century to 19th Century." Ph.D. diss., University of Pennsylvania, 1997.

Harding, Sandra, ed. *The 'Racial Economy of Science': Toward a Democratic Future*. Bloomington: Indiana University Press, 1993.

Hardy, Jack. *The Clothing Workers: A Study of the Conditions and Struggles in the Needle Trades*. New York: International Publishers, 1935.

Harley, J. B. "Deconstructing the Map." *Cartographica* 26 (1989): 1–20.

———. "Maps, Knowledge, and Power." In *The Iconography of Landscape: Essays on the Symbolic Representation, Design, and Use of Past Environments,* ed. Denis Cosgrove and Stephen Daniels. New York: Cambridge University Press, 1988.

Hartley, Katha G. "*Spring Valley Water Works v. San Francisco:* Defining Economic Rights in San Francisco." *Western Legal History* 3, no. 2 (summer-fall 1990): 287–308.

Hartsock, Nancy. "Foucault on Power: A Theory for Women?" In *Feminism/ Postmodernism,* ed. Linda J. Nicholson. New York: Routledge, 1990.

Heap, Chad. "Slumming: The Politics of American Culture and Identity, 1910–1940." Ph.D. diss., University of Chicago, 2000.

Heuerkamp, C. "The History of Smallpox Vaccination in Germany: A First Step in the Medicalization of the General Public." *Journal of Contemporary History* 20 (1985): 617–35.

Higginbotham, Evelyn Brooks. "African American Women's History and the Metalangue of Race." *Signs* (winter 1992): 251–74.

Hill, Patricia. *The World Their Household: The American Woman's Foreign Mission Movement and Cultural Transformation, 1870–1920*. Ann Arbor: University of Michigan Press, 1985.

Hirata, Lucie Cheng. "Free, Indentured, Enslaved: Chinese Prostitutes in Nineteenth Century America." *Signs* 5, no. 1 (1979): 3–29.

Hirsch, Arnold R. *Making the Second Ghetto: Race and Housing in Chicago, 1940–1960*. New York: Cambridge University Press, 1983.

Hirst, Leonard Fabian. *The Conquest of Plague: A Study of the Evolution of Epidemiology.* Oxford: Clarendon Press, 1953.

Hirst, Paul. "The Genesis of the Social." *Politics and Power* 3 (1981): 67–82.

Hoare, Quintin, and Geoffrey Nowell Smith, eds. and trans. *Selections from the Prison Notebooks of Antonio Gramsci.* New York: International Publishers, 1971.

Hobson, Barbara Meil. *Uneasy Virtue: The Politics of Prostitution and the American Reform Tradition.* New York: Basic Books, 1987.

Holston, James, and Arjun Appadurai. "Cities and Citizenship." *Public Culture* 8 (1996): 187–204.

Holt, Thomas C. "Afterword: Mapping the Black Public Sphere." *The Black Public Sphere: A Public Culture Book,* 325–26. Chicago: University of Chicago Press, 1995.

———. "Marking: Race, Race-Making, and the Writing of History." *American Historical Review* 100, no. 1 (February 1995): 1–20.

———. "Reflections on Race-Making and Racist Practice: Toward a Working Hypothesis." Paper prepared for the Newberry Seminar in American Social History, Chicago, May 30, 1991.

Honig, Bonnie. "Immigrant America? How Foreignness Solves Democracy's Problems." *Social Text,* no. 56 (fall 1998): 1–27.

Hopkins, D. R. *Princes and Peasants: Smallpox in History.* Chicago: University of Chicago Press, 1983.

Hoy, Suellen. *Chasing Dirt: The American Pursuit of Cleanliness.* New York: Oxford University Press, 1995.

Humphreys, Margaret. *Yellow Fever and the South.* New Brunswick: Rutgers University Press, 1992.

Hune, Shirley. "Rethinking Race: Paradigms and Policy Formation." *Amerasia Journal* 21, nos. 1–2 (1995): 29–40.

Hunt, Michael. "The Hierarchy of Race." *Ideology and U.S. Foreign Policy,* 46–91. New Haven: Yale University Press, 1987.

Hunter, Tera W. *To 'Joy My Freedom: Southern Black Women's Lives and Labors after the Civil War.* Cambridge: Harvard University Press, 1997.

Hutchinson, E. P. *Legislative History of American Immigration Policy, 1798–1965.* Philadelphia: University of Pennsylvania Press, 1981.

Hyman, Dr. Tony. "'Look for the Union Label': A Guide to Union Labels for Collectors." *Antique Trader Weekly* (March 11, 1987): 68–71.

Illeto, Reynaldo. "Cholera and Origins of American Sanitary Order in the Philippines." In *Discrepant Histories: Translocal Essays on Filipino Cultures,* ed. Vincente Rafael, 51–82. Philadelphia: Temple University Press, 1995.

Ingram, Gordon Brent, Anne-Marie Bouthillette, and Yolanda Ritter, eds. *Queers in Space: Communities, Public Places, Sites of Resistance.* Seattle: Bay Press, 1997.

Issel, William, and Robert Cherny. *San Francisco, 1865–1932: Politics, Power, and Urban Development.* Berkeley and Los Angeles: University of California Press, 1986.

Jacobson, Matthew Frye. *Whiteness of a Different Color: European Immigrants and the Alchemy of Race.* Cambridge: Harvard University Press, 1998.

Jaschok, Maria. *Concubines and Bondservants: A Social History.* London: Zed Books, 1988.

Johnson, Donald E., et al., eds. *Needs Assessment: Theory and Methods.* Ames: Iowa State University Press, 1987.

Johnson, Susan L. "Sharing Bed and Board: Cohabitation and Cultural Difference in Central Arizona Mining Towns, 1863–1873." In *Women's West,* ed. Susan Armitage and Elizabeth Jameson. Norman: University of Oklahoma Press, 1987.

Jones, Gareth Stedman. *Outcast London: A Study of the Relationship between the Classes in Victorian Society.* Oxford: Clarendon Press, 1971.

Jones, James Boyd. "A Tale of Two Cities: The Hidden Battle against Venereal Disease in Civil War Nashville and Memphis." *Civil War History* 31, no. 3 (September 1985): 270–76.

Jordan, Winthrop D. *White over Black: American Attitudes towards the Negro, 1550–1812.* New York: W. W. Norton, 1968.

Kahn, Judd. *Imperial San Francisco: Politics and Planning in an American City, 1897–1906.* Lincoln: University of Nebraska Press, 1979.

Kalisch, Philip A. "The Black Death in Chinatown: Plague and Politics in San Francisco, 1900–04." *Arizona and the West* 14 (1972): 113–36.

Kaplan, Amy. "Left Alone with America: The Absence of Empire in the Study of American Culture." In *Cultures of U.S. Imperialism,* ed. Amy Kaplan and Donald E. Pease. Durham, N.C.: Duke University Press, 1993.

———. "Manifest Domesticity." *American Literature* 70, no. 3 (September 1998): 581–606.

Kelley, Robin D. G. *Yo Mama's Disfunktional: Fighting the Culture Wars in Urban America.* Boston: Beacon Press, 1998.

Kerber, Linda. "The Meanings of Citizenship." *Dissent* 44 (1997): 33–37.

Kettner, James. *The Development of American Citizenship, 1608–1870.* Chapel Hill: University of North Carolina Press, 1978.

Kim, Elaine. "Such Opposite Creatures: Men and Women in Asian American Literature." *Michigan Quarterly Review* 29, no. 1 (winter 1990): 68.

Klaus, Alisa. *Every Child a Lion: The Origins of the Infant Health Policy in the United States and France, 1890–1920.* Ithaca: Cornell University Press, 1993.

Klee, Linnea. "The 'Regulars' and the Chinese: Ethnicity and Public Health in 1870s San Francisco." *Urban Anthropology* 12, no. 2 (summer 1983): 181–207.

Koshar, Rudy. "Foucault and Social History: Comments on Combined Underdevelopment." *American Historical Review* 98, no. 2 (April 1993): 354–63.

Koven, Seth, and Sonya Michel. *Mothers of a New World: Maternalist Politics and the Origins of Welfare States.* New York: Routledge, 1993.

Kraut, Alan M. *Silent Travelers: Germs, Genes, and the "Immigrant Menace."* New York: Basic Books, 1994.

Kudlick, Cathy. *Cholera in Postrevolutionary Paris.* Berkeley and Los Angeles: University of California Press, 1996.

Ladd-Taylor, Molly. *Mother Work: Women, Child Welfare, and the State, 1890–1930.* Urbana: University of Illinois Press, 1994.

Lai, David Cheunyan. *Chinatowns: Towns within Cities in Canada*. Vancouver: University of British Columbia Press, 1988.

Lai, Him Mark. "Chinese Language Sources Bibliography Project: Preliminary Findings." *Amerasia Journal* 5, no. 2 (1978): 95–107.

———. *From Chinese to Chinese Americans*. Hong Kong: Joint Publishing, 1992.

———. "Historical Development of the Chinese Consolidated Benevolent Association/Huiguan System." *Chinese America: History and Perspectives* (San Francisco) (1987): 13–51.

Lai, Him Mark, Genny Lim, and Judy Yung. *Island: Poetry and History of Chinese Immigrants on Angel Island, 1910–1940*. Seattle: University of Washington Press, 1980.

Langer, P. "Sociology—Four Images of Organised Diversity: Bazaar, Jungle, Organism, and Machine." In *Cities of the Mind: Images and Themes of the City in Social Science*, ed. Lloyd Rodwin and Robert M. Hollister. London: Plenum Press, 1984.

Laqueur, Thomas W. "Bodies, Details, and the Humanitarian Narrative." In *The New Cultural History*, ed. Lynn Hunt, 176–204. Berkeley and Los Angeles: University of California Press, 1989.

Latour, Bruno. *The Pasteurization of France*. Trans. Alan Sheridan and John Law. Cambridge: Harvard University Press, 1988.

Lears, T. J. Jackson. "The Concept of Cultural Hegemony: Problems and Possibilities." *American Historical Review* 56 (June 1985).

Leavitt, Judith Waltzer. *The Healthiest City: Milwaukee and the Politics of Health Reform*. Princeton: Princeton University Press, 1982.

———. *Typhoid Mary: Captive to the Public's Health*. Boston: Beacon, 1996.

———. "'Typhoid Mary' Strikes Back: Bacteriological Theory and Practice in Early Twentieth Century Public Health." *ISIS: International Review Devoted to the History of Science and Its Cultural Influences* 83, no. 4 (1992): 608–29.

Lee, Robert G. *Orientals: Asian Americans in Popular Culture*. Philadelphia: Temple University Press, 1999.

Lee, Rose Hum. "The Decline of Chinatowns in the United States." *American Journal of Sociology* 54 (1949): 422–32.

Lerner, Barron H. *Contagion and Confinement: Controlling Tuberculosis along Skid Row*. Baltimore: Johns Hopkins University Press, 1998.

Levine, Philippa. "Modernity, Medicine, and Colonialism: The Contagious Diseases Ordinances in Hong Kong and the Straits Settlements." *Positions: East Asian Critique* 6, no. 3 (winter 1998): 675–706.

Light, Ivan. "From Vice District to Tourist Attraction: The Moral Career of American Chinatowns, 1880–1940." *Pacific Historical Review* 43, no. 3 (1974): 382.

Link, Vernon B. *A History of Plague in the United States of America*. Public Health Monograph No. 26. Publication No. 392. Washington, D.C.: Government Printing Office, 1955.

Lipsitz, George. "The Possessive Investment in Whiteness: Racialized Social De-
    mocracy and the 'White Problem' in American Studies." *American Quarterly*
    47, no. 3 (September 1995): 369–87.
Lipson, Loren George. "Plague in San Francisco in 1900: The United States Ma-
    rine Hospital Service Commission to Study the Existence of Plague in San
    Francisco." *Annals of Internal Medicine* 77 (1972): 303–10.
Loo, Chasla M. *Chinatown: Most Time, Hard Time.* New York: Praeger,
    1991.
Lorde, Audre. "The Uses of the Erotic: The Erotic as Power." In *Sister/Outsider:
    Essays and Speeches.* Trumansburg, N.Y.: Crossing Press, 1984.
Lorwin, Louis L. [Louis Levine]. *The Women's Garment Workers.* New York:
    B. W. Heubsch, 1924; reprint, New York: Arno and the New York Times,
    1969.
Lowe, Lisa. *Immigrant Acts: On Asian American Cultural Politics.* Durham,
    N.C.: Duke University Press, 1996.
———. "The International within National: American Studies and Asian Amer-
    ican Critique." *Cultural Critique* 30 (fall 1998): 29–47.
Ma, Eve Armentrout. "Urban Chinese at the Sinitic Frontier: Social Organiza-
    tion in the United States Chinatowns, 1840–1898." *Modern Asian Studies*
    17 (1983): 107–35.
Macpherson, Kerrie L. *A Wilderness of Marshes: The Origins of Public Health
    in Shanghai, 1843–1893.* Hong Kong: Oxford University Press, 1987.
Maltz, Earl. *Civil Rights, the Constitution, and Congress, 1863–1869.* Law-
    rence: University of Kansas Press, 1990.
Marcus, Alan I. "Physicians Open Up a Can of Worms: American Nationality
    and Hookworm in the United States, 1893–1909." *American Studies* 30,
    no. 2 (1989): 103–21.
———. *Plague of Strangers: Social Groups and the Origins of City Services in
    Cincinnati, 1819–1870.* Columbus: Ohio State University Press, 1991.
Marez, Curtis. "The Coquero in Freud: Psychoanalysis, Race, and International
    Economies of Distinction." *Cultural Critique* 26 (1994): 65–93.
———. "The Other Addict: Reflections on Colonialism and Oscar Wilde's
    Opium Smoke Screen." *English Literary History* 64 (spring 1997): 257–87.
Markel, Howard. *Quarantine! East European Jewish Immigrants and the New
    York City Epidemics of 1892.* Baltimore: Johns Hopkins University Press,
    1997.
Marks, Lara, and Michael Worboys, eds. *Migrants, Minorities, and Health: His-
    torical and Contemporary Studies.* London: Routledge, 1997.
Marshall, Barbara. *Engendering Modernity: Feminism, Social Theory, and So-
    cial Change.* Cambridge, England: Polity Press, 1994.
Martyn, Byron Curti. "Racism in the United States: A History of Miscegenation
    Legislation and Litigation." Ph.D. diss., University of Southern California,
    1979.
Matthews, Lillian Ruth. *Women in Trade Unions in San Francisco.* Berkeley and
    Los Angeles: University of California Press, 1913.
McBride, David. *From Tuberculosis to AIDS: Epidemics among Urban Blacks
    since 1900.* Albany: State University of New York Press, 1991.

McCauley, Elizabeth Anne. "Taber and Company's Chinatown Photographs: A Study in Prejudice and Its Manifestations." *Bulletin of the University of New Mexico Art Museum*, no. 13 (1980–81): 9–17.

McClain, Charles J. "*In Re Lee Sing:* The First Residential-Segregation Case." *Western Legal History* 3, no. 2 (summer-fall 1990): 179–96.

———. *In Search of Equality: The Chinese Struggle against Discrimination in Nineteenth-Century America.* Berkeley and Los Angeles: University of California Press, 1994.

———. "Of Medicine, Race, and American Law: The Bubonic Plague Outbreak of 1900." *Law and Social Inquiry* 13, no. 3 (1988): 447–513.

McClelland, Keith. "Some Thoughts on Masculinity and the 'Respectable Artisan' in Britain, 1850–1880." *Gender and History* 1, no. 2 (summer 1989): 164–77.

McDonald, Terence J. *The Parameters of Urban Fiscal Policy: Socioeconomic Change and Political Culture, 1860–1906.* Berkeley and Los Angeles: University of California Press, 1986.

McKeown, Thomas. *The Modern Rise of Population.* New York: Academic Press, 1976.

McLeod, Alexander. *Pigtails and Gold Dust: A Panorama of Chinese Life in Early California.* Caldwell, Idaho: Caxton Printers, 1948.

Mears, Eliot G. *Resident Orientals on the American Pacific Coast.* New York: Arno Press, 1978.

Meckel, Richard A. *Save the Babies: American Public Health Reform and the Prevention of Infant Mortality, 1850–1920.* Baltimore: Johns Hopkins University Press, 1990.

Mehta, Uday S. "Liberal Strategies of Exclusion." In *Tensions of Empire: Colonial Cultures in a Bourgeois World,* ed. Frederick Cooper and Ann Laura Stoler, 59–86. Berkeley and Los Angeles: University of California Press, 1997.

Melosi, Martin V. "Out of Sight, Out of Mind: The Environment and the Disposal of Municipal Refuse, 1860–1920." *Historian* 35 no. 4 (1973): 621–40.

———. *The Sanitary City: Urban Infrastructure in America from Colonial Times to the Present.* Baltimore: Johns Hopkins University Press, 2000.

———. "Sanitary Services and Decision Making in Houston, 1876–1945." *Journal of Urban History* 20 (May 1994): 365–406.

Meyerowitz, Joanne. *Women Adrift: Independent Wage Earners in Chicago, 1880–1930.* Chicago: University of Chicago Press, 1988.

Miles, Robert. *Racism.* New York: Routledge, 1989.

Miller, Peter, and Nikolas Rose. "Political Rationalities and Technologies of Government." In *Texts, Contexts, and Concepts,* ed. S. Hanninen. Helsinki: Finnish Political Science Association, 1989.

Miller, Stuart Creighton. *The Unwelcome Immigrant: The American Image of the Chinese, 1785–1882.* Berkeley and Los Angeles: University of California Press, 1969.

Mink, Gwendolyn. "The Lady and the Tramp: Gender, Race, and the Origins of the American Welfare State." In *Women, the State, and Welfare,* ed. Linda Gordon. Madison: University of Wisconsin Press, 1990.

———. *The Wages of Motherhood: Inequality in the Welfare State, 1917–1942.* Ithaca: Cornell University Press, 1995.

Monkkonen, Eric J. *America Becomes Urban: The Development of U.S. Cities and Towns, 1780–1980.* Berkeley and Los Angeles: University of California Press, 1988.

Montejano, David. *Anglos and Mexicans in the Making of Texas, 1836–1986.* Austin: University of Texas Press, 1988.

Morantz, Regina. "Making Women Modern: Middle-Class Women and Health Reform in Nineteenth-Century America." *Journal of Social History* 10 (1977): 490–507.

Morman, Edward. "Scientific Medicine Comes to Philadelphia: Public Health Transformed, 1854–1899." Ph.D. diss., University of Pennsylvania, 1986.

Morrison, Toni. *Playing in the Dark: Whiteness and the Literary Imagination.* Cambridge: Harvard University Press, 1992.

Mosse, George L. *Nationalism and Sexuality: Middle Class Morality and Sexual Norms in Modern Europe.* Madison: University of Wisconsin Press, 1985.

Moulin, Anne Marie. *Le Dernier Langage de la Medicine: Histoire de lmmunologie de Pasteur au SIDA.* Paris: Presses Universitaires de France, 1991.

Muench, Christopher. "Chinese Medicine in America: A Study in Adaptation." *Caduceus: A Museum Quarterly for Health Sciences* (spring 1988): 4–35.

———. "One Hundred Years of Medicine: The Ah-Fong Physicians of Idaho." In *Chinese Medicine on the Golden Mountain: An Interpretive Guide,* ed. Henry G. Schwartz, 51–80. Seattle: Wing Luke Memorial Museum, 1984.

Mullan, Fitzhugh. *Plagues and Politics: The Story of the United States Public Health Service.* New York: Basic Books, 1989.

Mumford, Kevin J. *Interzones: Black / White Sex Districts in Chicago and New York in the Early Twentieth Century.* New York: Columbia University Press, 1997.

Musto, David F. "Quarantine and the Problem of AIDS." *Milbank Quarterly* 64, suppl. 1 (1986): 97–117.

Negt, Ooskar, and Alexander Kluge. *Public Sphere and Experience: Toward an Analysis of the Bourgeois and Proletarian Public Sphere.* Minneapolis: University of Minnesota Press, 1993.

Nelson, William. *The Fourteenth Amendment: From Political Principle to Judicial Doctrine.* Cambridge: Harvard University Press, 1988.

Ngai, Mae. "The Architecture of Race in American Immigration Law: A Reexamination of the Immigration Act of 1924." *Journal of American History* 86, no. 1 (June 1999): 67–92.

———. "Illegal Aliens and Alien Citizens: United States Immigration Policy and Racial Formation, 1924–1945." Ph.D. diss., Columbia University, 1998.

Novak, William J. *The People's Welfare: Law and Regulation in Nineteenth Century America.* Chapel Hill: University of North Carolina Press, 1996.

Nugent, Angela. "Organizing Trade Unions to Combat Disease: The Workers' Health Bureau, 1921–1928." *Labor History* 26 (summer 1985): 423–46.

"'Nuisance Bill' Approaches First Committee Meeting." *S.F. Frontiers* 15, no. 25 (April 10, 1997).

Nye, Robert A. "The Bio-Medical Origins of Urban Sociology." *Journal of Contemporary History* 20, no. 4 (1985): 659–75.

———. *Crime, Madness, and Politics: The Medical Concept of National Decline.* Princeton: Princeton University Press, 1984.

Okihiro, Gary Y. *Margins and Mainstreams: Asians in American History and Culture.* Seattle: University of Washington Press, 1994.

Oldenburg, Veena. *The Making of Colonial Lucknow, 1856–1877.* Princeton: Princeton University Press, 1984.

Omatsu, Glenn. "The 'Four Prisons' and the Movements of Liberation: Asian American Activism from the 1960s to the 1990s." In *The State of Asian America: Activism and Resistance in the 1990s,* ed. Karin Aguilar-San Juan. Boston: South End Press, 1994.

Omi, Michael, and Howard Winant. *Racial Formation in the United States from the 1960s to the 1990s.* New York: Routledge, 1986.

Onesti, Silvio J., Jr. "Plague, Press, and Politics." *Stanford Medical Bulletin* 13, no. 1 (February 1955): 1–10.

Ong, Aiwha. "Cultural Citizenship as Subject Making: New Immigrants Negotiate Racial and Cultural Boundaries." *Current Anthropology* 37, no. 5 (December 1996): 737–62.

———. "Making the Biopolitical Subject: Cambodian Immigrants, Refugee Medicine, and Cultural Citizenship in California." *Social Science and Medicine* 40, no. 9 (1995): 1243–57.

Ong, Paul Man. "Chinese Labor in Early San Francisco: Racial Segmentation and Industrial Expansion." *Amerasia Journal* 8, no. 1 (1981): 69–92.

———. "The Chinese, Laundry Laws, and the Use and Control of Urban Space." M.A. thesis, University of Washington, 1975.

———. "An Ethnic Trade: The Chinese Laundries in Early California." *Journal of Ethnic Studies* 8, no. 4 (1980): 95–113.

Osborne, Thomas. "Security and Vitality: Drains, Liberalism, and Power in the Nineteenth Century." In *Foucault and Political Reason: Liberalism, Neo-Liberalism, and the Rationalities of Government,* ed. Andrew Barry, Thomas Osborne, and Nikolas Rose, 99–122. Chicago: University of Chicago Press, 1996.

Osumi, Megumi Dick. "Asians and California's Anti-Miscegenation Laws." In *Asian and Pacific American Experiences: Women's Perspectives,* ed. Nobuya Tsuchida, 2–8. Minneapolis: Asian Pacific American Learning Resource Center and General College, University of Minnesota, 1982.

Packard, Randall. *White Plague, Black Labor: Tuberculosis and the Political Economy of Health and Disease in South Africa.* Pietermaritzburg: University of Natal Press, 1989.

Palumbo-Liu, David. *Asian/American: Historical Crossings of a Racial Frontier.* Stanford: Stanford University Press, 1999.

Pan, Erica Y. Z. *The Impact of the 1906 Earthquake on San Francisco's Chinatown.* New York: Peter Lang, 1995.

Pascoe, Peggy. "Miscegenation Law, Court Cases, and Ideologies of Race in Twentieth Century America." *Journal of American History* 83, no. 1 (June 1996): 44–69.

———. "Race, Gender, and Intercultural Relations: The Case of Interracial Marriage." *Frontiers* 12, no. 1 (1991): 5–18.

———. *Relations of Rescue: The Search for Female Moral Authority in the American West, 1874–1939.* New York: Oxford University Press, 1990.

Patton, Cindy. *Inventing AIDS.* New York: Routledge, 1990.

———. "Refiguring Social Space." In *Social Postmodernism: Beyond Identity Politics,* ed. Linda Nicholson and Steven Seidman, 216–49. New York: Oxford University Press 1995.

Peffer, George Anthony. "Forbidden Families: Emigration Experiences of Chinese Women under the Page Law, 1875–1882." *Journal of American Ethnic History* 6 (1986): 28–46.

———. *If They Don't Bring Their Women: Chinese Female Immigration before Exclusion.* Urbana: University of Illinois Press, 1999.

Pernick, Martin S. "Eugenics and Public Health in American History." *American Journal of Public Health* 87, no. 11 (November 1997): 1767–72.

———. "Politics, Parties, and Pestilence: Epidemic Yellow Fever in Philadelphia and the Rise of the First Party System." In *Sickness and Health in America: Readings in the History of Medicine and Public Health,* ed. Judith Waltzer Leavitt and Ronald L. Numbers. Madison: University of Wisconsin Press, 1985.

Perry, Stewart E. *San Francisco Scavengers: Dirty Work and the Pride of Ownership.* Berkeley and Los Angeles: University of California Press, 1978.

Peterson, Jon. "The Impact of Sanitary Reform on American Urban Planning." *Journal of Social History* 13 (fall 1979): 83–103.

Pillors, Brenda E. "The Criminality of Prostitution in the United States: The Case of San Francisco, 1854–1919." Ph.D. diss., University of California at Berkeley, 1986.

Poovey, Mary. *Making a Social Body: British Cultural Formation, 1830–1864.* Chicago: University of Chicago Press, 1995.

Porter, Dorothy. "'Enemies of the Race': Biologism, Environmentalism, and Public Health in Edwardian England." *Victorian Studies* 34, no. 2 (winter 1991): 158–71.

Porter, Dorothy, and Roy Porter. "The Politics of Prevention: Anti-Vaccination and Public Health in Nineteenth-Century England," *Medical History* 32 (1988): 231–32.

Power, J. Gerard. "Media Dependency, Bubonic Plague, and the Social Construction of the Chinese Other." *Journal of Communication Inquiry* 19, no. 1 (spring 1995): 89–110.

Prakash, Gyan. "Subaltern Studies as Postcolonial Criticism." *American Historical Review* 99, no. 5 (December 1994): 1475–90.

Prashad, Vijay. "Native Dirt/Imperial Ordure: The Cholera of 1832 and the Morbid Resolutions of Modernity." *Journal of Historical Sociology* 7, no. 3 (September 1994): 243–60.

Pratt, Mary Louise. *Imperial Eyes: Travel Writing and Transculturation.* New York: Routledge, 1992.

Quock, Dr. Collin P. *The Dawning.* San Francisco: Chinese Hospital Medical Staff Archives, 1978.

————, comp. *Following the Dawn*. San Francisco: Chinese Hospital Medical Staff Archives, 1979.

Radford, Gail. *Modern Housing for America: Policy Struggles in the New Deal Era*. Chicago: University of Chicago Press, 1997.

Rafael, Vincente L. "Colonial Domesticity: White Women and United States Rule in the Philippines." *American Literature* 67 (December 1995): 639–66.

————. "White Love: Surveillance and Nationalist Resistance in U.S. Colonization of the Philippines." In *Cultures of U.S. Imperialism*, ed. Don Pease and Amy Kaplan. Durham, N.C.: Duke University Press, 1994.

Read, J. Marion, and Mary E. Mathes. *History of the San Francisco Medical Society, 1850–1900*. San Francisco: San Francisco Medical Society, 1958.

Reddy, Chandan R. "Homes, Houses, Non-Identity: Paris Is Burning." In *Burning Down the House: Recycling Domesticity*, ed. Rosemary Maragoly George, 355–79. Boulder, Colo.: Westview Press, 1998.

Reid, Roddey. *Families in Jeopardy: Regulating the Social Body in France, 1750–1910*. Stanford: Stanford University Press, 1993.

Reiser, Stanley J. "The Emergence of the Concept of Screening for Disease." *Millbank Memorial Fund Quarterly* 56:4 (1978): 403–25.

Riley, Denise. *"Am I That Name?": Feminism and the Category of "Women" in History*. Minneapolis: University of Minnesota Press, 1988.

Risse, Guenter B. "'A Long Pull, a Strong Pull, and All Together': San Francisco and the Bubonic Plague, 1907–1908." *Bulletin of the History of Medicine* 66 (summer 1992): 263–64.

————. "The Politics of Fear: Bubonic Plague in San Francisco, California, 1900." In *New Countries and Old Medicine: Proceedings of an International Conference on the History of Medicine and Health*, ed. Linda Bryder and Derek A. Dow, 1–19. Auckland, New Zealand: Pyramid Press, 1995.

Rodgers, Daniel. "Exceptionalism." In *Imagined Histories: American Historians Interpret the Past*, ed. Anthony Moho and Gordon S. Wood, 21–40. Princeton: Princeton University Press, 1998.

Roediger, David. *The Wages of Whiteness: Race and the Making of the American Working Class*. London: Verso, 1991.

Rogaski, Ruth. "From Protecting Life to Defending the Nation: The Emergence of Public Health in Tianjin, 1859–1953." Ph.D. diss., Yale University, 1996.

Rogers, Naomi. "Germs with Legs: Flies, Disease, and the New Public Health." *Bulletin of the History of Medicine* 63, no. 4 (1989): 599–617.

Rosaldo, Renato. "Cultural Citizenship." *Cultural Anthropology* 7 (1994).

Rose, Nikolas. "The Death of the Social? Re-figuring the Territory of Government." *Economy and Society* 25, no. 3 (August 1996): 327–56.

————. "Governing Advanced Liberal Democracies." In *Foucault and Political Reason: Liberalism, Neo-Liberalism, and the Rationalities of Government*, ed. Andrew Barry, Thomas Osborne, and Nikolas Rose, 37–64. Chicago: University of Chicago Press, 1996.

————. "Governing by Numbers." *Accounting Organization and Society* 16, no. 7 (1991): 673–92.

Rosen, Christine Meisner. *The Limits of Power: Great Fires and the Process of City Growth in America*. Cambridge: Cambridge University Press, 1986.

Rosen, George. *A History of Public Health*. New York: MD Publications, 1958.
———. *Preventive Medicine in the United States, 1900–1975: Trends and Interpretations*. New York: Science History Publications, 1975.
Rosen, Ruth. *The Lost Sisterhood: Prostitution in America, 1900–1918*. Baltimore: Johns Hopkins Press, 1982.
Rosenberg, Charles E. *The Care of Strangers: The Rise of America's Hospital System*. New York: Basic Books, 1987.
———. *The Cholera Years: The United States in 1832, 1849, and 1866*. Chicago: University of Chicago Press, 1962.
———. "Deconstructing Disease." *Reviews in American History* 14 (1986): 110–15.
———. "Disease and Social Order in America: Perceptions and Expectations." *Milbank Quarterly* 64, suppl. 1 (1986): 34–55.
———. "Illness, Society, and History." In *Framing Disease: Studies in Cultural History*, ed. Charles E. Rosenberg and Janet Golden. New Brunswick: Rutgers University Press, 1992.
Rosencrantz, Barbara. *Public Health and the State: Changing Views in Massachusetts, 1842–1936*. Cambridge: Harvard University Press, 1972.
Rosenstirn, Julius. *The Municipal Clinic of San Francisco*. New York: William Wood, 1913.
Rosner, David, and Gerald Markowitz. "Safety and Health as a Class Issue: The Worker's Health Bureau of America during the 1920s." In *Dying for Work*, ed. David Rosner and Gerald Markowitz, 53–64. Bloomington: Indiana University Press, 1987.
Rothman, Sheila. *Living in the Shadow of Death: Tuberculosis and the Social Experience of Illness in American History*. New York: Basic Books, 1994.
Rouse, Joseph. "Foucault and the Natural Sciences." In *Foucault and the Critique of Institutions*, ed. John Caputo and Mark Yount. University Park: Pennsylvania State University Press, 1993.
Rubin, Gayle. "Thinking Sex: Notes for a Radical Theory on the Politics of Sexuality." In *Pleasure and Danger: Exploring Female Sexuality*, ed. Carol Vance. Boston: Routledge and Kegan Paul, 1984.
Ryan, Mary. *Women in Public: Between Banners and Ballots, 1825–1880*. Baltimore: Johns Hopkins University Press, 1990.
Salyer, Lucy E. "Captives of the Law: Judicial Enforcement of Chinese Exclusion Laws, 1891–1905." *Journal of American History* 76 (1989): 91–117.
———. *Laws Harsh as Tigers: Chinese Immigrants and the Shaping of Modern Immigration Law*. Chapel Hill: University of North Carolina Press, 1995.
Sandmeyer, Elmer. *The Anti-Chinese Movement in California*. Urbana: University of Illinois Press, 1973.
Santiago-Valles, Kelvin. "On the Historical Links between Coloniality and the Violent Production of the Native Body and the Manufacture of Pathology." *Centro* 7, no. 1 (1995): 108–18.
Saxton, Alexander. *The Indispensable Enemy: Labor and the Anti-Chinese Movement in California*. Berkeley and Los Angeles: University of California Press, 1971.

———. *The Rise and Fall of the White Republic: Class Politics and Mass Culture in Nineteenth Century America.* New York: Verso, 1990.

Schell, Robert. "Tender Ties: Women and the Slave Household, 1652–1834." In *The Societies of Southern Africa in the 19th and 20th Centuries.* University of London Institute of Commonwealth Studies no. 17. London: University of London, 1992.

Schultz, Stanley K., and Clay McSchane. "To Engineer the Metropolis: Sewers, Sanitation, and City Planning in Late Nineteenth-Century America." *Journal of American History* 65, no. 2 (1978): 389–411.

Scott, Anne Firor. "Women's Voluntary Associations: From Charity to Reform." In *Lady Bountiful Revisited: Women, Philanthropy, and Power,* ed. Kathleen D. McCarthy. New Brunswick: Rutgers University Press, 1990.

Scott, Joan Wallach. *Gender and the Politics of History.* New York: Columbia University Press, 1988.

Shah, Nayan. "Paradoxes of Inclusion and Exclusion in American Modernity: Formations of the Modern Self, Domicile, and Domesticity." Paper presented to the conference "Project to Internationalize the Study of American History," Joint Project of New York University and the Organization of American Historians, Villa La Pietra, Florence, Italy, July 4–7, 1999.

———. "San Francisco's Chinatown: Race and the Cultural Politics of Public Health, 1854–1952." Ph.D. diss., University of Chicago, 1995.

Shumsky, Neil Larry. *The Evolution of Political Protest and the Workingmen's Party of California.* Columbus: Ohio State University Press, 1991.

———. "The Municipal Clinic of San Francisco: A Study in Medical Structure." *Bulletin of the History of Medicine* 52 (1978): 542–59.

———. "Tacit Acceptance: Respectable Americans and Segregated Prostitution, 1870–1910." *Journal of Social History* 19 (summer 1986): 665–79.

———. "Tar Flat and Nob Hill: A Social History of Industrial San Francisco during the 1870s." Ph.D. diss., University of California at Berkeley, 1972.

Shumsky, Neil Larry, and Larry M. Springer. "San Francisco's Zone of Prostitution, 1880–1934." *Journal of Historical Geography* 7, no. 1 (1981): 71–89.

Sibley, David. *Geographies of Exclusion: Society and Difference in the West.* London: Routledge, 1995.

Silverstein, Arthur M. *A History of Immunology.* San Diego: Academic Press, 1989.

Singer, Linda. *Erotic Welfare: Sexual Theory and Politics in the Age of Epidemic.* New York: Routledge, 1993.

Sivin, Nathan. "The History of Chinese Medicine: Now and Anon." *Positions: East Asian Critique* 6, no. 3 (1998): 731–62.

———. "Science and Medicine in Imperial China—the State of the Field." *Journal of Asian Studies* 47 (1988).

Sklar, Kathryn Kish. *Catherine Beecher: A Study in American Domesticity.* New Haven: Yale University Press, 1973.

———. "The Historical Foundations of Women's Power in the Creation of the American Welfare State, 1830–1930." In *Mothers of a New World: Mater-*

*nalist Politics and the Origins of Welfare States,* ed. Seth Koven and Sonya Michel, 43–93. New York: Routledge, 1993.

Skocpol, Theda. *Protecting Soldiers and Mothers: The Political Origins of Social Policy in the United States.* Cambridge: Harvard University Press, 1992.

Smith, Rogers M. *Civic Ideals: Conflicting Visions of Citizenship in U.S. History.* New Haven: Yale University Press, 1998.

Solis-Cohen, Rosebud T. "The Exclusion of Aliens from the United States for Physical Defects." *Bulletin of the History of Medicine* 21 (1947): 33–50.

Soo, Annie. "The Life and Career of Minnie Fong Lee." *Chinese America: History and Perspectives* (San Francisco) (1991): 67–74.

Spedden, Ernest Radcliffe. *The Trade Union Label.* Baltimore: Johns Hopkins University Press, 1910.

Spivak, Gayatri Chakravorty. "Can the Subaltern Speak?" In *Marxism and the Interpretation of Culture,* ed. Cary Nelson and Lawrence Grossberg, 271–313. Urbana: University of Illinois Press, 1988.

———. "The Making of Americans: The Teaching of English, the Future of Colonial Studies." *New Literary History* 21 (1990): 28.

———. "Subaltern Studies: DeConstructing Historiography." In *Other Worlds.* New York: Methuen, 1987.

Spongberg, Mary. *Feminizing Venereal Disease: The Body of the Prostitute in Nineteenth-Century Medical Discourse.* New York: New York University Press, 1997.

Stallybrass, Peter, and Allon White. *The Politics and Poetics of Transgression.* London: Methuen, 1986.

Stanley, Amy Dru. "Conjugal Bonds and Wage Labor: Rights of Contract in the Age of Emancipation." *Journal of American History* 75 (September 1998): 471–500.

Stanton, William. *The Leopard's Spots: Scientific Attitudes toward Race in America, 1815–59.* Chicago: University of Chicago Press, 1960.

Starr, Paul. *The Social Transformation of American Medicine: The Rise of the Sovereign Profession and the Making of a Vast Industry.* New York: Basic Books, 1982.

Stepan, Nancy Leys. *Idea of Race in Science: Great Britain, 1880–1960.* Hampden, Conn.: Archon Books, 1982.

———. *In the Hour of Eugenics: Race, Gender, and Nation in Latin America.* Ithaca: Cornell University Press, 1991.

Stephens, John. "A Quantitative Study of San Francisco's Chinatown, 1870 and 1880." In *The Life and Influence and the Role of the Chinese in the U.S., 1776–1960.* San Francisco: Chinese Historical Society, 1976.

Stern, Alexandra Minn. "Buildings, Boundaries, and Blood: Medicalization and Nation-Building on the U.S.–Mexico Border, 1910–1930." *Hispanic American Historical Review* 79, no. 1 (February 1999): 41–82.

Stolberg, Benjamin. *Tailor's Progress: The Story of a Famous Union and the Men Who Made It.* New York: Doubleday, Doran, and Company, 1944.

Stoler, Ann Laura. *Race and the Education of Desire: Foucault's History of Sex-*

*uality and the Colonial Order of Things.* Durham, N.C.: Duke University Press, 1995.

Sugrue, Thomas J. *Origins of the Urban Crisis: Race and Inequality in Postwar Detroit.* Princeton: Princeton University Press, 1996.

Sullivan, Rodney. "Cholera and Colonialism in the Philippines, 1899–1903." In *Disease, Medicine, and Empire: Perspectives on Western Medicine and the Experience of European Expansion,* ed. Roy MacLeod, 284–300. London: Routledge, 1988.

Sutphen, Mary P. "Not What, but Where: Bubonic Plague and the Reception of Germ Theories in Hong Kong and Calcutta, 1894–1897." *Journal of the History of Medicine and Allied Sciences* 52, no. 1 (January 1997): 81–113.

Swan, Jim. "Mater and Nannie: Two Mothers and the Discovery of the Oedipus Complex." *American Imago* 31, no. 1 (spring 1974): 1–64.

Swanson, Maynard W. "The Sanitation Syndrome: Bubonic Plague and Urban Native Policy in the Cape Colony, 1900–1909." *Journal of African History* 17, no. 3 (1977): 387–410.

Takaki, Ronald. *Iron Cages: Race and Culture in 19th Century America.* Seattle: University of Washington Press, 1979.

———. *Strangers from a Different Shore.* New York: Little, Brown, and Company, 1989.

Tarr, Joel A. "Sewerage and the Development of the Networked City in the United States, 1850–1930." In *Technology and the Rise of the Networked City in Europe and America,* ed. Joel A. Tarr and Gabriel DuPuy. Philadelphia: Temple University Press, 1988.

Tarr, Joel A., and Gabriel DuPuy. Introduction to *Technology and the Rise of the Networked City in Europe and America,* ed. Joel A. Tarr and Gabriel DuPuy. Philadelphia: Temple University Press, 1988.

Taylor, J. "Haffkine's Plague Vaccine." *Indian Medical Research Memoirs.* Memoir no. 27 (1933): pp. 3–7.

Terry, Charles E., and Mildred Pellens. *The Opium Problem.* New York: n.p., 1928.

Terry, Jennifer. "Theorizing Deviant Historiography." *Differences* 3, no. 2 (1991): 55–74.

Terry, Jennifer, and Jacqueline Urla, eds. *Deviant Bodies: Critical Perspectives on Difference in Science and Popular Culture.* Bloomington: University of Indiana Press, 1995.

Ting, Jennifer. "Bachelor Society: Deviant Heterosexuality and Asian American Historiography." In *Privileging Positions: The Sites of Asian American Studies,* ed. Gary Okihiro et al., 271–79. Pullman: Washington State University Press, 1995.

Tomes, Nancy J. *The Gospel of Germs: Men, Women, and the Microbe in American Life.* Cambridge: Harvard University Press, 1998.

———. "The Private Side of Public Health: Sanitary Science, Domestic Hygiene, and the Germ Theory, 1870–1900." *Bulletin of the History of Medicine* 64 (1990): 509–39.

Tomes, Nancy J., and John Harley Warner. "Introduction to the Special Issue on Rethinking the Reception of the Germ Theory of Disease: Comparative Perspectives." *Journal of the History of Medicine and Allied Sciences* 52 (January 1997): 7–16.

Tong, Benson. *Unsubmissive Women: Chinese Prostitutes in Nineteenth-Century San Francisco.* Norman: University of Oklahoma Press, 1994.

Trauner, Joan B. "The Chinese as Medical Scapegoats in San Francisco, 1870–1905." *California History* 57 (1978): 70–87.

Triechler, Paula A. *How to Have Theory in an Epidemic: Cultural Chronicles of AIDS.* Durham, N.C.: Duke University Press, 1999.

Tsai, Shih-shan Henry. *China and Overseas Chinese in the United States, 1868–1911.* Fayetteville: University of Arkansas Press, 1983.

Turner, Bryan S. "Contemporary Problems in the Theory of Citizenship." In *Citizenship and Social Theory,* ed. Bryan S. Turner. London: Sage, 1993.

Tygiel, Jules Everett. "Workingmen in San Francisco, 1880–1901." Ph.D. diss., University of California at Los Angeles, 1977.

Unschuld, Paul U. *Medicine in China: A History of Ideas.* Berkeley and Los Angeles: University of California Press, 1985.

Valverde, Mariana. *The Age of Light, Soap, and Water: Moral Reform in English Canada, 1885–1925.* Toronto: McClelland and Stewart, 1991.

Verbrugge, Martha H. *Able-Bodied Womanhood: Personal Health and Social Change in Nineteenth Century Boston.* New York: Oxford University Press, 1988.

———. "The Gospel and Science of Health: Hygienic Ideology in America, 1830–1920." *Reviews in American History* 11, no. 4 (December 1983): 507.

Vose, Clement E. *Caucasians Only: The Supreme Court, the NAACP, and the Restrictive Covenant Cases.* Berkeley and Los Angeles: University of California Press, 1959.

Wald, Priscilla. "Cultures and Carriers: Typhoid Mary and the Science of Social Control." *Social Text,* nos. 52–53 (1997): 181–214.

Walkowitz, Judith. *City of Dreadful Delight: Narratives of Sexual Danger in Late Victorian London.* Chicago: University of Chicago Press, 1992.

———. *Prostitution in Victorian Society: Women, Class, and the State.* New York: Cambridge University Press, 1980.

Wang, Ling-chi. "The Structure of Dual Domination: Toward a Paradigm for the Study of Chinese Diaspora in the U.S." *Amerasia Journal* 21, nos. 1–2 (1995): 149–70.

Ware, Vron. *Beyond the Pale: White Women, Racism, and History.* London: Verso, 1992.

Warner, John Harley. "From Specificity to Universalism in Medical Therapeutics: Transformation in 19th Century United States." In *Sickness and Health in America: Readings in the History of Medicine and Public Health,* ed. Judith Waltzer Leavitt and Ronald L. Numbers, 87–102. Rev. ed. Madison: University of Wisconsin Press, 1985.

Warner, Michael. *Fear of a Queer Planet: Queer Politics and Social Theory.* Minneapolis: University of Minnesota Press, 1993.

Watney, Simon. *Practices of Freedom: Selected Writings on HIV/AIDS.* Durham, N.C.: Duke University Press, 1994.

Weeks, Jeffrey. *Invented Moralities: Sexual Values in the Age of Uncertainty.* New York: Columbia University Press, 1995.

———. *Making Sexual History.* London: Polity Press, 2000.

———. *Sex, Politics, and Society.* London: Longman, 1981.

Wei, William. *The Asian American Movement.* Philadelphia: Temple University Press, 1993.

Weiss, Marc. "The Real Estate Industry and the Politics of Zoning in San Francisco, 1914–1928." *Planning Perspectives* 3 (1988): 311–24.

White, Luise. *The Comforts of Home: Prostitution in Colonial Nairobi.* Chicago: University of Chicago Press, 1990.

———. "Prostitution, Differentiation, and the World Economy: Nairobi, 1899–1939." In *Connecting Spheres: Women in the Western World, 1500 to the Present,* ed. Marilyn Boxer and Jean Quataert. New York: Oxford University Press, 1987.

———. "Prostitution, Identity, and Class Consciousness during World War II." *Signs: Journal of Women in Culture and Society* 11, no. 2 (winter 1986): 255–73.

Winkler, Gail Caskey, and Roger W. Moss. "How the Bathroom Got White Tiles . . . and Other Victorian Tales." *Historic Preservation* 36, no. 1 (1984): 33, 35.

Wong, K. Scott, and Sucheng Chan. *Claiming America: Constructing Chinese American Identities during the Exclusion Era.* Philadelphia: Temple University Press, 1999.

Woo, Wesley. "Protestant Work among the Chinese in the San Francisco Bay Area, 1850–1920." Ph.D. diss., Graduate Theological Union, Berkeley, California, 1983.

Woodward, C. Vann. *Strange Career of Jim Crow.* New York: Oxford University Press, 1955.

Wright, Carroll, and William C. Hunt. *History and Growth of the United States Census.* Washington, D.C.: Government Printing Office, 1900.

Wright, Gwendolyn. *Building the Dream: A Social History of Housing in America.* Cambridge: MIT Press, 1981.

———. *Moralism and the Model Home: Domestic Architecture and Cultural Conflict in Chicago, 1873–1913.* Chicago: University of Chicago Press, 1980.

Wu, Judy Tzu-Chun. "Mom Chung of the Fair-Haired Bastards: A Thematic Biography of Doctor Margaret Chung (1889–1959)." Ph.D. diss., Stanford University, 1997.

Wu, William. *The Yellow Peril: Chinese Americans in American Fiction, 1850–1940.* Hamden, Conn.: Archon Books, 1982.

Yew, Elizabeth. "Medical Inspection of the Immigrant at Ellis Island: 1891–1924." *Bulletin of the New York Academy of Medicine* 56 (1980): 488–510.

Yip, Christopher Lee. "San Francisco's Chinatown: An Architectural and Urban History." Ph.D. diss., University of California at Berkeley, 1985.

Young, Robert J. C. *Colonial Desire: Hybridity in Theory, Culture, and Race.* London: Routledge, 1990.

Yu, Connie Young. "A History of San Francisco Chinatown Housing." *Amerasia Journal* 8, no. 1 (1981): 93–109.

———. "Rediscovered Voices: Chinese Immigrants and Angel Island." *Amerasia Journal* 4, no. 2 (1977): 123–39.

Yuan, D. Y. "Voluntary Segregation: A Study of New York Chinatown." *Phylon: The Atlanta University Review of Race and Culture* 24 (1963): 255–65.

Yung, Judy. *Unbound Feet: A Social History of Chinese Women in San Francisco.* Berkeley and Los Angeles: University of California Press, 1995.

# Index

Compositor: G & S Typesetters, Inc.
Text: 10/13 Sabon
Display: Sabon
Printer and Binder: Thomson-Shore, Inc.